T φA

# AGING AND MOTOR BEHAVIOR

*Edited by*
**Andrew C. Ostrow, Ph.D.**
West Virginia University

Benchmark Press, Inc.
Indianapolis, Indiana

Library of Congress Cataloging in Publication Data:

OSTROW, ANDREW C. 1946-

AGING AND MOTOR BEHAVIOR


Cover Design: Gary Schmitt
Copy Editor: Laura Culliton


Library of Congress Catalog Card number: 86-71567


ISBN: 0-936157-10-0


Printed in the United States of America
10 9 8 7 6 5 4 3 2 1

The Publisher and Author disclaim responsibility for any adverse effects or consequences from the misapplication or injudicious use of the information contained within this text.

To my wife Lynne
whose love, devotion, and support
have made aging seem as robust
as a bottle of fine Bordeaux wine.

# Contents

Contributors . . . . . . . . . . . . . . . . . . . . . . . . . . . . . . . . . . . . . . . . . . . . . ix

Preface . . . . . . . . . . . . . . . . . . . . . . . . . . . . . . . . . . . . . . . . . . . . . . . xiii

PART I     AGING, AROUSAL, AND MOTOR
PERFORMANCE . . . . . . . . . . . . . . . . . . . . . . . . . . . . . . .   1
Introduction . . . . . . . . . . . . . . . . . . . . . . . . . . . . . . . . .   1

Chapter 1   The Relationship Between Level of Arousal and
Cognitive Operations During Motor Behavior
in Young and Older Adults
*Lars Bäckman and Bo Molander* . . . . . . . . . . . . . . . . . . . . .   3

PART II    AGING, PSYCHOMOTOR SLOWING, AND
AEROBIC EXERCISE . . . . . . . . . . . . . . . . . . . . . . . . . .   35
Introduction . . . . . . . . . . . . . . . . . . . . . . . . . . . . . . . . .   35

Chapter 2   Aerobic Function, Information Processing, and Aging
*Tonya Toole and Tami Abourezk* . . . . . . . . . . . . . . . . . . . .   37

Chapter 3   Aerobic Exercise Training and Improved Neuro-
psychological Function of Older Individuals
*Robert E. Dustman, Robert O. Ruhling, Evan M. Russell,*
*Donald E. Shearer, H. William Bonekat, John W. Shigeoka,*
*James S. Wood, and David C. Bradford* . . . . . . . . . . . . . . . .   67

PART III   AGING AND MOTOR MEMORY . . . . . . . . . . . . . . .   85
Introduction . . . . . . . . . . . . . . . . . . . . . . . . . . . . . . . . .   85

Chapter 4   Memory Retrieval in the Adult Population
*Tami Benham and Melissa Heston* . . . . . . . . . . . . . . . . . . .   87

Chapter 5   The Effects of Regular Aerobic Exercise on
Short-Term Memory Efficiency in the Older Adult
*Tami Abourezk* . . . . . . . . . . . . . . . . . . . . . . . . . . . . . . .   105

PART IV      AGING, MENTAL HEALTH, AND EXERCISE .... 115
                   Introduction ..................................... 115

Chapter 6    Exercise, Aging, and Psychological Well-Being:
                   The Mind-Body Question
                   *Bonnie G. Berger and Lillian Mushabac Hecht* ............ 117

Chapter 7    The Effects of Age on Physiological and
                   Psychological Responses to a Training and
                   Detraining Program in Females
                   *Peggy A. Richardson and Beth S. Rosenberg* .............. 159

Chapter 8    The Psychological Effects of Chronic Exercise
                   in the Elderly
                   *Jeffrey S. Hird and Jean M. Williams* ................... 173

Chapter 9    An Exercise Program for Nursing Home Residents
                   *Wendy Blankfort-Doyle, Howard Waxman,*
                   *Kathleen Coughey, Frank Naso,*
                   *Erwin A. Carner, and Elaine Fox* ...................... 201

PART V       AGING AND EXERCISE MOTIVATION ......... 217
                   Introduction ..................................... 217

Chapter 10   Personal Investment in Exercise Among
                   Middle-Aged and Older Adults
                   *Joan L. Duda and Marlene K. Tappe* ................... 219

Chapter 11   Personal Investment in Exercise Among Adults:
                   The Examination of Age and Gender-Related
                   Differences in Motivational Orientation
                   *Joan L. Duda and Marlene K. Tappe* ................... 239

Chapter 12   A Social Cognitive Theory of Older Adult
                   Exercise Motivation
                   *David A. Dzewaltowski* ............................. 257

PART VI      AGING AND MOTOR SKILL ENHANCEMENT 283
                   Introduction ..................................... 283

Chapter 13   An Information Processing Approach for
                   Teaching Motor Skills to the Elderly
                   *Mark H. Anshel* .................................... 285

**PART VII**   **METHODOLOGICAL ISSUES** .................. 305

**Chapter 14**   **Evaluating the Influence of Physiological Health on Sensory and Motor Performance Changes in the Elderly**
*Wojtek J. Chodzko-Zajko and Robert L. Ringel* ............ 307

**Chapter 15**   **A Longitudinal Analysis of Anticipatory Judgment in Older Adult Motor Performance**
*Kathleen M. Haywood* ............................. 325

**Index** ...................................................... 337

# Contributors

**TAMI ABOUREZK** received the Master of Science degree in movement science and physical education at Florida State University in 1986. She is currently a candidate for the doctoral degree with an emphasis in motor behavior at Florida State University. Ms. Abourezk enjoys playing tennis, running, and snorkeling.

**MARK ANSHEL** is an associate professor in the Department of Human Movement and Sport Science at the University of Wollongong, New South Wales, Australia. Dr. Anshel's research interests and publications have centered on aging and motor short-term memory, coding strategies and movement extent, and the effects of arousal on warm-up decrement. He has served as a consultant to the United States Olympic ski team and as recreation director of programs for the elderly.

**LARS BÄCKMAN** is a research scientist with the Stockholm Gerontology Research Center, Karolinska Institute, Stockholm, Sweden. Dr. Bäckman's research has appeared as significant publications in journals such as *Experimental Aging Research, Memory and Cognition*, and *Psychology and Aging*. He is a member of a number of professional organizations including the American Psychological Association, the Gerontological Society of America, and the New York Academy of Sciences. Dr. Bäckman enjoys long-distance running and he was a member of the team that won bronze and silver medals in the Swedish championships in miniature golf in 1983 and 1984, respectively.

**TAMI BENHAM** is an associate instructor at Indiana University. Ms. Benham received the Master of Science degree at Indiana University in 1987 and is currently working on completing the doctoral degree at that institution. She has presented invited papers and workshops on motor development at state and national levels. Ms. Benham is an avid sports fan, and sports photography serves as her main hobby.

**BONNIE BERGER** is Professor and Director of the Sport Psychology Laboratory at Brooklyn College in New York. Dr. Berger has published extensively in the sport psychology field including six book chapters and over 35 journal articles. She also is active in many professional organizations. Dr. Berger is an avid jogger, downhill skier, weight training enthusiast, and swimmer.

**WENDY BLANKFORT-DOYLE** is clinical researcher and coordinator in the Department of Psychiatry and Human Behavior at Thomas Jefferson University in Philadelphia. She received the master's degree from the University of San Francisco in 1982. Ms. Blankfort-Doyle is a consultant to a number of area nursing homes on implementing physical activity and exercise programs. She enjoys tennis, horseback riding, and traveling.

**WOJTEK CHODZKO-ZAJKO** is an assistant professor in the area of Health, Physical Education, and Recreation at the University of Alabama. Dr. Chodzko-Zajko's research interests have centered on exercise and sensory-motor performance changes in old age. He is a member of the Gerontological Society of America and the American College of Sports Medicine, and he is a participant in a wide variety of sport activities.

**JOAN DUDA** is an associate professor at Purdue University. Dr. Duda's major research focus has been on gender and age-linked variations in motivational orientation and the relationship to perceived competence and behavior in sport and exercise settings. She has published 22 refereed research papers, and has made over 60 presentations at national and international professional meetings. Dr. Duda has participated at the intercollegiate and semi-professional levels in softball, basketball, and tennis.

**ROBERT DUSTMAN** is Director of the Neuropsychology Laboratories, Veterans Administration Medical Center at Salt Lake City, Utah. Dr. Dustman's research has centered on lifespan changes in cortical evoked potentials and EEG, aerobic fitness and cognitive efficiency, and central inhibitory deficits associated with aging. Dr. Dustman enjoys playing squash, downhill skiing, hiking, and pleasure reading.

**DAVID DZEWALTOWSKI** is an assistant professor in the Department of Physical Education and Leisure Studies at Kansas State University. His research interests have centered on the psychosocial correlates of exercise motivation and aging. Dr. Dzewaltowski is a distance runner and former track and field and cross-country competitor.

**KATHLEEN HAYWOOD** is an associate professor in the Department of Physical Education at the University of Missouri-St. Louis. Dr. Haywood has published a textbook on *Life Span Motor Development*. She is currently chair of the Motor Development Academy of the American Alliance for Health, Physical Education, Recreation, and Dance. Dr. Haywood is a member of the Professional Archer's Association, and she is an avid tennis player and jogger.

**LILLIAN HECHT** is a research specialist in the sport psychology laboratory at Brooklyn College in New York. Dr. Hecht has investigated the physical parameters, blood chemistries, and hemotological changes following a marathon race in elite and non-elite male and female runners. She is a member of the American College of Sports Medicine, and enjoys cross-country skiing and tennis.

**MELISSA HESTON** is an associate instructor at the Smith Research Center, Indiana University. Ms. Heston completed the Master of Science degree at Indiana University in 1982, and is currently a doctoral candidate at that institution. She has participated in numerous conferences and workshops focusing on developmental movement programs for young children. Ms. Heston enjoys swimming, canoeing, white water rafting, theater, opera, and reading science fiction.

**JEFFREY HIRD** is completing the master's degree at Arizona State University. He is a student member of the American Psychological Association, and the Association for the Advancement of Applied Sport Psychology. He played on the collegiate baseball team for the University of Arizona when the team won the NCAA championship in 1985.

**BO MOLANDER** is a senior lecturer in the Department of Psychology at the University of Umea, Sweden. Dr. Molander has published research in the *Scandinavian Journal of Psychology*, the *British Journal of Psychology* and *Psychology of Aging*. Dr. Molander has served as Director of Undergraduate Studies, Department Chairman, and is a member of the International Society of Sport Psychology. Dr. Molander enjoys listening to classical organ music, reading science fiction by American writers, and participating in miniature golf competitions.

**ANDREW OSTROW** is a professor in the Department of Sport and Exercise Studies at West Virginia University. Dr. Ostrow has published extensively in the area of age stereotyping of physical activity participation, and he has published a book on *Physical Activity and the Older Adult: Psychological Perspectives*. He is currently co-investigator of a research grant focusing on physical fitness in relation to older driver performance, funded by the AAA

Foundation for Traffic Safety. Dr. Ostrow is a former collegiate tennis player and tennis teaching professional, and he enjoys competing in racquet sports, being married, and raising two daughters, two cats, and one dog.

**PEGGY RICHARDSON** is professor in the Department of Physical Education at North Texas State University. Dr. Richardson has published one book and 36 articles related to stress, psychological momentum, achievement motivation and attribution, sex differences in physical skills, and motor skill acquisition. Dr. Richardson is a member of numerous professional organizations, and is a consultant to the Women's Sports Foundation. She enjoys competing in regional tennis tournaments, and has interests in swimming, golf, and sports journalism.

**ROBERT RINGEL** is Professor of Audiology and Speech Science, and Vice-President and Dean of the Graduate School at Purdue University. Dr. Ringel has published extensively in the areas of oral perception and sensation, and the auditory and acoustic correlates of aging. Dr. Ringel's accomplishments are listed in *Who's Who*, and he is a participant in a wide variety of sport activities.

**BETH ROSENBERG** was formerly an assistant professor in the Department of Physical Education at North Texas State University. She currently is a medical student at the Medical College of Pennsylvania in Philadelphia. Dr. Rosenberg has published in *Medicine and Science in Sport and Exercise*, and she is a member of the American College of Sports Medicine and the American Association of Cardiovascular and Pulmonary Rehabilitation. Dr. Rosenberg enjoys hiking/backpacking, cycling, swimming, and running, and she is a competitor in local shortcourse triathlons.

**MARLENE TAPPE** is an assistant professor at Purdue University. Dr. Tappe has published and presented in the areas of the motivational aspects of health-related behaviors and health education program evaluation. She currently serves as a health education consultant, and is an active participant in volleyball and other sport activities.

**TONYA TOOLE** is an associate professor and Director of the Motor Behavior Laboratory at Florida State University. Dr. Toole has published extensively in the areas of motor learning, memory, and control. She is a consulting editor for the *Research Quarterly for Exercise and Sport*, Academic Press, and Prentice-Hall. Dr. Toole directs a wellness program for older adults through the Area Agency on Aging. She enjoys competing in golf, choral singing, snorkeling, jogging, swimming, and gardening.

**HOWARD WAXMAN** is an associate professor and research director in the Department of Psychiatry and Human Behavior at Thomas Jefferson University in Philadelphia. Dr. Waxman has published over 30 scientific papers on aging and mental health. He is a regular runner and swimmer.

**JEAN WILLIAMS** is an associate professor in the Exercise and Sport Sciences Department at the University of Arizona. Dr. Williams is co-editor of *Cognitive Sport Psychology* and editor of *Applied Sport Psychology: Personal Growth to Peak Performance*. She has published extensively in the areas of group dynamics, socialization and sport, psychological effects of exercise, and the effects of stress on performance and injuries. Dr. Williams is currently secretary-treasurer of the Association for the Advancement of Applied Sport Psychology, past president of the NASPE Sport Psychology Academy, and consulting editor for six journals. She enjoys camping, fishing, golfing, and reading.

# Preface

Interest in the field of gerontology has increased dramatically among physical educators and allied health professionals during the last decade. This interest has been kindled, in part, by demographic trends pointing toward an aging society, and the concomitant concerns that people will be able to lead healthful, productive, and independent lives during their later years. It is now recognized that participation in exercise and related movement activities on a regular basis plays an important role in ensuring that aging does not become synonymous with decline, deprivation, and despair.

Programs in physical education, physical therapy, and the exercise sciences have introduced service activities and formal training related to physical activity and aging. Research in this area has increased markedly. The general public has become more aware of the importance of participating in physical activity throughout life.

The book I wrote, *Physical Activity and the Older Adult: Psychological Perspectives* (1984), was the first to summarize the findings of research related to aging and motor behavior. The book integrated knowledge from the areas of motor control and learning, exercise physiology, personality theory, sociology, and life-span development in order to better understand the role of physical activity in the lives of older adults. I felt that a logical sequence to this book was the publication of an edited book highlighting current research on aging and motor behavior.

*Aging and Motor Behavior* is organized around a number of important theoretical papers synthesizing research on the psychological aspects of physical activity and aging. Each contributing author was asked to summarize and integrate existing research on topics in the behavioral sciences that are central to understanding the interplay between physical activity, the older adult, and aging processes. More importantly, the contributors were encouraged to offer creative suggestions for future theoretical, methodological, and empirical research directions. Each chapter either incorporates or is followed by original, data-based research investigations.

Part I explores deficits in cognitive capacities underlying the commonly reported finding of a decline with age in adult motor performance under stressful conditions. In a series of fascinating studies of miniature golf competitors in Sweden, the authors examine the greater vulnerability of older players to impairments in memory and attention during stressful motor performance.

Part II examines morphological and physiological changes that occur in the central nervous system that contribute to declines in speed of processing with advancing age. A major emphasis is highlighting research literature on the value of aerobic exercise, by its trophic effects on the central nervous system, in delaying commonly observed age-related declines in psychomotor speed and neuromuscular coordination. Part III follows by focusing on age-related deficits in motor memory, and the potential role of aerobic exercise in ameleriorating short-term memory retention in older adults.

Part IV explores what is known about the effects of exercise participation on the mental health of older people. Conceptual and methodological research concerns are addressed. Behavioral guidelines for developing exercise programs for the elderly also are outlined. Given the potential mental health benefits of exercise participation for older people, Part V focuses on the development of several theoretical frameworks for understanding the motivational orientation of older adults toward exercise participation. Part VI follows by identifying a number of important instructional strategies for enhancing motor skill among older people. Part VII then focuses on several methodological issues germane to aging and motor behavior.

This is an appropriate reference textbook for upper-division and first-year graduate students who are taking courses related to gerontology, primarily in fields such as psychology, physical education, and life-span human development. Students in nursing, physical therapy, and social work will find this textbook to be an important supplement to their training in gerontology. This textbook is also an excellent reference source for those who are preparing to become leaders of older-adult physical activity programs.

Although I was responsible, in part, for soliciting, evaluating, and editing the manuscripts, developing an organizational framework for the text, and writing the introductions to each part of the book, the content and quality of the textbook resides primarily with the contributing authors. I am deeply grateful for their commitment to making this reference textbook an important scholarly contribution to an emerging and important field of study. I also would like to thank Dr. Douglas Larish, Arizona State University, and Dr. Tonya Toole, Florida State University, for their assistance in evaluating the manuscripts. A special thanks to Carol Ann Straight who is an incredibly good secretary and friend, and who made my job as editor a lot easier. I would also be remiss if I did not acknowledge the encouragement and assistance I received from Irving L. Cooper, Publisher, Benchmark Press. Mr. Cooper had the vision to recognize the need for gerontological-related textbooks in the exercise and sport sciences. Finally, I am deeply grateful to my family, Lynne, Jennifer, and Olivia, whose love and support made the publication of this book all the more enjoyable.

**Andrew C. Ostrow, Editor**

# Part I
# Aging, Arousal, and Motor Performance

## INTRODUCTION

Little is known about the cognitive factors underlying stressful motor performance, particularly as these factors are mediated by aging. It has been proposed that an optimal level of central nervous system activity underlies skillful performance, and that increasing autonomic activity (arousal), to an extent, promotes optimal central nervous system activity. The inverted-U hypothesis, originally based on the work of Yerkes and Dodson (1908) on mice, has frequently been cited to explain theoretically the relationship of arousal to motor performance. This hypothesis suggests that a curvilinear relationship (inverted U) exists between arousal and gross motor performance. The hypothesis predicts that, up to a certain point, increasing arousal facilitates performance; once an optimal level of arousal is reached, further increases in arousal lead to performance decrements.

A number of mediating variables affect this hypothesized arousal-performance relationship (cf. Bird & Cripe, 1986). Individual difference variables such as the performer's skill level, trait anxiety, and previous experience in competitive motor activity affect this predicted curvilinear relationship, particularly under competitive conditions. One of the least understood individual difference variables affecting this relationship is age.

Cognitive based interpretations of the inverted-U hypothesis center on the disruptions in the ability of the performer to process information effectively from the environment under conditions of high arousal. Excessive arousal may lead to greater distractibility, an excessive narrowing of attentional focus, and a redirection of attention toward task-irrelevant cues (Landers, 1980; Nideffer, 1981). Thus, explanations for a decline in older adult motor performance under stressful conditions should consider deficits in cognitive processing that may mediate this decline.

In a stimulating paper, Bäckman and Molander discuss a series of recent field and laboratory research studies that explore the interplay between age, arousal, and miniature golf performance. As the authors noted, they chose to study miniature golf because (1) precision sports can be studied under both field and laboratory conditions without losing their meaning, (2) precision sport performances are sensitive to variations in performer arousal, (3) successful performances in miniature golf are based on the proficient utilization of a variety of cognitive abilities. In a series of studies examining the performances of young and older miniature golfers under training and competitive conditions, Bäckman and Molander found that while stressful responses to competition were evoked in both age groups, only the performances of the older golfers were impaired.

After systematically ruling out a number of plausible hypotheses for this age-related decline in motor performance under high-stress conditions, the authors explore the greater vulnerability of the older players to impairments in memory and attention during stressful performance. In a series of carefully controlled experiments they found that age (rather than motor skill proficiency) accounted for the inability of older players to recall the nature of their golf shots taken under competitive conditions. They also found that older players, when concentrating on addressing and striking the ball, showed greater deficits in attention during competition (as indicated by heart rate changes). Furthermore, the authors found that older miniature golf competitors had a deficit in the selective aspect of attention; they exhibited (relative to younger competitors) a disproportionate disruption in both memory and golf performance when asked to listen to a radio broadcast of a soccer game while competing in miniature golf (i.e., under a condition of meaningful background stimuli).

1

Backman and Molander conclude by reviewing a number of methodological and theoretical issues pertinent to this area of investigation including the role of cognitive training in ameleriorating older adults' competitive performance in miniature golf.

## REFERENCES

Bird, A.M., & Cripe, B.K. (1986). *Psychology and sport behavior*. St. Louis: Times Mirror/Mosby.
Landers, D.M. (1980). The arousal-performance relationship revisited. *Research Quarterly for Exercise and Sports, 51*, 77-90.
Nideffer, R.M. (1981). *The ethics and practice of applied sport psychology*. Ithaca, NY: Mouvement Publications.
Yerkes, R.M., & Dodson, J.D. (1908). The relation of strength of stimulus to rapidity of habit-formation. *Journal of Comparative Neurology of Psychology, 18*, 459-482.

# 1

## The Relationship Between Level of Arousal and Cognitive Operations During Motor Behavior in Young and Older Adults

LARS BÄCKMAN

BO MOLANDER

## ABSTRACT

Although the knowledge concerning the relationships among cognitive, emotional, and motor applications of behavior are of practical importance in everyday life, research on these relationships is sparse. This state of affairs exists particularly with respect to the area of aging research. In this chapter we discuss how precision sport tasks may be fruitfully employed in adult developmental research on the interplay of cognitive, stress, and sensory-motor factors. Several field studies are presented in which young and older adults who are highly skilled miniature golfers are examined under various levels of arousal; that is, under training and competitive conditions. The results from these studies indicate that older players show impaired motor and cognitive performance in tournaments; whereas young players perform as well in high-stress competitive activities as in relaxed training conditions. It is suggested that this age decrement may be attributed to an age-related deficit in compensating for the detrimental effects of stressful competitive conditions, due to an age decrement in task-relevant cognitive capacities. A series of laboratory studies supporting this contention are presented. Finally we discuss some methodological and theoretical implications of a research approach, in which field and laboratory studies are combined, and where the meaningfulness and ecological relevance of the tasks are salient features.

## INTRODUCTION

Few would disagree with the postulate that skilled motor behavior requires the appropriate control of a variety of cognitive functions (e.g., Kerr, 1983; Saltzman & Kelso, 1983; Schneider & Fisk, 1983), and that many real-life activities in which precise motor behavior is integral (e.g., driving a car, sports, working at a conveyor belt) may be stressful.

The general experimental literature indicates a strong interest among researchers in studying the interaction of stress and cognitive factors (e.g., Broadbent, 1971; Eysenck, 1984; Mandler, 1975), cognitive and motor factors (e.g., Kelso, 1982; Magill, 1983; Prinz & Sanders, 1984), and stress and motor factors (e.g., Cratty, 1973; Singer, 1980). However, except for some research concerning the psychology of sport (e.g., Hatfield & Landers, 1983; Hatfield, Landers & Ray, 1984; Landers, 1985), not much is known about the interactions between cognitive and stress factors as related to motor activities.

This state of affairs becomes even more obvious with respect to adult developmental research. The relationship between basic psychological research and psychological aging has been characterized as a "front wheel-back wheel" relationship (Salthouse, 1982). That is, whereas researchers on aging (as well as their colleagues in other more applied domains) typically adopt theories, methods, and research paradigms from the area of basic research, influences the other way around are rarely seen (Bäckman, in press). Thus, it is no surprise that research addressing the issue of cognitive and emotional determinants of motor performance in aging adults is lacking in the most cited reviews and textbooks within this area (Kausler, 1982; Poon et al. 1980; Poon, Rubin & Wilson, in press; Salthouse, 1982, 1985; however, see Ostrow, 1984 for an exception).

In this chapter, we discuss a series of recent field and laboratory experiments which attempt to elucidate this neglected interplay. For several reasons, we have selected a precision sport, viz. miniature golf, as the experimental task in this research. First, precision sports may be studied under field conditions, as well as under restricted laboratory conditions. Second, participants are presumably highly motivated, because precision sports are competitive. Third, precision sports may reflect performance variations caused by changes in levels of arousal, due to the requirement of precise motor behavior (cf. Welford, 1977). Finally, successful motor performance in these sports rests on proficient utilization of a variety of cognitive abilities such as attention and memory.

In addition to the presentation of a series of field and laboratory studies examining younger and older miniature golf players during training and various types of competitions, we introduce a theoretical framework for the understanding of adult age-related differences in coping with high-stress and noise conditions during motor behavior. Finally, we discuss some conceptual and methodological implications of an ecological approach to aging research.

## MOTOR PERFORMANCE AND LEVEL OF AROUSAL

### Field Experiments

Bäckman and Molander (1986a) reported three field experiments in which highly skilled miniature golf players varying in age were examined in three types of activities: training, minor local competitions (MCs), and large national competitions (LCs). These three activities took place at the miniature golf course in Umeå, Sweden. In all three experiments, measures of motor performance (number of shots) and arousal (heart rate and subjective ratings of anxiety) were registered. We hypothesized that the three types of activity represented three points on an arousal continuum; that is, training was supposed to represent an event of low arousal, MCs were supposed to be events of intermediate arousal, whereas LCs were expected to be events of high arousal.

A miniature golf course typically consists of 18 tracks that vary in appearance and difficulty, and in the experiments reported by Bäckman and Molander (1986a) each player was observed in four rounds, each comprising 18 tracks, for all three activities. The order of the competitions was MC, LC, LC, MC. The competitive events always consisted of two rounds. Training data were collected during the period of the competitions (two months), training rounds being relatively randomly distributed over the period.

Heart rate (HR) and ratings of anxiety (RA) were registered twice per round: immediately before the subject started the round and immediately after he or she had played the ninth track (one half of the round). On the RA scale, (1) was defined as completely relaxed and (10) as very nervous. In the first experiment, young (5 men; mean age = 27.4 years; range = 22-32 years) and older (3 men and 2 women; mean age = 50.2 years; range = 47-58 years) adult players served as subjects. In miniature golf competitions the players are grouped into separate classes: youths (ages 7-14), junior players (ages 15-18), young adult players (ages 19-45), and older adult players (age 46 and above). In all experiments reported in this chapter, subjects are sampled from these age classes. The results of the first experiment are displayed in Table 1-1.

As can be seen in this table, both age groups showed an increase of HR and RA from training through MCs to LCs. Although the older play-

TABLE 1.1. *Mean Heart Rate, Mean Rated Anxiety, and Mean Number of Shots as a Function of Age and Type of Activity.*

| | Type of activity | | | | | | | | |
| | Training | | | Minor competitions | | | Large competitions | | |
| Group | HR | RA | NS | HR | RA | NS | HR | RA | NS |
|---|---|---|---|---|---|---|---|---|---|
| Young ($n=5$) | 71.83 | 2.30 | 36.20 | 74.33 | 2.83 | 35.70 | 93.91 | 5.35 | 35.70 |
| Old ($n=5$) | 83.08 | 2.75 | 43.45 | 83.53 | 4.33 | 44.45 | 98.28 | 5.88 | 47.55 |

*Note.* HR = heart rate (beats per min); RA = rated anxiety; NS = number of shots per round. Each activity comprised four 18-track rounds.

From "Adult Age Differences in the Ability to Cope With Situations of High Arousal in a Precision Sport" by L. Bäckman and B. Molander, 1986, *Psychology and Aging, 1*, p. 135. Copyright 1986 by the American Psychological Association. Adapted by permission.

ers showed somewhat higher values than their younger counterparts for both these measures, analyses of variance (ANOVAs) only indicated effects of the task variable ($ps < .01$). However, the results of the measure of motor performance (number of shots) told a different story. As can be seen in Table 1-1, the young players performed at about the same level regardless of type of activity, whereas the older players deteriorated from training through MCs to LCs. This pattern of results was confirmed by an interaction between age and type of activity ($p < .06$).

The reliabilities of HR and RA within each activity were assessed by correlating the values obtained during play (after the ninth track) in the first two rounds. The Pearson coefficients calculated on HR were .67, .77, and .67, for training, MC, and LC, respectively. For the RA measure the corresponding correlations were .92, .91, and .92, respectively. In the present experiment as well as in the experiments discussed below, HR values were highest before the start of the round and decreased slightly during play. However, this decrement was about the same for the older players as for the young players, which indicates that the difference in motor performance between the age groups is not due to a difference in condition, given that HR is taken as an index of the player's condition.

The relations between HR, RA, and number of shots (NS) over the three activities were calculated for each subject and group. For the young players, the mean individual Pearson correlations ($z$ transformed) for HR-RA, HR-NS, and RA-NS were .79 ($p < .001$), −.19 ($p > .05$), and −.03 ($p > .05$), respectively. The corresponding values for the older players were .44 ($p < .001$), .35 ($p < .01$), and .29 ($p < .05$), respectively. The correlations between HR and NS and between RA and NS showed a pattern consistent with the results of the ANOVAs. That is, the two arousal measures and NS correlated significantly only for the older group. Since the correlational analyses and the ANOVAs showed similar patterns with respect to the relationships among the three dependent measures in all experiments presented in this chapter, our discussion of these relationships is henceforth confined to the ANOVAs.

In the second experiment, three groups of players were studied under the same conditions as those of the first experiment: youth players (4 boys; mean age = 12.0 years; range = 10-13 years), juniors (5 boys; mean age = 17.2 years; range = 16-18 years), and five young adults (3 men and 2 women; mean age = 32.4 years; range = 22-44 years). The results of this experiment are portrayed in Table 1-2.

As indicated in Table 1-2, all three groups of players showed an increase of HR and RA from training through MCs to LCs ($ps < .01$). In addition, although substantial differences in the level of motor performance among groups were observed, none of the groups exhibited any deterioration in motor performance in LCs in the same way as did the older adults of Experiment 1.

**TABLE 1.2.** *Mean Heart Rate, Mean Rated Anxiety, and Mean Number of Shots as a Function of Age and Type of Activity.*

| | Type of activity | | | | | | | | |
| | Training | | | Minor competitions | | | Large competitions | | |
| Group | HR | RA | NS | HR | RA | NS | HR | RA | NS |
|---|---|---|---|---|---|---|---|---|---|
| Younger adults ($n=5$) | 76.83 | 2.23 | 41.55 | 90.65 | 3.75 | 40.50 | 95.05 | 5.23 | 40.30 |
| Juniors ($n=5$) | 74.23 | 2.00 | 37.75 | 72.48 | 2.90 | 37.25 | 88.28 | 5.43 | 37.15 |
| Youths ($n=4$) | 78.34 | 3.09 | 45.13 | 80.34 | 4.44 | 45.63 | 90.38 | 5.47 | 44.69 |

*Note.* HR = heart rate (beats per min); RA = rated anxiety; NS = number of shots per round. Each activity comprised four 18-track rounds.

From "Adult Age Differences in the Ability to Cope With Situations of High Arousal in a Precision Sport" by L. Bäckman and B. Molander, 1986, *Psychology and Aging, 1*, p. 136. Copyright 1986 by the American Psychological Association. Adapted by permission.

The third experiment was basically a replication of Experiment 1. Two new samples of young adults (5 men and 1 woman; mean age = 27.7 years; range = 23-35 years) and older adults (3 men and 2 women; mean age = 51.0 years; range = 48-59 years) were examined during four training rounds and in one LC comprising four rounds. Arousal and motor performance data for this experiment are presented in Table 1-3.

Table 1-3 shows that both HR and RA increased from training to the LC in a similar way for both age groups ($ps<.05$). Further, the motor performance data also replicated exactly those of Experiment 1: whereas the older adults performed worse in the LC than in training, no difference in motor performance among these two activities was observed on

**TABLE 1.3.** *Mean Heart Rate, Mean Rated Anxiety, and Mean Number of Shots as a Function of Age and Type of Activity.*

| | Type of activity | | | | | |
| | Training | | | Large competition | | |
| Group | HR | RA | NS | HR | RA | NS |
|---|---|---|---|---|---|---|
| Young ($n=6$) | 76.13 | 3.02 | 39.42 | 84.10 | 4.35 | 38.84 |
| Old ($n=5$) | 81.50 | 2.56 | 40.50 | 88.74 | 5.08 | 46.40 |

*Note.* HR = heart rate (beats per min); RA = rated anxiety; NS = number of shots per round. Each activity comprised four 18-track rounds.

From "Adult Age Differences in the Ability to Cope With Situations of High Arousal in a Precision Sport" by L. Bäckman and B. Molander, 1986, *Psychology and Aging, 1*, p. 137. Copyright 1986 by the American Psychological Association. Adapted by permission.

the part of the young adults. This pattern of results brought about a significant Age × Type of Activity interaction ($p < .02$).

The results of these three field experiments are straightforward and may be summarized in two basic points. First, all of the players showed a similar increase of arousal from training through MCs to LCs, as indicated by the measures of HR and RA. These data thus support our initially described hypothesis that the three activities represent three points on an arousal continuum. Second, whereas all groups of younger players performed equally well in all three activities, the older players performed consistently worse in LCs compared to training or MCs. However, although the effects demonstrated by Bäckman and Molander (1986a) appear to be stable, there are still reasons to be cautious with respect to the generality of the findings. In Bäckman and Molander (1986a) the players were only examined in the most common types of competitions, MCs and LCs. It is possible that these competitions do not bring about optimal variations of arousal when compared to, for example, the Swedish championships; the fact that the competitions used by Bäckman and Molander (1986a) took place on the home course strengthens this suspicion (cf. Silva, 1985). In addition, players from Umeå miniature golf club were studied exclusively; other clubs may develop and foster different attitudes to competitive activity.

To approach these issues and to further assess the generality of the described results, we conducted two more field studies. In the first of these, we examined only young adult players (9 men; mean age = 22.3 years; range = 17-32 years) from Umeå miniature golf club in two training rounds and in two rounds at the 1984 Swedish championships at Katrineholm. Results showed an identical pattern as that observed previously from this group of subjects: there was an increase of HR and RA from training to competition ($ps < .01$), but no decline in motor performance under high-stress competitive conditions ($p > .10$).

In the second follow-up investigation, we compared three groups of older adults (14 men and 1 woman) from three different regions in Sweden (mean ages = 51.0 years, 53.0 years, and 58.0 years, respectively; ranges = 46-60 years, 46-58 years, and 46-70 years, respectively) with two groups of younger adults (11 men), representing different clubs (mean ages = 21.8 years and 28.1 years, respectively; ranges = 18-26 years and 23-36 years, respectively). These players were tested in two training rounds and in two rounds at the 1986 Swedish championships at Grimsås. Again, the same basic pattern of results was observed: all of the players exhibited a similar increase of HR and RA from training to competition ($p < .01$), and the older players performed significantly worse in competition compared to training ($p < .01$).

In sum, the results from this series of field experiments suggest that there is an age-related decline in motor performance under high-stress conditions. This age-related decline appears to be general in the sense that it appears in competitions of varying importance; it holds for players from different clubs; and it occurs regardless of whether the competition is arranged at the home course or away. The inability of older players to perform optimally under conditions of high arousal may have a variety of different origins: (a) a low level of skill; (b) insufficient experience of competition; (c) a low/high level of competitive anxiety; and (d) a disproportionate heightening of level of arousal during competition. However, none of these explanations are supported by data, and the relevant evidence is summarized below.

With respect to the skill variable, the results of Bäckman and Molander (1986a, Experiment 2) indicated that the motor performance of young adults and youths did not deteriorate in large, national competitions, despite the fact that these players performed at about the same level during relaxed training conditions, as did the older adults of the Bäckman and Molander (1986a, Experiments 1 & 3) study. In addition, the young and older adults of the Bäckman and Molander (1986a, Experiment 3) study performed equally well during training, whereas the performance of the older adults deteriorated in competition. Thus, it may be concluded that level of skill is not a critical factor for maintaining a high level of motor performance under stressful conditions, at least not for the range of highly skilled players examined by Bäckman and Molander (1986a).

The factor of experience in competition may have affected the observed age effect in at least two ways. First, it may be that the older adults are less experienced than the young adults regarding miniature golf competitions of the type investigated. Second, it might be argued that competition is more of a reality for the young than for older individuals, and that this Age × Everyday Competition interaction may be a causative factor. The results pertaining to the first of these aspects of competitive experience are straightforward: there were no reliable differences ($ps > .10$) in experience of competition (measured as number of years of competitive experience in miniature golf) between the age groups examined by Bäckman and Molander (1986a, Experiments 1 and 3). Also, despite the fact that one group of older players in the previously described follow-up investigation had greater competitive experience than all three of the younger control groups ($p < .05$), they nevertheless deteriorated in motor performance during competition.

Although it seems likely that young and older adults differ in the extent to which they participate in various types of competitions, we do not believe that this is an important factor for the described results: all of the older players examined here devote hundreds of hours each year to training and competition. They compete in as many miniature golf competitions as the young players, and they have as much (or more) competitive experience as the young players. However, an interesting implication of this state of affairs is that the older players studied here may be less representative of their cohort than are the young players regarding competitive activities. Consequently, the observed age differences may be an underestimation of existing population differences among younger and older cohorts in their ability to cope with high-stress conditions when precise motor behavior control is required.

To assess potential age-related differences in how the competitive situation is perceived, accepted, and appraised; that is, competitive anxiety, the Sport Competition Anxiety Test or SCAT (Martens, 1977) was administered to all players examined in our field studies. Note that this measure reflects competitive anxiety in general (trait anxiety), whereas the ratings of anxiety we registered throughout the experimental series reflect task-and situation-specific anxiety (state anxiety). The SCAT data did not reveal any differences among the different age groups ($ps > .10$), which may allow for the conclusion that young and older players were equally prone to competitive anxiety.

There is some evidence from the literature on verbal learning, arousal, and aging to suggest that older adults are more stressed than younger adults by arousal-inducing task demands (see Elias & Elias, 1977 for a review). Eisdorfer and colleagues (see Eisdorfer, 1968; Eisdorfer, Nowlin & Wilkie, 1970; Eisdorfer & Wilkie, 1977; Powell, Eisdorfer & Bogdanoff, 1964) have demonstrated that older adults exhibit a disproportionate heightening of level of arousal (as indicated by measures of heart rate, galvanic skin response, and free fatty acid levels) during learning and testing of verbal information, and that it is possible to increase the learning performance of older adults via some modification of autonomic nervous system activity by means of drug therapy. If age-related differences in arousal-induced anxiety exist, closed-skill motor activities such as miniature golf may reveal these differences because of the requirement of precise motor action (cf. Welford, 1977).

However, a strictly arousal-based explanation of the results from the field studies described above seems to be implausible: all of the groups examined showed a similar increase in level of arousal (as indicated by measures of heart rate and subjective ratings of anxiety), and there was no selective heightening of arousal on the part of the older players in any of the studies. Hence, it appears that level of arousal per se may not be a general factor explaining the reported age decline in motor performance under high-stress conditions. Rather, the data suggest that there is an age-specific inability to cope with the situational demands of miniature golf events with high levels of arousal. In the next section, we elaborate this notion by introducing a theoretical framework for the understanding of adult age differences in coping with situations of high arousal during motor performance.

## A THEORETICAL FRAMEWORK

This framework rests upon two basic assumptions. First, in agreement with several theorists (e.g., Broadbent, 1971; Easterbrook, 1959; Eysenck, 1984; Mandler, 1975) we assume that the way in which cognitive operations, such as attention and remembering, are carried out varies as a function of level of arousal, and that the functioning of attentional and memory processes may be impaired under conditions of nonoptimal levels of arousal. Some authors (e.g., Lindsay & Norman, 1977) have argued that not only attentional and memory processes, but also decision making operations—as, for example, the ability to decide how to alter an erroneous response—may deteriorate in high-stress conditions.

During a round of miniature golf, as with many other closed-skill motor activities, there are a variety of cognitive operations that have to be carried out in order to achieve good performance. For example, the player has to remember which shots were good and which shots were bad during previous rounds in order to maintain the good shots and adjust the bad ones on a later round. The player also has to make several decisions appropriately before each track is played, (e.g., speed and length of the swing, selection of ball, estimation of angles, etc.). In addition, the player has to make adequate decisions on how to improve upon an erroneous shot; that is, to perceive, assess, and interpret the visual information from a miss, so that the motor behavior pattern may be changed accordingly in readiness for the next shot. The ability to focus selectively on important features of the stimulus array, while simultaneously ignoring irrelevant information (e.g., other players, sounds, traffic, audience) constitutes another example of a task-relevant cognitive operation during miniature golf.

Conceivably, the aforementioned cognitive activities are critical to successful miniature golf performance, and in agreement with previous theorizing and research on arousal and cognition (e.g., Broadbent, 1971; Eysenck, 1984); it may be argued that the increase of arousal during competition makes these task-relevant operations more difficult to carry out.

Second, we assume that, under certain conditions, the individual possesses the ability to compensate for the detrimental effects of nonoptimal levels of arousal via internally guided operations, such as concentration and narrowing of attention (cf. Broadbent, 1971). We interpret the lack of deterioration in motor performance during competition, observed in all of the groups of players except the older adult group, as a demonstration of this compensatory behavior. In other words, the young players perform equally well under high and low stress conditions, due to cognitively mediated compensatory efforts. Analogously, the age decrement in competition is attributed to an age-related deficit in compensating for the negative effects of stressful competitive conditions.

There is considerable evidence to suggest that the aging process is accompanied by deficits in many cognitive abilities that are critical to successful miniature golf performance, such as attention, memory, effortful processing, decision making, and problem solving (see Hasher & Zacks, 1979; Kausler, 1982; Rabbitt, 1977; Salthouse, 1982, 1985 for reviews). Age deficits in these basic cognitive capacities may lead to a reduced proficiency for the compensatory activity assumed to exist under situations of high arousal. Specifically, older players may play well, sometimes even at the level of their younger counterparts, under relaxed conditions by investing more of their capacity in the task at hand; but when task difficulty increases through increased stress they may no longer be able to match the young players by investing more of their already mobilized capacities (see Crowder, 1980 for a similar line of reasoning in the context of memory aging).

Next, we describe three experiments from our laboratory that corroborate our position that older adults decline in motor performance under high-stress conditions reflects an age-related loss in task-relevant cognitive abilities. These experiments deal with (a) motor and memory performance under higher and lower stress conditions; (b) attentional processing during concentration; and (c) the ability to cope with increased cognitive demands in the form of irrelevant background noise.

## REPLICATIONS AND EXTENSIONS IN THE LABORATORY

### Motor Performance, Arousal, and Memory for Shots

In the first laboratory study (Bäckman and Molander 1986b), we sought to qualify the aforementioned theoretical framework by measuring one task-relevant cognitive ability in young and older adult miniature golf players in training and competition. We selected the ability to pick up critical features of the game as the parameter to be measured. Clearly, many cognitive operations used to encode critical aspects of the game are difficult to quantify. However, one task-relevant ability that may be experimentally detectable is to remember the nature of one's own shots. As mentioned, it is important to remember how a certain track was played during a previous round, in order to maintain the shot if it was good (or adjust it if it was bad) on a later round. We reasoned that an outcome showing a selective impairment in this cognitive measure for older players during competitive conditions would support our framework: if older adults, due to an age-related decline in basic cognitive capacities (e.g., attention, memory), have a deficit in the ability to compensate for the negative effects of nonoptimal levels of arousal during motor behavior, then it seems reasonable to expect the same pattern in a critical cognitive measure as in motor performance.

Besides the inclusion of this cognitive task, the Bäckman and Molander (1986b) study extended the field studies in two ways. First, in addition to highly skilled players, groups of young and older less accomplished players were also examined. As discussed, the highly skilled older players investigated in the field studies may be unrepresentative of their cohort in the sense that competition is more a fact of their daily lives compared to their age-mates. Given that younger adults, in general, take part in more competitive events than older adults, this problem of representativeness should not be as pronounced for the highly skilled young players. Thus, if experience in competition and level of skill counteract some of the detrimental effects of the aging process on the ability to cope with situations of high arousal, an exacerbation of age effects should be expected for less accomplished players.

Second, the Bäckman and Molander (1986b) study yielded comparisons between laboratory data and previous results from the field. Such a validation is of utmost importance because field studies of the type described involve a variety of sources of variance that are difficult to control (e.g., effects of time of day, changes in weather, and effects of distracting events such as traffic and a cheering audience). Further, it is very difficult to control for potential differences among players with respect to how many rounds they have played on the particular courses upon which the field experiments took place. All these factors are easily controlled in a laboratory setting.

Bäckman and Molander (1986b) used four groups of players: highly skilled young adults (4 men and 2 women; mean age = 25.5 years; range = 22-32 years), highly skilled older adults (3 men and 3 women; mean age = 50.7 years; range = 47-58 years), moderately skilled young adults (6 men; mean age = 27.7 years; range = 22-35 years), and moderately skilled older adults (5 men and 1 woman; mean age = 51.5 years; range = 46-55 years). The highly skilled players were randomly selected among the players showing the best scores within their age groups in recent competitions arranged by the local miniature golf club. The moderately skilled players were randomly selected among those players whose recent scores were judged to be typical for the advanced beginner. That is, these players mastered the elementary aspects of the game, but had not yet reached the level of skill of the highly skilled players. All of the players were tested in three rounds of training and three rounds of competition (MC). Unlike the field experiments, however, each round comprised only 10 tracks.

To create as realistic a competitive atmosphere as possible in the laboratory, monetary prizes equivalent to those of "real competitions" in the field were awarded to the best players in each of the four groups of players. In addition, spectators and journalists accompanied the competition. In this study, number of shots, HR, RA, and number of shots correctly recalled were registered. Also, the SCAT questionnaire was administered to all participants. However, no differences among groups on ratings of competitive trait anxiety as assessed by this questionnaire were obtained. The two arousal measures were registered after the fifth track in each round was played (after half the round). The reliabilities of the HR and RA measures were assessed in the same way as in the Bäckman and Molander (1986a) field study, that is by calculating the values obtained after the half the round in the first two rounds in each activity. The Pearson correlation coefficients for HR were .83 and .82 for training and competition, respectively. The corresponding coefficients for RA were .78 and .78 respectively. The fact that the reliabilities of the HR values were higher than those obtained in the Bäckman and Molander (1986a) field studies suggests that some of the error variance was reduced in the laboratory setting.

During all rounds, three observers recorded the qualitative nature of players' first shots for each of the 10 tracks. In the memory task that followed the completion of the training and competitive activity, subjects were provided with drawings of the 10 tracks and requested to describe the nature of their first shots on the second round of training or competition for each track (good shot: hole in one or not; miss: left or right, weak or hard; or combination error: aiming and distance error).

The results of the Bäckman and Molander (1986b) study are presented in Table 1-4.

Several aspects of the results should be highlighted. First, although

**TABLE 1.4.** *Mean Heart Rate, Mean Rated Anxiety, Mean Number of Shots, and Mean Number of Shots Recalled as a Function of Age, Level of Skill, and Type of Activity.*

| | Type of activity | | | | | | | |
| | Training | | | | Competition | | | |
| Group | HR | RA | NS | SR | HR | RA | NS | SR |
|---|---|---|---|---|---|---|---|---|
| Highly skilled | | | | | | | | |
| Young (n=6) | 72.12 | 2.37 | 21.60 | 9.00 | 88.98 | 4.43 | 20.68 | 9.33 |
| Old (n=6) | 89.33 | 3.77 | 25.02 | 8.33 | 95.10 | 5.70 | 26.12 | 7.00 |
| Moderately skilled | | | | | | | | |
| Young (n=6) | 73.17 | 3.38 | 29.50 | 7.67 | 88.10 | 4.47 | 30.72 | 9.03 |
| Old (n=6) | 92.38 | 3.38 | 33.02 | 6.33 | 102.85 | 3.98 | 38.07 | 4.67 |

*Note.* HR = heart rate (beats per min); RA = rated anxiety; NS = number of shots per round. SR = shots recalled. Each activity comprised three 10-track rounds.

From "Effects of Adult Age and Level of Skill on the Ability to Cope With High-Stress Conditions in a Precision Sport" by L. Bäckman and B. Molander, 1986, *Psychology and Aging, 1*, p. 335. Copyright 1986 by the American Psychological Association. Adapted by permission.

the older adults showed significantly higher HR than the young adults ($p<.05$), there was no interaction of age and type of activity for either arousal measure ($ps>.10$). Thus, in agreement with the results from the field experiments, young and older adults showed a similar increase of HR and RA from training to competition. The nominal values of these arousal measures were about the same as those of the field experiments, indicating that realistic training and competitive conditions were created in the laboratory.

Second, the data on number of shots also replicated previous results: whereas no differences in level of motor performance between younger and older players at any of the two skill levels were obtained during training ($ps>.10$), the older players deteriorated in competition compared to training ($p<.05$), whereas the young did not ($p>.10$). In addition, the data analysis showed that the moderately skilled players deteriorated from training to competition ($p<.05$), in contrast to the highly skilled players ($p>.10$). Although the interactions of both age and type of activity and skill and type of activity were significant for number of shots ($ps<.05$), the interaction among age, skill, and type of activity fell far short of significance ($p>.20$). Thus, it may be concluded that age and skill have additive rather than multiplicative effects on the ability to maintain motor precision under high-stress conditions.

Third, and most important, in terms of age effects the data of the memory task paralleled, almost exactly, those of the motor task: whereas the young adults recalled as many shots from both activities ($p>.10$), the older players recalled fewer shots from competition than from training ($p<.05$). However, in contrast to the analysis on number of shots, this analysis did not reveal the Skill × Type of Activity interaction to be significant ($p>.05$).

These parallel results for motor and memory performance support our contention that older adults' deterioration in motor performance under situations of high arousal is due to deficits in task-relevant cognitive abilities. Due to these deficits older players may be less proficient than young players in compensating for the negative effects of nonoptimal levels of arousal during competitive play. It should be noted, however, that a lower level of skill was not associated with a selective impairment in memory of shots from competition, although the moderately skilled players deteriorated in motor performance during competition. This discrepancy suggests that the motor decline caused by a low level of skill is not mediated by the same factors as that caused by the aging process. In other words, the cognitive origin of the motor decline in high-stress conditions may be uniquely associated with the adult aging process.

Finally, it may be noted that this laboratory study yielded the same pattern of data as did the field experiments with respect to HR, RA, and motor performance. The fact that similar results have been obtained under restricted laboratory and field conditions may be taken as evidence for both the validity and the reliability of the reported findings.

## Attentional Processes During Concentration

The results of the Bäckman and Molander (1986b) laboratory study suggest that young and older adults may differ in their ability to attend to critical events during situations of high arousal. However, not only the memory data (see Table 1-4), but also patterns of individual HR variability point to the existence of attentional differences between young and older players. An inspection of the within-subject HR standard deviations in the Bäckman and Molander (1986b) study revealed that the variation increased from training to competition for the young adult players, whereas the older players demonstrated a decrease in this measure from training to competition. Similar patterns were found in Experiment 1 and 3 in the Bäckman and Molander (1986a) field study. Analyses of the within-subject HR variability data showed that the interactions between age and type of activity were significant in both field and laboratory studies ($ps<.05$), whereas no significant main effects of age were obtained ($ps>.10$).

It is well known that changes in the focusing of attention are accompanied by phasic changes in HR (e.g., Graham & Clifton, 1966; Marsh & Thompson, 1977, for reviews). It is also known that phasic HR variability is affected by the attentional demands of a task, such that the variability tends to increase when attentional demands increase (Porges, 1972; Porges & Raskin, 1969). Thus, the Age × Type of Activity interaction for the within-subject HR variability data observed by Bäckman and Molander (1986a, 1986b) suggests that the attentional focusing on the part of the older players is more narrow during high-arousal competitive events than during training. Young players, on the other hand, manage to keep their attention at least as flexible in competition as in training.

This interpretation is supported by our own informal observations of the behavior of the players during competitions. The young players kept track of the scores of their competitors and payed greater attention to whatever was happening around the course, whereas the older players seemed to be less attentive and more uninterested in this respect. However, in the Bäckman and Molander (1986a, 1986b) studies HR was measured when each player waited for his turn to play (just before the start of the round, and after playing half the round), and it is possible that the HR variation reflected differences between young and older players in motor activity and mobility during the waiting time, rather than differences in attentional processing.

Recently we performed a second laboratory experiment (Molander

& Bäckman, 1987a), in which possible age differences in motor activity were more stringently controlled. Here we tried to examine the variations in attention more directly than in the earlier studies. This was accomplished by measuring HR continuously during training and competitive activity. Of particular interest was the continuous measurement in those situations where the attentional capacity of the player was most necessary, and motor activity was reduced to a minimum. Such situtions arise when the player concentrates on addressing and striking the ball. The task during the concentration phase, then, may be considered as a complex, self-paced decision task: where the player focuses the attention on internal and external stimuli, and where the stimuli eliciting the motor response are under the player's control.

Lacey and associates (e.g., Lacey, 1959; Lacey et al., 1963) have demonstrated that HR decreases in situations which require the subject to attend to external stimuli, and this effect is obtained both when the response-eliciting events are experimenter-controlled and subject-controlled (Lacey & Lacey, 1978). In contrast, Lacey et al. (1963) found that situations which require an internal focusing of attention, as in problem solving, give rise to HR acceleration. The miniature golf task is complex and it is not obvious how HR should change during periods of deep concentration. Although miniature golf players have to solve problems, remember the qualitative nature of earlier shots, and make decisions during play, it is also very important that they focus their attention on visual external stimuli (e.g., position of obstacles, angle of club head, the length and slope of the track). It is not known whether the focusing of attentional processes during the concentration phase has an internal or an external locus, or some combination of these two loci.

There is a widespread opinion among miniature golfers and among golfers as well that conscious cognitive activity during deep concentration negatively affects motor performance (Cochran, 1979). Furthermore, observations in other precision sports such as rifle-shooting and archery show that HR tends to decrease during preparation and concentration phases (see Landers, 1985). Thus, there are some empirical reasons for expecting HR to show a deceleration rather than an acceleration during the concentration phases in miniature golf. It should be noted, though, that the evidence for HR deceleration during concentration in precision sport activities has been obtained exclusively in young adults (see Landers, 1985 for a review on shooting). It is possible that there might be a tendency toward a more internal focusing of attention as the individual grows older. In view of the plethora of studies showing cognitive deficits in the elderly (Kausler, 1982; Salthouse, 1982), it seems reasonable to assume that the task of concentration involves more cognitive problems, and thus more problem-solving activity for older players than for young players. That is, in an attempt to compensate for their cognitive deficits, the older players may consciously try to retrieve all the steps that are necessary for making a good shot.

The purpose of this next experiment, then, was to examine the relationship between the direction of attention (as indicated by HR change during concentration) and motor performance in highly skilled young adults (5 men and 1 woman; mean age = 29.5 years; range = 22 – 36 years of age) and older adults (4 men and 2 women; mean age = 50.0 years; range = 47 – 58 years of age). The players were observed under relaxed training conditions as well as under competitive conditions (MCs). For both types of activity, HR was registered continuously during the concentration phases by means of a telemetry system. Also, subjective ratings of anxiety (RA) and number of shots were registered. The concentration phase was defined as the time interval elapsing from the start of addressing the ball to the start of the backswing. Thus, the influence of motor activity on HR was minimized.

In accordance with the Bäckman and Molander (1986a, 1986b) findings, we expected the motor performance scores to show an Age × Type of Activity interaction pattern, such that the older adults deteriorate from training to competition, whereas the young adults perform at about the same level in both activities. Also, we expected that the age-related differences in motor performance would be accompanied by differences in attentional processes between the age groups (as indicated by HR changes). Specifically, it was expected that the magnitude of HR change during the concentration phases would be less in competition than in training for the older adults, whereas the change would be about the same in both activities for the young adults. That is, the same Age × Type of Activity interaction pattern was expected for the HR data as for the data on motor performance.

The results of this experiment are presented in Tables 1-5 and 1-6. Table 1-5 shows means for HR, RA, and number of shots for the two groups of players in each of the activities. The HR and RA values in this

**TABLE 1.5.** *Mean Heart Rate, Mean Rated Anxiety, and Mean Number of Shots as a Function of Age and Type of Activity.*

| | Type of activity | | | | | |
| | Training | | | Competition | | |
| Group | HR | RA | NS | HR | RA | NS |
|---|---|---|---|---|---|---|
| Young (n=6) | 72.00 | 2.67 | 22.33 | 83.50 | 3.37 | 20.00 |
| Old (n=6) | 90.50 | 4.17 | 25.33 | 99.33 | 5.33 | 28.50 |

*Note.* HR = heart rate (beats per min); RA = rated anxiety; NS = number of shots. Each activity comprised one 10-track round.

table were obtained in the same way as in the earlier laboratory experiment; that is, after half the round had been completed.

There was a significant increase of HR and RA for both age groups from training to competition ($ps < .01$) and there were no Age × Type of Activity interactions for these measures ($ps > .10$). However, such an interaction was found for the motor performance measure: the older players performed worse in competition compared to training ($p < .05$), whereas the young players performed equally well in both conditions ($p > .10$). The present experiment thus confirmed the findings from our previous studies that the performance of older players deteriorates during competitive conditions, and that this age-related deterioration is not due to a disproportionate heightening or lowering of arousal in the older players.

Assessment of the HR change during concentration was carried out by measuring HR second-by-second in the period extending from three seconds before the start of the concentration phase to three seconds after the end of the phase, and where the three-second periods preceding (PRE) and following (POST) the phase served as baselines. Mean HR for the first (C1) and last (CL) second of the concentration phase, as well as for the PRE and POST periods are presented in Table 1-6. These means are based on the first shot on each track, which was considered to be more attention-demanding and critical for good performance than the succeeding shots played. However, calculations based on all the shots showed essentially the same results as those presented in Table 1-6.

The difference between PRE and CL was selected as one measure of HR change during concentration, and t-tests showed that this difference

**TABLE 1.6.** *Mean Heart Rate (beats per min) During Concentration as a Function of Age and Type of Activity.*

| Group | Type of activity | |
|---|---|---|
| | Training | Competition |
| Young (n=6) | | |
| PRE | 83.88 | 100.71 |
| C1 | 83.88 | 101.02 |
| CL | 78.73 | 92.28 |
| POST | 78.90 | 93.22 |
| Old (n=6) | | |
| PRE | 100.30 | 108.10 |
| C1 | 101.87 | 109.72 |
| CL | 104.27 | 109.07 |
| POST | 104.08 | 108.80 |

*Note.* PRE = the three-second period preceding the start of the concentration phase; C1 = the first second of the concentration phase; CL = the last second of the concentration phase; POST = the three-second period following the end of the concentration phase.

was significant for both young and older adults in training, but only for the young adults in competition ($ps<.05$). The CL-POST difference was nonsignificant for both groups and both activities ($ps>.10$), indicating that the deceleration or the acceleration of HR declined as soon as the stroke was executed and the concentration phase was terminated. As illustrated in Table 1-6, the older adults demonstrated an accelerating HR during concentration in training and a weak tendency towards deceleration in competition. The young players showed decelerating HR in both activities. An analysis of the magnitude of HR change, as indicated by the PRE—CL measure, yielded a significant Age × Type of Activity interaction ($p<.04$), such that the magnitude decreased from training to competition for the older players, whereas the magnitude increased from training to competition for the young players. A similar interaction pattern was found for the analysis of the within-subject variation of HR change: the older players showed decreasing variation from training to competition, whereas the younger players showed increasing variation from training to competition.

The results of this experiment support our hypothesis that the decline in motor performance of older players during competition is attributable to aging loss in task-relevant cognitive abilities, and that this loss is especially devastating during high-stress conditions. In the Bäckman and Molander (1986b) study it was shown that the decline in motor performance was accompanied by a decline in memory for shots. The results of the present experiment suggest that these declines may, in part, be due to attentional deficits in the older players.

It is evident from Table 1-6 and from the statistical analyses that the two age groups show different HR patterns during concentration. This result is at variance with the results in the relatively few psychological studies that have addressed the question of adult age differences in cardiac patterns (e.g., Faucheux et al., 1983; Morris & Thompson, 1969; Riege, Cohen & Wallach, 1980). In general, these studies have found HR-changes in the same direction (either deceleration or acceleration, depending on type of task) for young and older subjects, but that the change is less pronounced for older than for young individuals. However, the tasks used in the cited studies seem to demand either internal focusing of attention (e.g., intelligence tests, recognition memory) or external focusing of attention (e.g., simple reaction-time tasks). It is possible that the rather restricted nature of these tasks, in contrast to the complex nature of the miniature golf task, which allows for both internal and external focusing, tends to mask qualitative age-related differences in direction of attention.

Our interpretation of the obtained age differences is that younger and older players adopt different attentional strategies during the concentration phase, and that the attentional processing on the part of the

*AGING AND MOTOR BEHAVIOR*

older players is more efficient during relaxed training conditions than in competitive conditions where nonoptimal levels of arousal prevail. The strategy associated with the internal focusing of attention in the older players may be construed as an attempt to compensate for various age-related cognitive deficits. This compensatory effort is relatively successful during "normal" conditions, but under stressful conditions the effort may tend to dissipate and, as a consequence, neither an internal nor an external strategy can be efficiently adopted.

## Background Noise During Competitive Play

During the concentration phases, the attention of the miniature golf players may be both selective and focused. According to a commonly accepted definition, selective attention refers to the differential processing of simultaneous sources of information, separating the relevant from the irrelevant stimuli. The sources of information may be internal (memory, knowledge) as well as external (environmental objects and events). In contrast, attention is said to be focused when only some of the present stimuli are relevant for successful task performance (Johnston & Dark, 1986).

A popular hypothesis within the area of cognitive aging holds that the ability to focus selectively on relevant stimuli while ignoring irrelevant stimuli is impaired in older people (Kausler, 1982; Salthouse, 1982). This hypothesis was supported by our laboratory experiments (Bäckman & Molander, 1986b; Molander & Bäckman, 1987a) where the process of selective or focused attention in the older players appeared to be disrupted during conditions of high arousal. However, in competitive activity the players have to ignore not only irrelevant internal stimuli resulting from possible anxiety or nervousness, but also different kinds of external background noise, such as other players, traffic sounds, audience and loudspeakers, some of which are irrelevant for the playing activity. From the hypothesis of impaired selected attention in older people one should therefore expect the external background noise to be more devastating for the performance of older players than for the performance of young players.

There is reason to believe that each player's level of arousal in competitive activity may increase further if the intensity of the background noise is high (Broadbent, 1971; Poulton, 1978), but it is also possible that the player's focusing of attention is affected differently by the different types of noise prevailing during tournaments. For example, the sounds from loudspeakers and audience may be much more attention-demanding than traffic sounds.

In a third laboratory experiment (Molander & Bäckman, 1987b), the effects of two different noise conditions during competition on the motor and cognitive performance of new samples of highly skilled players was investigated. Young (5 men and 1 woman; mean age = 27.8 years; range = 19-36 years) and older (4 men and 2 women; mean age = 53.2 years; range = 49 - 59 years) normal hearing adult miniature golf players participated in competitions (MCs), in which the background sound was either tape-recorded traffic noise or a radio broadcasting of a soccer game. The loudness of the noise on the tapes was set to a relatively low level (62 dBA) in order to minimize the influence of noise intensity per se on the level of arousal. Thus, both noise conditions were equal with respect to loudness and differed only in the sense that the traffic condition was less meaningful than the radio broadcasting condition. We registered HR and number of shots in this experiment, and memory for shots was also tested as in the Bäckman and Molander (1986b) study.

Several authors (e.g., Baker & Holding, 1986; Cohen & Weinstein, 1982; Loeb, 1986) have argued that the information load imposed under noise exposure is affected more by the meaning of the noise than by the intensity of the sound, and that the predictability of the noise source is an important factor that must be considered. In line with this reasoning, and on the basis of our contention that older players' performance decline in competition is associated with age-related deficits in cognitive functioning, we expected the older players to exhibit a disproportionate disruption in both motor and memory performance in the radio broadcasting condition. Further, since competitions were arranged for both noise conditions, and since the two conditions were equal with respect to loudness, no effect of condition for HR was expected. As shown in Table 1-7, both these sets of predictions were confirmed. Whereas the older participants played less well and remembered fewer shots in the radio broadcasting than in the traffic condition ($ps < .05$), the young participants performed almost as well for both measures in both noise conditions ($ps > .10$). No significant effects were obtained for the HR measure ($ps > .10$).

The fact that the older players showed impaired memory performance in the radio broadcasting condition as compared to the traffic noise condition is consistent with the hypothesis that older adults have a

**TABLE 1.7.** *Mean Heart Rate, Mean Number of Shots, and Mean Number of Shots Recalled as a Function of Age and Type of Background Noise.*

| | Type of background noise | | | | | |
| | Traffic sounds | | | Radio broadcasting | | |
| Group | HR | NS | SR | HR | NS | SR |
|---|---|---|---|---|---|---|
| Young ($n=6$) | 81.38 | 39.00 | 14.92 | 81.84 | 39.83 | 13.25 |
| Old ($n=6$) | 82.15 | 47.17 | 14.50 | 81.73 | 53.17 | 11.67 |

*Note.* HR = heart rate (beats per min); NS = number of shots; SR = shots recalled. Each background noise condition comprised one 18-track round.

deficit in the selective aspect of attention (e.g., Layton, 1975; Madden, 1983; Rabbitt, 1965). However, such age effects have only been obtained when the irrelevant stimuli have to be searched to find the relevant stimuli (e.g., Ford et al., 1979; Wright & Elias, 1979). As shown in Table 1-7, age effects were found in the present experiment although the players were not explicitly instructed to listen to the noise. Neither did the task require that the irrelevant noise stimuli be searched. However, in the Wright and Elias (1979) study tachistoscopically presented letters were used, and in the Ford et al., (1979) study subjects listened to tones of high and low frequencies. It seems highly likely, then, that the difference between the present results and previous findings is due to differences in the meaningfulness of the irrelevant background stimuli.

It is worth noting that the motor performance measure and the memory measure revealed the same age impairment in the radio broadcasting condition. This result, if considered together with the result of the Bäckman and Molander (1986b) study, in which an age-related impairment was found for both these measures in competition compared to training, may reflect a general age deficit in the ability to cope with increased cognitive demands (Salthouse, 1985).

Although the experiments reported by Bäckman and Molander (1986b) and Molander and Bäckman (1987b) were not designed to examine the interaction between different types of stressors, the results of these experiments indicate that both high levels of arousal and meaningful noise are detrimental to motor and cognitive performance in older players; in both cases, the effects of the stressors appear to affect attentional functioning in a detrimental manner.

It should be noted that the negative effects of the radio broadcasting condition were not associated with an increased level of arousal. This result is somewhat difficult to reconcile with theories which assume that negative or positive effects of noise are caused by changes in arousal (e.g., Broadbent, 1971; Poulton, 1979). The present findings seem to be much more easily accommodated by theories which assume that noise acts to reduce processing capacity because it provides a source of competing demand (e..g, Boggs & Simon, 1968; Weinstein, 1974) or composite theories (e.g., Fisher, 1984), which assume that any one stress has a variety of potential targets of influence.

## CONCLUSIONS

The research described in this chapter indicates that there is an age-related decline in the ability to cope with situations of high arousal and distracting events during performance in a motor task such as miniature golf. The age deficit was observed in motor and cognitive performance during high-stress competitive conditions and when task-irrelevant, but meaningful, background noise was presented. The age-related decline observed under these two different conditions may reflect a general age deficit in the ability to cope with increased cognitive demands.

The results of these studies thus support the previously described framework for the relationship of aging, arousal, and cognitive operations during motor performance. Although young adults are capable of compensating for the detrimental effects of nonoptimal levels of arousal or increased noise through compensatory cognitive efforts, the loss in basic cognitive capacities with aging hinders older adults from compensating efficiently for increased cognitive demands during task performance. This postulate received further support by the Molander and Bäckman (1987a) study, which demonstrated qualitative age differences in the direction of attention during concentration, suggesting a breakdown of attentional focus in older players during high stress.

In the remainder of the chapter we would like to discuss some general aspects of the described research. In our view, there are four issues especially worth emphasizing in this context: (a) the relationship of field and laboratory experiments; (b) the nature of age-related performance differences; (c) the generality of the results; and (d) the potential reversibility of the age-related decline.

## THE LAB-LIFE RELATIONSHIP

During recent years, basic cognitive psychology (e.g., Baddeley & Wikins, 1984; Neisser, 1982) as well as the experimental psychology of human aging (e.g., Bäckman, in press; Dixon, 1983; Kausler, 1983; Poon, Rubin & Wilson, in press) and motor behavior (e.g., Goode & Magill, 1986; Reed, 1982; Stelmach, 1982) have been criticized for a lack of ecological validity and for being too concerned with arbitrary laboratory trivia. In many cases, the argument goes, experimental paradigms in, for example, memory research, are not very representative of the encoding and retrieval requirements of the natural environment, and pleas have been made both to employ more ecologically relevant tasks and materials, and to examine the behavior under study within natural settings.

As far as experimental aging research is concerned, this criticism has been quite effective. A comparison of a current major journal in this field (e.g., *Journal of Gerontology*) with the same journal 10 or 15 years ago reveals that most of the research on paired-associate learning, the Sternberg paradigm, or anagram solving have been replaced with research on tasks such as prose comprehension, television recall, or memory for action events. The last three tasks all constitute examples of attempts to mirror the cognitive reality of everyday life in the laboratory. Such laboratory models of real-life situations are extremely important in that they enable validations of empirical laws derived from research on standard laboratory tasks. However, examples of validations from these supposedly ecologically relevant tasks to their real-life origins (or vice versa) are essentially lacking. In other words, the ecological approach to experimental aging research has been quite successful in developing laboratory analogies to real-life situations, but less so when it comes to studying behaviors of young and older adults as they are manifested in the natural environment.

We argue that precision sports such as sharp-shooting, bowling, billiards, archery, golf, or miniature golf constitute an interesting task category if the purpose is to examine real-life emotional, cognitive, and motor behaviors without necessarily relaxing methodological criteria. Most people would probably agree that precision sports are ecologically valid, and many of the aforementioned instances of this task category may be studied in the laboratory without losing significance, or without altering essential aspects of the game in any important respect; therefore, precision sports are well suited for the type of life to lab validations described above. We hope that the field and laboratory studies presented in this chapter illustrate this possibility.

## THE NATURE OF AGE-RELATED DIFFERENCES

The dominant research design in investigations on psychological aspects of aging, the cross-sectional design, may have considerable external validity in that it indicates the general nature of the age-performance relationship present in the actual populations, but, at the same time, the internal validity of the results obtained with this type of design may be questionable. By this we mean that it is often very difficult to identify true causative factors of age-related performance differences on the basis of cross-sectional data (see Kausler, 1982). This difficulty may be because representative age groups typically differ not only in chronological age, but also in a number of potentially important non-age attributes (educational level, task-relevant experience). The confounding between age and non-age attributes makes it difficult to identify which variable (or variables) accounts for most of the variance, thereby restricting internal validity.

Researchers have tried to solve this problem by matching young and older adult subjects with respect to non-age attributes known to covary both with age and performance scores on the task at hand. Although such balanced designs may provide us with unconfounded data (whatever age differences that occur may be attributed to true ontogenetic change in performance), the balancing procedure may instead threaten the external validity of the results. For example, as noted by Salthouse (1982), it is commonplace in studies on aging to match young and older participants on the basis of years of schooling to avoid differential influence of this factor on the dependent variable. Educational trends have changed drastically, however, over the last 50-100 years, and individuals with the same level of education are probably not equally representative of their respective cohort. Specifically, an older adult with college education is likely to have come from a more highly educated family than a young college graduate. The matching procedure may thus create differential representativeness in the two age groups and impair external validity.

In addition, whereas some non-age attributes, such as number of years of schooling and verbal ability may be dealt with easily in a matching procedure, others such as motivation and task-relevant knowledge may continue to resist an effective balancing, especially between groups of young and older individuals.

Several authors (e.g., Baltes & Schaie, 1976; Comfort, 1976; Cornelius, 1984; Langer et al., 1979; Popkin, Schaie & Krauss, 1983; Schaie, 1978) have argued that motivational factors and task-relevant experience influence performance differences between young and older adults. Hultsch and Pentz (1980) claimed that traditional learning and memory tasks, which require verbatim recall of verbal materials, are not perceived as meaningful by many older adults. These authors noted that the incidence of older adults' questions regarding the relevance of such tasks are striking compared to that of young adults, and that this age difference may reflect something more than uncooperativeness and obstinacy among the elderly: the absence of understanding of the relevance of the task from the point of view of the aged (see also Erickson, Poon & Walsh-Sweeney, 1980). If these observations are valid, there are strong reasons for assuming motivational differences, favoring the young, in many laboratory tasks used in aging research (cf. Thompson & Nowlin, 1973).

With respect to age differences in task-relevant experience or skill, Bäckman and Nilsson (1984) suggested that the majority of standard cognitive tasks correspond with the demands of formal education, which obviously favors performance of younger subjects who are enrolled in university classes or recently finished school. Analogously, older subjects, who left school several decades ago, may be at a disadvantage in the bulk of cognitive tasks due to a lack of task-relevant experience (see also Gardner & Monge, 1977; Wiersma & Klausmeier, 1965). There are also those investigations that have emphasized the converse, viz. older adults' ability to compensate for age-related performance decline via task-relevant experience in, for example, chess (Charness, 1981), reading (Hultsch & Dixon, 1983), and typing (Salthouse, 1984). Thus, intrinsic variables such as motivational level and prior knowledge may lead to an overestimation of age differences, but with appropriate selection procedures they may also reduce age-related performance differences.

The research on miniature golf and aging presented in this chapter is

AGING AND MOTOR BEHAVIOR

relevant to the above discussion in several respects. By using a task for which it is possible to assess subjects' task-relevant experience (experience of competition, frequency of playing), level of skill, and motivation, the confounding of age and these important non-age attributes may be minimized. Consequently, the described results from the miniature golf task may reflect relatively uncontaminated age-related differences.

Viewed from a different perspective, the reported research provides a conservative test of potential age-related differences. As noted, it is commonly held among theorists on cognitive aging that a high level of skill or prior knowledge can compensate for age-related performance decline; our older subjects showed deficits in motor and cognitive performance during conditions of high-stress and meaningful noise, despite the fact that they were highly skilled, highly motivated, and had equal or more competitive experience compared to the young. The true nature of the reported age-related differences is further strengthened by the fact that our older subjects had a mean age just above 50 years of age in all of the studies. In many studies on aging, for example in the area of intelligence research, an age-related decline may not be observed until 65 years of age or later (Botwinick, 1977, Salthouse, 1982).

Thus, the robust differences between 25-year-old and 50-year-old miniature golf players in motor and cognitive performance clearly suggest that the differences are due to the adult aging process: the relatively short cross-sectional time span should minimize the negative influences of biological aging (e.g., sensory deficits, disease) and simultaneously reduce the impact of uncontrolled generational factors, thereby minimizing the probability of making Type 1 errors.

## THE GENERALITY OF RESULTS

The age-related decline in miniature golf performance in situations of high arousal and high cognitive demand appears to be a reliable effect. It has occurred (a) with a large number of samples of young and older players at various levels of skill; (b) in competitions of varying degree of importance; (c) independent of type of miniature golf course (difficult/less difficult, home course or away); (d) independent of club association; and (e) in the field as well as in the laboratory. Thus, it may be concluded that this age deterioration is general as far as miniature golf is concerned.

However, it is reasonable to argue that the observed pattern of results is not restricted to miniature golf or even to precision sports in general. Many authors have suggested that the adult aging process is accompanied by a loss in physiological adaptability (e.g., Marx, 1974; Timiras, 1972), and it has been indicated that the older individual may be less able than the younger to cope with a stress or environmental change, due to age changes in the neuroendocrine system. These changes may originate from an age-related reduction in functional activity of the endocrine glands or metabolic rate, or from age changes in the responsiveness of target tissue or organs to hormonal action, or from a combination of these factors (Eisdorfer & Wilkie, 1977).

Thus, there are reasons to believe that an age-related deficit in the ability to cope with stress and increased cognitive demands would be found across a wide variety of task situations and demands. However, since studies addressing this issue are essentially lacking in the literature, it is an important task to replicate the reported findings with other types of tasks. This may include real-life tasks which require precise motor action (e.g., other precision sports) as well as standard motor and cognitive tasks.

## THE POTENTIAL REVERSIBILITY OF THE AGE-RELATED DECLINE

Another avenue for future investigation is to examine the reversibility of the observed age-related decline. Within other domains of psychological research on aging (e.g., intelligence, memory), knowledge concerning older adults' potential of performance or plasticity of functioning has proven to be extremely important for the theoretical understanding of adult development (see Baltes, 1987; Bäckman, in press, for reviews).

In the present context, one may investigate whether it is possible to enhance the level of motor and cognitive performance in older adults in high-stress and noise conditions through different forms of intervention (e.g., cognitive training, relaxation techniques, pharmacological treatments). Although both relaxation training (Yesavage, Rose & Spiegel, 1982) and pharmacological therapy, for example, by means of administration of beta adrenergic blocks (Eisdorfer, Nowlin & Wilkie, 1970), may be effective in improving older adults' cognitive performance, the results from the research described in this chapter suggest that the most interesting form of intervention in the present case is that of cognitive training.

This is because (a) no selective heightening of arousal on the part of older adults has been observed in any of our studies; and (b) our theoretical framework for the understanding of older adults' performance decline in competition emphasizes the cognitive origin of the decline. Thus, we hypothesize that in order to maximize the possibility of reducing or eliminating older adults' performance deficit, the cognitive operations utilized during task performance may have to be altered.

One way of accomplishing this is to influence the way in which attention is directed during the phase of concentration. As suggested by the results of Molander and Bäckman (1987a), there may be qualitative adult age-related differences in focusing of attention during concentration in this situation, such that older adults may tend to focus more on internal stimuli (as indicated by an acceleration of HR), whereas young adults may tend to direct their attentional resources towards external stimuli (as indicated by a deceleration of HR).

The results of motor performance from the Molander and Bäckman (1987a) study suggest that the attentional strategy employed by older adults is less effective in competition than in training, whereas the attentional focus of young adults is associated with good performance in both types of activities. Accordingly, if it would be possible through extended practice to change the attentional strategy typically employed by an older individual during task performance from an internal to an external focus of attention, and further, if this change would be associated with an improvement of motor performance in high-stress conditions, then we would have another piece of evidence that it is, in fact, possible to teach an older individual to reactivate a latent, but normally inactive cognitive skill (Dixon & Bäckman, in press).

## GENERAL SUMMARY

In this chapter, we have described a series of field and laboratory experiments examining the multiple relationships among the factors of adult age, level of arousal, and cognitive operations during motor behavior. The motor behavior of interest is that of playing miniature golf.

Several arguments were put forward as to why precision sports such as miniature golf constitute an interesting task category for research addressing these relationships: (a) it is possible to compare field and laboratory data; (b) participants' motivational level is high; (c) the requirement of precise motor behavior makes the task sensitive in detecting performance variation caused by changes in level of arousal; and (d) successful performance rests on proficient utilization of a variety of task-relevant cognitive abilities.

With respect to the field studies, a quite consistent pattern of results has been obtained. Whereas older adult miniature golf players routinely performed worse in high-stress competitive conditions than in relaxed training conditions, several groups of younger players (youths, juniors, and young adults) performed equally well in both conditions. In addition, all groups of players examined exhibited a similar increase of level of arousal from training to competition. The age-related decline in motor performance could not be explained by age differences in heightening of arousal, level of skill, competitive anxiety, or competitive experience.

We entertain the hypothesis that older players' selective decline in motor performance during competition reflects an age-specific inability to compensate for the detrimental effects of the nonoptimal levels of arousal that prevail in competitive activity. There are several cognitive abilities that are critical to successful miniature golf performance, many of which are related to basic attentional, memory, and problem solving operations. It is well known that the adult aging process is associated with deficits in these cognitive abilities. Cognitive deficits may hinder older players from compensating efficiently for the high-stress conditions in competition. During relaxed training conditions, older players may "catch up" by investing more of their capacity in the task, but when task difficulty increases through increased stress, they may no longer be able to match their younger counterparts, by investing more of their already mobilized cognitive capacities.

This theoretical account received empirical support from three laboratory studies, which replicated the pattern of results from the field studies with respect to motor performance. In addition, the results of the first of these studies showed that older players' decline in motor performance during competition was paralleled by a similar decline in a task-relevant cognitive ability, namely, to remember the qualitative nature of one's own shots.

In a second laboratory study, we obtained age-related differences in patterns of heart rate change during concentration, such that older players showed accelerating heart rate and young players showed decelerating heart rate. These age-related changes in autonomic nervous system activity may reflect a tendency among older players to focus attention on internal stimuli, and a tendency among young players to attend to external stimuli during concentration. Results of motor performance suggest that the attentional strategy adopted by the young players was more effective during competition than that adopted by the older players.

The third laboratory study demonstrated that it is possible to obtain an age-related decline in motor and cognitive performance not only in high-stress conditions, but also when a division of attentional resources is required, by presenting meaningful, but task-irrelevant background noise during play. These results suggest that the age-related decline in motor and cognitive performance observed throughout the series of field and laboratory studies reflects a general aging deficit in the ability to cope with increased cognitive demands.

Further, some general theoretical and methodological implications of the described research were discussed. Here, we emphasized the importance of employing experimental tasks which may be studied both in the field without relaxing methodological criteria, and in the laboratory without violating principles of ecological relevance and representativeness. In addition, we made the point that the age-related differences reported in our research were obtained despite the fact that the older participants were highly skilled, highly motivated, and had equal or more competitive experience compared to the young. Also, we discussed the generality of our findings both within the realm of precision sport tasks, and as related to motor and cognitive tasks in general. Finally, the issue of whether the age-related decline in motor and cognitive performance is reversible or not was approached, by exemplifying how older adults may be trained so as to reduce or eliminate the age-related performance deficit.

## REFERENCES

Bäckman, L. (in press. Varieties of memory compensation of older adults in episodic remembering. In L.W. Poon, D.C. Rubin & B.A. Wilson (Eds.), *Everyday cognition in adulthood and late life.* New York: Cambridge University Press.

Bäckman, L., & Molander, B. (1986a). Adult age differences in the ability to cope with situations of high arousal in a precision sport. *Psychology and Aging, 1,* 133-139.

Bäckman, L., & Molander, B. (1986b). Effects of adult age and level of skill on the ability to cope with high-stress conditions in a precision sport. *Psychology and Aging, 1,* 334-336.

Bäckman, L., & Nilsson, L.G. (1984). Aging effects in free recall: An exception to the rule. *Human Learning, 3,* 53-69.

Baddeley, A.D., & Wilkins, A. (1984). Taking memory out of the laboratory. In J.E. Harris & P.E. Morris (Eds.), *Everyday memory, actions, and absent-mindedness* (pp. 1-17). London: Academic Press.

Baker, M.A., & Holding, D.H. (1986, November). Noisiness and meaningfulness. Paper presented at the 27th Annual Meeting of the Psychonomic Society, New Orleans, LA.

Baltes, P.B. (1987). Theoretical propositions of life-span developmental psychology: On the dynamics between growth and decline. *Developmental Psychology, 23,* 611-626.

Baltes, P.B., and Schaie, K.W. (1976). On the plasticity of intelligence in adulthood and old age: Where Horn and Donaldson fail. *American Psychologist, 31,* 720-725.

Boggs, D.H., & Simon, J.R. (1968). Differential effect of noise on tasks of varying complexity. *Journal of Applied Psychology, 52,* 148-153.

Botwinick, J. (1977). Intellectual abilities. In J.E. Birren & K.W. Schaie (Eds.), *Handbook of the psychology of aging* (pp. 580-605). New York: Van Nostrand.

Broadbent, D.A. (1971). *Decision and stress.* New York: Academic Press.

Charness, N. (1981). Aging and skilled problem solving. *Journal of Experimental Psychology: General, 110,* 21-38.

Cochran, A.J. (1979). The golfer. In W.T. Singleton (Ed.), *The study of real skills. Compliance and excellence* (Vol. 2) (pp. 198-221). Lancaster: MTP Press Ltd.

Cohen, S., & Weinstein, N. (1982). Nonauditory effects of noise on behavior and health. In G.W. Evans (Ed.), *Environmental stress* (pp. 45-74). New York: Cambridge University Press.

Comfort, A. (1976). *A good age.* New York: Simon & Schuster.

Cornelius, S.W. (1984). Classic pattern of intellectual aging: Test familiarity, difficulty, and performance. *Journal of Gerontology, 39,* 201-216.

Cratty, B.J. (1973). *Movement behavior and motor learning* (3rd ed.). Philadelphia: LEA & Febiger.

Crowder, R.G. (1980). Echoic memory and the study of aging memory systems. In L.W. Poon, J.L. Fozard, L.S. Cermak, D. Arenberg & L.W. Thompson (Eds.), *New directions in memory and aging* (pp. 181-204). Hillsdale, NJ: Erlbaum.

Dixon, R.A. (1983). How to avoid aging effects in free recall. *Scandinavian Journal of Psychology, 24,* 335-337.

Dixon, R.A., & Bäckman, L. (in press). Reading and memory for prose in adulthood: Issues of expertise and compensation. In S.R. Yussen & M.C. Smith (Eds.), *Reading across the life span.* New York: Springer.

Easterbrook, J.A. (1959). The effect of emotion on cue utilisation and the organisation of behavior. *Psychological Review, 66,* 183-201.

Eisdorfer, C. (1968). Arousal and performance: Experiments in verbal learning and a tentative theory. In G.A. Talland (Ed.), *Human aging and behavior* (pp. 189-216). New York: Academic Press.

Eisdorfer, C., Nowlin, J., & Wilkie, F. (1970). Improvement of learning in the aged by modification of autonomic nervous system activity. *Science, 170,* 1327-1329.

Eisdorfer, C., & Wilkie, F. (1977). Stress, disease, aging, and behavior. In J.E. Birren & K.W. Schaie (Eds.), *Handbook of the psychology of aging* (pp. 251-275). New York: Van Nostrand.

Elias, M.F., & Elias, P.K. (1977). Motivation and activity. In J.E. Birren & K.W. Schaie (Eds.), *Handbook of the psychology of aging* (pp. 357-383). New York: Van Nostrand.

Erickson, R.C., Poon, L.W., & Walsh-Sweeney, L. (1980). Clinical memory testing of the elderly. In L.W. Poon, J.L. Fozard, L.S. Cermak, D. Arenberg & L.W. Thompson (Eds.), *New directions in memory and aging* (pp. 379-402). Hillsdale, NJ: Erlbaum.

Eysenck, M.W. (1984). *A handbook of cognitive psychology.* London: Erlbaum.

Faucheux, B.A., Dupuis, C., Baulon, A., Lille, F., & Bourlière, F. (1983). Heart rate reactivity during minor mental stress in men in their 50s and 70s. *Gerontology, 29,* 149-160.

Fisher, S. (1984). *Stress and the perception of control*. London: Erlbaum.

Ford, J.M., Hink, R.F., Hopkins, W.F.,III., Roth, W.T., Pfefferbaum, A., & Kopell, B.S. (1979). Age effects on event-related potentials in a selective attention task. *Journal of Gerontology, 34*, 388-395.

Gardner, E.G., & Monge, R.H. (1977). Adult age differences in cognitive abilities and educational background. *Experimental Aging Research, 3*, 337-383.

Goode, S., & Magill, R.A. (1986). Contextual interference effects in learning three badminton serves. *Research Quarterly for Exercise and Sport, 57*, 308-314.

Graham, F.K., & Clifton, R.K. (1966). Heart-rate change as a component of the orienting response. *Psychological Bulletin, 65*, 305-320.

Hasher, L., & Zacks, R.T. (1979). Automatic and effortful processes in memory. *Journal of Experimental Psychology: General, 108*, 356-388.

Hatfield, B.D., & Landers, D.M. (1983). A new direction for sports psychology. *Journal of Sport Psychology, 5*, 243-259.

Hatfield, B.D., Landers, D.M., & Ray, W.J. (1984). Cognitive processes during self-paced motor performance: An electroencephalographic profile of skilled marksmen. *Journal of Sport Psychology, 6*, 55-70.

Hultsch, D.F., & Dixon, R.A. (1983). The role of pre-experimental knowledge in text processing in adulthood. *Experimental Aging Research, 9*, 17-22.

Hultsch, D.F., & Pentz, C.A. (1980). Encording, storage, and retrieval in adult memory: The role of model assumptions. In L.W. Poon, J.L. Fozard, L.S. Cermak, D. Arenberg & L.W. Thompson (Eds.), *New directions in memory and aging* (pp. 73-94). Hillsdale, NJ: Erlbaum.

Johnston, W.A., & Dark, V.J. (1986). Selective attention. *Annual Review of Psychology, 37*, 43-75.

Kausler, D.H. (1982). *Experimental psychology and human aging*. New York: John Wiley.

Kausler, D.H. (1983, August). *Episodic memory and human aging*. Paper presented at the 91st Annual Meeting of the American Psychological Association, Anaheim, CA.

Kelso, J.A.S. (Ed.). (1982). *Human motor behavior: An introduction*. Hillsdale, NJ: Erlbaum.

Kerr, B. (1983). Memory, action, and motor control. In R.A. Magill (Ed.), *Memory and control of action* (pp. 47-65). Amsterdam: North-Holland.

Lacey, J.I. (1959). Psychophysiological approaches to the evaluation of psychotherapeutic process and outcome. In E.A. Rubinstein & M.B. Parloff (Eds.), *Research in psychotherapy* (pp. 160-208). Washington, D.C.: American Psychological Association.

Lacey, J.I., Kagan, J., Lacey, B., & Moss, H.A. (1963). The visceral level: Situational determinants and behavioral correlates of autonomic response patterns. In M.H. Knapp (Ed.), *Expression of the emotions in man* (pp. 161-196). New York: International Universities Press.

Lacey, J.I., & Lacey, B.C. (1978). Two-way communication between the heart and the brain. Significance of time within the cardiac cycle. *American Psychologist*, 99-113.

Landers, D.M. (1985). Psychophysiological assessment and biofeedback: Applications for athletes in closed-skill sports. In J.H. Sandweiss & S.L. Wolf (Eds.), *Biofeedback and sports science* (pp. 63-105). New York: Plenum Press.

Langer, E.J., Rodin, J., Beck, P., Weinman, C., & Spitzer, L. (1979). Environmental determinants of memory improvement in late adulthood. *Journal of Personality and Social Psychology, 37*, 2002-2013.

Layton, B. (1975). Perceptual noise and aging. *Psychological Bulletin, 82*, 875-883.

Lindsay, P.H., & Norman, D.A. (1977). *Human information processing* (2nd ed.). New York: Academic Press.

Loeb, M. (1986). *Noise and human efficiency*. Chichester: Wiley.

Madden, D.J. (1983). Aging and distraction by highly familiar stimuli during visual search. *Developmental Psychology, 19*, 499-507.

Magill, R.A. (Ed.). (1983). *Memory and control of action*. Amsterdam: North-Holland.

Mandler, G. (1975). *Mind and emotion*. New York: Wiley.

Marsh, G.R., & Thompson, L.W. (1977). Psychophysiology of aging. In J.E. Birren & K.W. Schaie (Eds.), *Handbook of the psychology of aging* (pp. 219-248). New York: Van Nostrand.

Martens, R. (1977). *Sport Competition Anxiety Test*. Champaign, IL: Human Kinetics Publishers.

Marx, J. (1974). Aging research (II): Pacemakers for aging? *Science, 186*, 1196-1197.

Molander, B., & Bäckman, L. (1987a). Adult age differences in heart rate patterns during concentration in a precision sport: Implications for attentional functioning. Manuscript submitted for publication.

Molander, B., & Bäckman, L. (1987b). Adult age differences in coping with irrelevant background noise during miniature golf competition. Unpublished manuscript.

Morris, J.D., & Thompson, L.W. (1969). Heart rate changes in a reaction time experiment with young and aged subjects. *Journal of Gerontology, 24*, 269-275.

Neisser, U. (1982). Memory: What are the important questions? In U. Neisser (Ed.), *Memory observed* (pp. 3-19). San Francisco: Freeman.

Ostrow, A.C. (1984). *Physical activity and the older adult: Psychological perspectives*. Princeton: Princeton Book Co.

Poon, L.W., Fozard, J.L., Cermak, L.S., Arenberg, D., & Thompson, L.W. (Eds.). (1980). *New directions in memory and aging*. Hillsdale, NJ: Erlbaum.

Poon, L.W., Rubin, D.C., & Wilson, B.A. (Eds.). (in press). *Everyday cognition in adulthood and late life*. New York: Cambridge University Press.

Popkin, S.J., Schaie, K.W., & Krauss, I.K. (1983). Age-fair assessment of psychometric intelligence. *Educational Gerontology, 9,* 47-55.

Porges, S.W. (1972). Heart rate variability and deceleration as indexes of reaction time. *Journal of Experimental Psychology, 92,* 103-110.

Porges, S.W., & Raskin, D.C. (1969). Respiratory and heart rate components of attention. *Journal of Experimental Psychology, 81,* 497-503.

Poulton, E.C. (1978). A new look at the effects of noise: A rejoinder. *Psychological Bulletin, 85,* 1068-1079.

Poulton, E.C. (1979). Composite model for human performance in continuous noise. *Psychological Review, 86,* 361-375.

Powell, A.H., Eisdorfer, C., & Bogdanoff, M.D. (1964). Physiologic response patterns observed in a learning task. *Archives of General Psychiatry, 10,* 192-195.

Prinz, W., & Sanders, A.F. (Eds.). (1984). *Cognition and motor processes.* Heidelberg: Springer-Verlag.

Rabbitt, P. (1965). An age-decrement in the ability to ignore irrelevant information. *Journal of Gerontology, 20,* 233-238.

Rabbitt, P. (1977). Changes in problem-solving ability in old age. In J.E. Birren & K.W. Schaie (Eds.), *Handbook of the psychology of aging* (pp. 606-625). New York: Van Nostrand.

Reed, E.S. (1982). An outline of a theory of action systems. *Journal of Motor Behavior, 14,* 98-134.

Riege, W.H., Cohen, M.J., & Wallach, H.F. (1980). Autonomic responsivity during recognition memory processing in three age groups. *Experimental Aging Research, 6,* 159-174.

Salthouse, T.A. (1982). *Adult cognition.* New York: Springer-Verlag.

Salthouse, T.A. (1984). Effects of age and skill in typing. *Journal of Experimental Psychology: General, 113,* 345-371.

Salthouse, T.A. (1985). *A theory of cognitive aging.* Amsterdam: North-Holland.

Saltzman, E.L., & Kelso, J.A.S. (1983). Toward a dynamical account of motor memory and control. In R.A. Magill (Ed.), *Memory and control of action* (pp. 17-38). Amsterdam: North-Holland.

Schaie, K.W. (1978). External validity in the assessment of intellectual development in adulthood. *Journal of Gerontology, 33,* 695-701.

Schneider, W., & Fisk, A.D. (1983). Attention theory and mechanisms for skilled performance. In R.A. Magill (Ed.), *Memory and control of action* (pp. 119-143). Amsterdam: North-Holland.

Silva, J. (1985, June). *Effects of an active audience on performance in sports.* Paper presented at the 3rd World Congress in Sport Psychology, Copenhagen, Denmark.

Singer, R.N. (1980). *Motor learning and human performance. An application to motor skills and movement behaviors* (3rd ed.). London: Collier MacMillan Publishers.

Stelmach, G.E. (1982). Information-processing framework for understanding human motor behavior. In J.A.S. Kelso (Ed.), *Human motor behavior. An introduction* (pp. 63-91). Hillsdale, NJ: Erlbaum.

Thompson, L.W., & Nowlin, J.B. (1973). Relation of increased attention to central and autonomic nervous system states. In L. Jarvik, C. Eisdorfer & J. Blum (Eds.), *Intellectual functioning in adults: Psychological and biological influences* (pp. 107-124). New York: Springer.

Timiras, P.S. (1972). *Developmental physiology and aging.* New York: Macmillan.

Weinstein, N.D. (1974). Effect of noise on intellectual performance. *Journal of Applied Psychology, 59,* 548-554.

Welford, A.T. (1977). Motor performance. In J.E. Birren & K.W. Schaie (Eds.), *Handbook of the psychology of aging* (pp. 450-496). New York: Van Nostrand.

Wiersma, W., & Klausmeier, H.J. (1965). The effect of age upon speed of concept attainment. *Journal of Gerontology, 20,* 398-400.

Wright, L.L., & Elias, J.W. (1979). Age differences in the effects of perceptual noise. *Journal of Gerontology, 34,* 704-708.

Yesavage, J.A., Rose, T.A., & Spiegel, D. (1982). Relaxation training and memory improvement in elderly normals. *Experimental Aging Research, 8,* 195-198.

## Author Notes

The research reported in this chapter was supported by grants from the Swedish Council for Research in Humanities and the Social Sciences, and the Swedish Sports Research Council.

Both authors contributed equally to this chapter.

# Part II
# Aging, Psychomotor Slowing, and Aerobic Exercise

## INTRODUCTION

One of the most persistent findings in the motor skills literature is the increasing slowness in performance with advancing age. This slowness is not limited to simple motor responses commonly reported in the reaction time literature, but affects complex forms of motor behavior as well.

More than 20 years ago, Birren (1965) reviewed literature on health and speed of behavior in the elderly. He concluded that there may be at least two factors related to aging that affect speed: a primary age factor and a factor of cortical integrity affected by disease, particularly those diseases leading to cell loss and reduced arterial blood flow. These observations served as a foundation for subsequent theoretical and experimental efforts to uncover and modify those factors responsible for increased psychomotor slowing with age.

Although there have been field-based assessments of psychomotor slowing with age (e.g., Stones & Kozma, 1980), traditionally this phenomenon has been studied in the laboratory using a reaction time-movement time paradigm. This approach has been useful in terms of evaluating under carefully controlled conditions those cognitive processes—such as decision making and response programming—responsible for the decline in speed with age. One of the most popular approaches to evaluating the decline in speeded response within this paradigm has been to conceptualize motor skill performance in terms of an information processing model. This approach has enabled researchers to explore the relative contributions of central and peripheral mechanisms responsible for the decline in psychomotor speed with age.

In the chapter that follows, Toole and Abourezk draw on Salthouse's (1985) processing rate theory as a basis for explaining age-related slowing in information processing speed. They also examine some of the morphological and physiological changes that occur with age in the central nervous system that contribute to declines in speed of processing.

One of the more fascinating lines of research that has emerged in the aging and motor behavior literature has centered on reports that aerobic exercise may prevent premature aging of the central nervous system, perhaps by modifications of the cardiovascular and neuroendocrine systems (Spirduso, 1983). Exercise has been shown to increase cerebral blood flow to areas of the brain that are involved in the programming, control, and execution of movements such as the prefrontal, somatosensory, primary motor regions, and the cerebellum (Fletcher, 1985). Thus, aerobic exercise, by its trophic effect on the central nervous system, may help stem commonly observed age-related declines in psychomotor speed.

Toole and Abourezk follow this line of research by documenting earlier reports centering on retrospective analyses of inactive and active individuals on laboratory-based assessments of movement speed. They also review more direct lines of research on the effects of aerobic exercise on information processing speed that were based on experimental manipulation. The research investigation by Dustman and his colleagues that follows illustrates nicely a comprehensive experimental investigation of the effects of exercise on older adult performance on a battery of neuropsychological tests.

The role of aerobic exercise in ameliorating information processing deficits in the elderly is important to study beyond laboratory investigations of movement speed. My colleagues and I at West Virginia University recently received funding* to investigate the role of aerobic activity as it relates to the proficiency in older adults to drive an automobile. Clearly, the relationship of exercise to speed of response holds great promise as an avenue of research within the domain of aging and motor behavior.

## REFERENCES

Birren, J.E. (1965). Age changes in speed of behavior: Its central nature and physiological correlates. In A.T. Welford & J.E. Birren (Eds.), *Behavior, aging, and the nervous system* (pp. 119-216). Springfield, IL: Charles C. Thomas.

Fletcher, L.M. (1985). *The relation of maximum oxygen uptake and hyperoxia to reaction and movement times in older men and women.* Unpublished master's thesis, Pennsylvania State University, University Park.

Salthouse, T.A. (1985). *A theory of cognitive aging.* Amsterdam: Elsevier Science.

Spirduso, W.W. (1983). Exercise as a factor in aging motor behavior plasticity. In H.M. Eckert & H.J. Montoye (Eds.), *Exercise and health* (pp. 89-100). Champaign, IL: Human Kinetics.

Stones, M.J. & Kozma, A. (1980). Adult age trends in record running performances. *Experimental Aging Research, 6,* 407-416.

* This project is currently being funded by a grant from the AAA Foundation for Traffic Safety.

*AGING AND MOTOR BEHAVIOR*

# 2

# Aerobic Function, Information Processing, and Aging

Tonya Toole

Tami Abourezk

## ABSTRACT

An overview of explanations for age-related slowing in information processing was presented. A recent processing rate theory (Salthouse, 1985) that utilizes a limited resources interpretation of aging was shown to account for age-related slowing in information processing speed as measured by reaction time as well as to explain overall cognitive functioning declines. The neurophysiological changes that occur with age that are possible causes of the behavioral slowing and cognitive functioning declines were also reviewed. Topics covered were neuronal, dendritic, and synaptic loss, and decreases in neurotransmitters, regional cerebral blood flow, and energy metabolism. Several hypotheses that incorporate these morphological and neurochemical changes into an explanation of behavioral slowing were discussed. The possible influence aerobic exercise and oxygen utilization have on CNS changes in the older adult was also considered. Recent experiments that have used exercise interventions to examine pre/post oxygen utilization measures provide some support for the ameliorative affects of exercise for information processing time as measured by reaction time. Other intervention investigations provide support for the benefits of exercise on other cognitive functioning tests. Finally, suggestions were made for potential experimental directions.

## INTRODUCTION

It is commonly known that as we age we experience slowed responses. The phenomenon of age-related slowing of behavior is often considered the most reliable finding in the gerontological literature (Salthouse, 1985). The nature of this slowing has been the topic of investigation for several years and many hypotheses have resulted. One shortcoming in the area of cognitive aging has been the lack of testable theories. The goal of this chapter is to review one of the most recent theories of cognitive aging as well as present an overview of neurophysiological evidence that could support the theory. Next, current investigations dealing with the effect of physical activity on information processing speed in the older adult will be presented. These studies will be discussed especially because they may make a significant contribution to the overall theory of cognitive aging reviewed in this chapter. This research on information processing speed and physical activity can also have lasting impact on our understanding about the integrity of the central nervous system. Lastly, we will suggest possible directions for future research.

## A THEORY OF COGNITIVE AGING: PROCESSING RATE THEORY

Many central phenomena occur when humans are required to respond rapidly and accurately. Those include perceiving or receiving of external stimulus, encoding and recognizing input, selectively attending to a limited number of stimuli, searching and retrieving from long-term memory, and using a working memory system to possibly integrate procedural or control directions with the new input and retrieved long-term information. Additionally, a response must be selected and the appropriate parameters for that specific response must be programmed.

Many years of experimentation have contributed to our knowledge about the age-related declines that occur within these central processing phenomena. For example, declines have been observed at the input stage in encoding or registration as well as attending to select input based on instructions held in short-term memory. Short-term storage, retrieval, and organization also are impaired with age. These are only a few of the deficiencies found in the processing of information. An examination of Table 2-1 will provide the reader with an overview of the extensive experimentation that has been conducted, resulting in many individual hypotheses to account for age differences in cognition. Emerging theory proposes that much of the overall cognitive decline with age is time based, and that most of these separate hypotheses can be integrated into one theory: the processing rate theory.

For many years there has been debate and speculation over a primary area dealing with age-related slowing of reaction time as well as other aspects of behavior that indicate slowing. The debate concerns whether specific processes or general resources were the cause of the slowing. These causes of slowing will be reviewed as they relate to this recent theory of cognitive aging, which supports the suppositions of the remainder of this chapter. This theory, the processing rate theory, has been presented by Salthouse (1985) in his book, *A Theory of Cognitive Aging*. As noted by Salthouse, " . . . because a reduction in speed is assumed to be the primary behavioral change associated with increased age, it can be hypothesized that the speed differences may be largely responsible for many of the age-related changes in cognitive performance" (p. 250). The reader is referred to many reviews on the absolute magnitude of the effects of age on speed of behavior (e.g., Birren, Woods, & Williams, 1979, 1980; Salthouse, 1985; Welford, 1977, 1984). The general finding for

**TABLE 2.1.** *Proposed Hypotheses for Age Differences in Cognition.*

| Age-Related Impairments are Attributable to: | Source: |
| --- | --- |
| Decline in Organization | Denney, 1974; Hultsch, 1971 |
| Decline in Logical Classification | Denney & Denney, 1973 |
| Decreased Proficiency of Elaborative Rehearsal | Kausler & Puckett, 1979 |
| Decrement in Memory-Driven Attentional Selectivity | Rabbitt, 1979b |
| Deficiencies in Both Input and Retrieval | Till & Walsh, 1980; Craik, 1968 |
| Deficit in Attending to Relevant Information | Madden, 1983 |
| Deficit in Encoding or Registration | Botwinick & Storandt, 1974; Craik & Masani, 1967; Taub, 1979 |
| Deficit in Retrieval | Craik & Masani, 1969; Schonfield & Robertson, 1966 |
| Deficit in Short-Term Storage | Craik, 1965, 1968; Drachman & Leavitt, 1972; Gordon & Clark, 1974; Inglis & Ankus, 1965; Welford, 1958 |
| Difficulty in Identifying or Utilizing Hierarchical Structure | Dixon, Simon, Nowak, & Hultsch, 1982 |
| Difficulty in Integration and Recoding of Information | Craik, 1968 |
| Faster Decay of Immediate Memory | Fraser, 1958 |
| Failure to Elaborate and Integrate Specific Context | Craik & Rabinowitz, 1984 |
| Failure to Use Context at Encoding and Retrieval | Shaps & Nilsson, 1980 |
| Greater Susceptibility to Interference | Caird, 1966; Craik & Masani, 1967; Talland, 1968; Welford, 1958 |
| Inability to Maintain Activity with New Input | Canestrari, 1968 |
| Inability to Maintain and Retrieve Meaningful Materials | Taub, 1979 |
| Inability to Recode, Integrate or Chunk Verbal Material | Craik & Masani, 1967 |
| Inefficient Spontaneous Use of Encoding and Retrieval Strategies | Perlmutter & Mitchell, 1982 |
| Less Distinctive Encoding | Hess & Higgins, 1983 |
| Loss of Flexibility of Active Control | Rabbitt, 1982 |

Adapted from *A Theory of Cognitive Aging* (pp. 180-182) by T.A. Salthouse, 1985, Amsterdam: Elsevier Science Publishers B.V. Copyright 1985 by Elsevier Science Publishers B.V. Used with permission.

many variables suggests that the proportional differences between those in their 60s and those in their 20s is between 20% and 60%. This suggests that the speed loss is between 5% and 15% per decade. Therefore, it is accepted that there is a general decline in speed with age. As we will discuss later in this chapter, there are exceptions to this general loss.

Figure 2-1 portrays the hypothesized relationships among the factors contributing to the processing rate theory. While the importance of the speed factor in the schematic is not apparent, speed is the major component that is directly related to age. In fact, it is the essence of the processing rate theory. The reader is referred to Salthouse (1985) for explicit

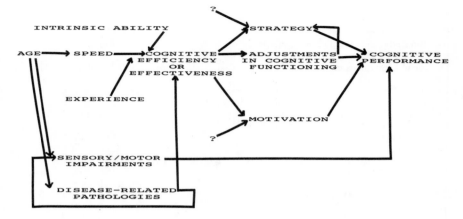

**FIGURE 2.1.** *Hypothesized relations among factors contributing to cognitive performance according to the processing rate theory of cognitive aging.*
From A Theory of Cognitive Aging *(p. 299) by T.A. Salthouse, 1985, Amsterdam: Elsevier Science Publishers B. V. Copyright 1985 by Elsevier Science Publishers B. V. Reprinted by permission.*

information on the contribution of the other variables of Intrinsic ability, Experience, and other factors.

One of the bases for his processing rate theory is a limited resources interpretation of age differences in cognitive functioning. He, as well as many other researchers (Birren, 1974; Craik & Byrd, 1982; Craik & Rabinowitz, 1984; Hasher & Zacks, 1979; Light, Zelinski, & Moore, 1982), advocate an integrated view of mental aging, that of a single, general mechanism of limited processing resources.

## General Limited Resources

One only needs to examine Table 2-1 to realize that a host of mental functions decline with age. Salthouse (1985), in contrast to the separate mechanisms explanation that is depicted in the table, advocates a more parsimonious account of cognitive decline that could incorporate age-related changes in many of these mental functions. Salthouse views time as a processing resource, and reduction in the available time processing resources is affected by age. It is an ". . . impairment at a subordinate level concerned with the supply of an 'ingredient' essential for most aspects of information processing" (p. 189). Therefore, he assumes that the quantity of resources decreases with age. "Many questions still remain concerning the interrelations of various speed measures both within and across age groups, but it is indisputable that the time required to perform nearly all behavior activities, which is presumably inversely related to the

*AGING AND MOTOR BEHAVIOR*

quantity of temporal resources available, increases with increasing age" (p. 200).

How could this limited resources proposal account for overall mental functioning decline, and how does this relate to the original comments in this chapter that response speed slows with age? Few researchers have been explicit about the nature of these resources or how they could be measured. According to Salthouse, resources could be categorized in terms of space, energy, and time characteristics. If the resource were spatially based, memory span and working memory capacity as well as recency-based measures would be affected with aging. An energy limitation would affect attentional capacity or mental energy, while a time limiting resource would affect speed of behavior with many tasks. It is this latter resource, that of a speed factor, that is the basis of Salthouse's (1985) Processing Rate Theory of Cognitive Aging.

He believes that two lines of evidence must be provided in order to support the general limited resource account. First, ". . . it must be shown that limitations of the relevant resource do in fact produce the types of differences one is trying to explain. And second, it must be demonstrated that the relevant resource does change in the predicted manner across the lifespan" (p. 200).

## Specific Processes

Others have advocated that age-related changes occur due to the decline of specific processes or separate mechanisms. This stance proposes that each ability would have a separate mechanism to account for the age decline. Again, Table 2-1 illustrates each one of the abilities and the proposed explanations for age declines. Many phenomena are dealt with separately and because of the specificity of the explanations, the phenomena are assumed to be unrelated. As one can learn from Table 2-1, these abilities include encoding or registration of stimuli, memory-driven attentional selectivity, organization, short-term storage, recording, integrating, or chunking, and retrieval, just to name a few. The specific process account of slowing views that the efficiency of one or all of these components declines with age, or that the effectiveness of a sequence of these components declines with age. While it appears that Salthouse does not attempt to rule out this specific process account of slowing, he does view the limited resource explanation to have the advantages of a more integrated and parsimonious account of cognitive slowing.

## Slowing of Behavior:
## Cause or Consequence of Cognitive Aging

The next question leading to the processing rate theory of cognitive aging is whether slowing is a cause or a consequence of cognitive aging.

Both psychological and physiological causes for age changes in speed have been proposed. According to Salthouse (1985), ". . . if the cause of the speed differences is psychological then it is reasonable to think of speed as a consequence of the other psychological factors, while if the cause is physiological then speed might be considered to be the determinant of other psychological phenomena" (p. 273). Those psychological factors which have been postulated to account for age-related slowing are strategy shifts, motivational loss, and lack of familiarity with experimental tasks. For the most part, when these variables are controlled within the experimental paradigm, they do not reduce the age-related speed reduction (e.g., Baron, Menich, & Perone, 1983; Botwinick, Brinley, & Robbin, 1958; Grant, Storandt, & Botwinick, 1978). Salthouse cites 20 studies on two pages alone that support this finding, whereas a few studies (e.g. Rabbitt, 1979a) failed to support it. Therefore the "speed as consequence" explanation appears untenable (Salthouse, 1985).

Many physiological explanations have been proposed to account for behavioral slowing with age. The processing rate theory of cognitive aging is not explicit about these physiological explanations but it does view them, in general, to be the primary basis and cause for age-related slowing in cognitive functioning. We will address some potential physiological explanations in subsequent sections.

How can the process rate theory be investigated? Salthouse has suggested a number of possibilities. First, research on speed and intelligence relationships needs to be conducted on task independent measures of processing speed such as by using the Digit Symbol Substitution Test from the Wechsler Adult Intelligence Scale. Second, researchers might carry out manipulations thought to simulate the effects of an altered rate of processing, and then determine their effects on cognitive functioning. One way to manipulate this has been attempted in our laboratory (Toole, Abourezk, Qasem, 1987). We assumed that an altered rate of processing, based on a general limited resource model, must affect all central processing and that $O_2$ enhancement to the CNS would benefit central processing for a speeded task. Our findings are presented later in this chapter. Another avenue might be to use task dependent measures of processing speed that measure the speed of component processes for these tasks. One might acquire measures of the duration of several components in a complex task and then enter these component times into a multiple regression equation. One could predict composite performances from these components if the general limited resource hypothesis is correct.

While recent research investigating the role of exercise for slowing of behavior has not been specifically directed toward the processing rate theory as proposed by Salthouse (1985), it will be reviewed in this chapter as potential evidence that could be related to the theory. How the exercise research might relate to some of Salthouse's suggested ways of testing processing rate theory will be addressed in the Future Directions Section. Before we review some of the recent exercise literature, we have chosen to present some of the evidence concerned with age-related CNS changes with explanations for psycho-motor slowing.

# NEUROPHYSIOLOGICAL AGE-RELATED CNS CHANGES

In an attempt to explain behavioral changes associated with advancing age, it is imperative to have an understanding of age-related central nervous system (CNS) alterations. The CNS is a highly integrated system that depends upon the functional unit, the neuron. The vast network of connections among the billions of neurons within the CNS represents the very essence of behavior. Thus we are assuming that a breakdown in communication among neurons, in the form of morphological and/or neurochemical changes, results in age-related phenomenon such as slowed behavior. Therefore, the following review will consist of research evidence centering around neurophysical changes within the CNS such as: neuronal, dendritic, and synaptic loss; neurotransmitters, cerebral blood flow, and energy metabolism. A final discussion will be devoted to some of the hypotheses which attempt to incorporate such morphological and neurochemical changes into an explanation of the age-related slowing of behavior.

## Morphological Changes

A common measure that reveals structural changes in the aging brain is neuronal count. The method of determining neuronal loss has progressed from the light microscope to the more advanced electron microscope. Regardless of the method utilized, advancement in age leads to neuronal loss in various regions of the brain.

Brody (1955) examined 20 human brains ranging in age from newborn to 95 years. He determined that the cell count in the cerebral cortex was the greatest for newborns compared to all other ages. But with increased age the number of neurons progressively decreased. The brain regions of interest were the pre-central and post-central gyri, superior temporal and inferior temporal gyri, and area striata. Brody reported that the greatest neuronal death was observed in the superior temporal gyrus followed by the pre-central gyrus, area striate, inferior temporal gyrus, and post-central gyrus. More recently, Henderson, Tomlinson, and Gibson (1980) confirmed Brodys' earlier findings. Utilizing an imaging analyzing computer they demonstrated at age 90 as compared to age 20, a 66% and 48% reduction of small and large neurons, respectively, occurred in the superior temporal region of the cerebral cortex. Again, the smallest loss of neurons was observed in the post-central gyrus.

Other areas of the CNS which exhibit an age-related decrement in neurons include the cerebellar cortex, substantia nigra, and locus ceruleus (Hall, Miller, & Corsellis, 1979; McGeer, 1978; Vijayashankar & Brody, 1979). These areas of the brain are associated with coordinated movement, motoric functions, and arousal, respectively. It must be noted that neuronal loss is not common in all regions of the CNS. For example, nuclei of the brainstem (i.e. ventral cochlear and inferior olive) fail to show neuronal loss with age (Konigsmark & Murphy, 1970; Monagle & Brody, 1974).

The loss of neurons in and of itself may not adequately explain behavioral changes with advanced age. However, one of the consequences of neuronal death is the loss of synaptic interconnections, which according to Bondareff (1985), is of functional importance; that is, a loss of interconnections could result in less efficient neuronal communication. Evidence to support the loss of neuronal interconnections is based on studies which investigated the effects of increased age on dendritic branches, dendritic spines and synapses. Feldman and Dowd (1975) observed an age-related decline in dendritic spines of the pyramidal neurons located in the cerebral cortex of rats. A 24% spine loss was exhibited on the terminal tuft while a 40% loss was seen on the oblique branches. Other spine reductions were counted in basal and apical dendrites. Scheibel et al. (1976), utilizing the Golgi method, qualitatively described dendritic changes seen in the 3rd layer pyramidal cells of 10 subjects aged 58 to 96 years. The authors reported a progressive loss of the basilar (horizontally oriented) dendrites. They noted that this reduction eventually led to a loss of apical shafts and cell death. It was suggested that degeneration of the basilar dendrites, due to their synaptic connections to layers two and four of the cortex, would ultimately affect higher order cortical activity.

In addition to the reduction in dendritic branches and the number of dendritic spines, there is also a loss of synapses with age. Glick and Bondareff (1979) indicated a 24% and 33% decrease in axodendritic synapses and dendritic spines, respectively, in the senescent rat (25 mo.). The area studied was the cerebellar cortex which, according to the authors, may help to explain age associated motor dysfunctions such as loss of coordinated movement or poor balance. Similarly, the density of synaptic zone (total length of synaptic zones per unit area) and the density of synapses of the cerebellar glomeruli in rats, decrease with age (Freddari & Giuli, 1980). Synaptic loss has also been observed in the hippocampus (Hasan & Glees, 1973) and the 3rd layer of the frontal cortex (Huhenlucher, 1979).

## Neurotransmitters

The integrated activity of the CNS is possible via the many connections among neurons and the chemical activity of those connections. Therefore, any age-related alterations in neurotransmitters at the synaptic level may shed some light on slowed behavior, as described below.

**Acetlycholine:** In order for a neuron to fire, the release of this transmitter is essential. It is an excitatory substance that depolarizes the postsynaptic membrane (Carlson, 1986). The amount of neurotransmitter released effects the time it takes the postsynaptic membrane to reach threshold (i.e. fire), ultimately effecting neuronal time. Because acetlycholine (ACH) rapidly hydrolyzes following death, the enzyme responsible for ACH biosynthesis, choline acetltransferase (CAT), is normally studied.

The effects of advancing age on CAT activity has been demonstrated in both humans and rats. McGeer and McGeer (1975) demonstrated a decrease in CAT activity in the cerebral cortex of humans. There appears to be a negative correlation between age and CAT activity up to 50 years of age. Perry et al. (1977) observed a pronounced decrement of CAT in the hippocampal region of elderly human brains. Research conducted by Meek et al. (1977) and Unsworth, Fleming, & Caron (1980) indicate lowered CAT in the telencephalon, cerebellum, and brainstem of rat and mouse brains.

**Dopamine:** The role of this neurotransmitter in movement is most evident when dopamergic neurons deteriorate, such is the case with Parkinson's disease. People who suffer from this disease exhibit symptoms of fine tremors, rigidity, and difficulty in movement initiation (Carlson, 1986). With advancing age, a decrease in dopamine is common in the caudate nucleus (Finch, 1973). As well, the enzymes necessary for the synthesis of dopamine, tyrosine hydroxylase, and dopa decarboxylase are reduced in several areas of the CNS. For example, McGeer and McGeer (1975) indicated a 50% decrease in both enzymes in the substantia nigra of 60-year-olds compared to 15-year-olds. Other locations within the human brain which exhibit decrements in one or both of these enzymes include the hypothalamus, amygdala, putamen, and caudate nucleus.

**Noradrenaline:** Similar to ACH, noradrenaline is an excitatory neurotransmitter that affects specific sympathetic nervous system organs (Carlson, 1986). An additional role of this transmitter substance is arousal and alertness. While McGeer et al. (1971) indicate that noradrenaline content remains unchanged in rat brain, Samorajski, Rolsten, and Ordy (1971) report a decrease. In human brain stem, however, the reduction is 40% (Robinson et al., 1972). Furthermore, these investigations suggested that monoamine oxidase, which plays a role in noradrenaline degeneration, appears to increase with age.

**Serotonin:** Where ACH increases the chance that a neuron will fire, serotonin acts as an inhibitor of neuronal firing. It too plays a role in arousal (Carlson, 1986). Finch (1973) reported that serotonin content is unchanged in the large hemisphere of rat brain. As well, serotonin is stable in human and animal brainstem (Robinson et al., 1972). More re-

cently, however, Ponzio et al. (1982) have reported a reduction in serotonin levels with advancing age.

In summary, the time that it takes a neuron(s) to fire may possibly be
affected by a reduction in actual density of neurons, dendrites, dendritic
spines, and synapses. A relationship between neuronal transmission time
and the production and release of neurotransmitters is also likely. Because firing of a neuron is both electrical (along the axon) and chemical
(across the synapse), a decrease in neurotransmitter substances could
manifest itself in synaptic delays (Welford, 1984), subsequently reducing
the conduction time from neuron to neuron.

The preceeding represented a brief review of the age-related alterations in neurons and neurotransmitters. For a more extensive review on
this topic the reader is referred to Frolkis and Bezrukov (1979).

## CEREBRAL BLOOD FLOW (CBF)
## AND ENERGY METABOLISM

Similar to all tissues of the body, such as skeletal muscle, the brain
also expends energy in order to function effectively. Dekoninck (1985)
describes brain energy metabolism as, "the level of energy utlized in the
brain . . ." (p. 147) Based on the notion that energy demands the brain to
mediate the flow of blood to that tissue (Roy & Sherrington, 1980), researchers have investigated possible age-related changes in cerebral
blood flow (CBF) and oxygen consumption. The basic assumption implied
is that an alteration in any of these parameters may be indicative of a decrement in energy metabolism, and therefore, slow central processing
down. Researchers have speculated that a reduction in energy metabolism could be a result of the morphological changes (i.e., neuronal loss)
observed in the aging CNS (Frolkis & Bezrukov, 1979). On the other
hand, Bondareff (1985) suggested that a reduction in metabolic processes
may lead to the death of neurons. Despite this contradiction, a decline in
brain metabolism may be evidence of a breakdown in neuronal communication.

Is there an age-related decline in CBF and/or energy metabolism?
Past research investigating this notion has included subjects who were
not representative of a normal population. Thus any observed decrements in cerebral blood flow and/or energy metabolism may have reflected pathological disorders. However, recent studies, which have employed the use of noninvasive scanning techniques, have reported reductions in regional cerebral blood flow and oxygen consumption in
normal aging subjects. Pantano et al. (1983) measured regional cerebral
blood flow (rCBF) and cerebral oxygen consumption (rCMRO2) by

means of positron computer tomography (PET) and steady-stage oxygen-15 inhalation. A total of 27 normal (free from any brain or vascular diseases) subjects ages 19-76 years were used. This noninvasive technique allowed the researchers to study the frontal and temporosylvian, sensory motor, parietooccipital, occipital cortex, and thalamic regions of the brain. The authors reported a 17% reduction in both rCBF and rCMRO2 in the frontal, temporosylvian, and parietooccipital areas of gray matter for the elderly subjects. Pantano et al. equate this reduction to a decrease in cortical metabolism as a result of neuronal loss or a decrease in metabolic activity of residual neurons. Several studies have reported similar findings (Frackowiak et al., 1980; Frackowiak et al., 1983; Lenzi et al., 1981).

## NEUROPHYSIOLOGICAL EXPLANATIONS FOR AGE-RELATED CNS SLOWING

The link between age induced neurophysiological changes and the slowing phenomenon is not clear. With the complexity of the CNS, it is extremely difficult, if not impossible, to accurately pinpoint which neural mechanism(s) is responsible for such behavior. Although documentation exists to support morphological and neurochemical changes associated with age, variations in methodology and subject selection may have resulted in some of the inconsistencies discovered. Regardless, it is well established that slowed behavior is common with age. Keeping this in mind, researchers have attempted to explain this behavioral decrement within a neurophysiological framework. The following hypotheses are examples of such attempts.

A theory of sensory detection has been proposed which suggests that the aging nervous system becomes increasingly "noisy" (random neural firing). This increase in background noise results in an increase in the time it takes the CNS to perceive incoming sensory signals. The CNS must differentiate between the afferent signal and random firing, subsequently reducing the signal to noise ratio (Birren, 1970; Swets, 1964; Welford, 1984). It is speculated that neural noise may be a result of hyperexcitability and/or aftereffects of prior stimulation of neurons (Birren, 1970). Welford (1984) indicated that spatial and temporal summation within the aging CNS may possibly be affected by decreases in the density of neurons and synapses, thus implying a weak sensory signal against a background of neural noise, resulting in an increase in processing time. Salthouse (1985) discussed this explanation of cognitive slowing as a type of dynamic mechanism that would be needed to account for his processing rate theory. While the two experiments reported by Salthouse (1980) support the signal-to-noise interpretation of aging, a recent one (Salthouse & Lichty, 1985) failed to be supportive. Therefore, Salthouse (1985) concluded that:

> The reduced signal-to-noise interpretation of the age-related slowing phenomenon must therefore be considered unverified at the present time because the available evidence is equivocal. Nevertheless, it is still a promising perspective because of its generality and plausibility, and hence it probably deserves more thorough investigation before being completely dismissed. (p. 283)

In addition to the signal to noise ratio notion, Birren (1970) proposed a second hypothesis for slowed behavior. He stated, ". . . the older nervous system may be in a less activated state so that any stimulus yields a slower response" (p. 132). Birren, Woods, and Williams (1979) further substantiated this notion by suggesting that the documented (Brody, 1955; Hall, Miller, & Corsellis, 1979; Henderson, Tomlinson, & Gibson, 1980; Vijayashankar & Brody, 1979) reduction in the number of neurons located in the reticular formation (i.e. locus ceruleus) may influence the arousal state of the CNS. According to Birren et al. (1979), this particular nucleus makes up a portion of the ascending reticular system, which projects fibers up to the cerebellum, cerebrum, and limbic system. Therefore, neuronal death within the locus ceruleus would eliminate some of the fibers innervating these areas of the CNS, consequently reducing the arousal level.

Research provided by McFarland (1952, 1963) indicated that with increased age there is either less oxygen available to the CNS due to ineffective transport, or available oxygen is less adequately utilized. He reports that young subjects exposed to hypoxic conditions demonstrated behavioral deficits in short-term memory, attention, and processing time. According to McFarland (1952, p. 353), ". . . the sensory and mental impairment which occurs in both normal and clinical subjects under experimental conditions of oxygen deprivation simulate very precisely the behavioral changes observed in the aging process."

The exact CNS mechanism(s) involved remains to be explained. However, the synapse and its neurochemical action, provides an attractive site within the CNS for which slowed behavior may be explained. Although the following studies would appropriately fit in the cerebral blood flow and energy metabolism section of this chapter, these research findings are mentioned here in order to illustrate the effects of diminished oxygen supply in the CNS. It is interesting to note several studies in which the inhibition of either oxygen or glucose reduced the amount of ACH produced in rat brain tissue (Gibson & Blass, 1976; Gibson & Peterson, 1982; Ksiezak & Gibson, 1981). In another study, Gibson, Peterson, and Sansone (1981) had rats inspire oxygen mixtures of 15% or 10%. Prior to being sacrificed, the rats were tested on their ability (use of paws and tail) and time (speed was the valued response) to traverse a string. In addition to a decrement on the string test (rats fell off the string within 0-15 seconds after being placed on it) at low levels of oxygen, a reduction in ACH was also measured. The authors proposed that the brain's sensitivity to a decrease in the availability of oxygen is reflected in ACH synthesis, and ultimately behavior.

A final hypothesis, one that fits well with Salthouse's processing rate theory, can be explained as a decrease in neuronal transmission time in the CNS. Welford (1984) reported that the measure of the brain's electrical activity (EEG) could account for the slowing down of central processes with aging. Frolkis and Bezrukov (1979) reported reductions in the alpha rhythms of elderly subjects (40-70 years of age). Giaquito and Nolfe (1983) utilized 48 normal older subjects, 60 years of age and older. They also included 100 healthy control subjects between the ages of 20-40 years. The authors not only reported significantly slower simple and choice reaction times (SRT's and CRT's) and flicker frequency fusion in the older individuals, but also a decrease in alpha rhythms. According to Giaquito and Nolfe, "the 'normal' aging brain keeps it capabilities but with a speed loss in processing" (p. 31). Frolkis and Bezrukov (1979) advocated that a combination of any or all morphological and neurochemical alterations in the aging CNS could account for the age-related slowing of alpha rhythms.

In summary, based on the literature presented, several CNS structures exhibit neuronal and synaptic loss with age. Dendrite and dendritic spines also appear to decrease in density. Furthermore, neurotransmitters and their enzymes are decreased in the aging brain tissue. Additionally, several investigations have reported a reduction in rCBF and rCMRO2, which may indicate a decrease in energy metabolism. Thus, this brief review was intended to present some of the neurophysiological changes that occur with increased age. In order to relate changes in the aging CNS to slowed information processing in the older adult, we have also presented several hypothesis which have attempted to explain slowed behavior, integrating age-related morphological and/or neurochemical alterations.

Assuming that a relationship between morphological and neurochemical CNS changes and slowed behavior in the elderly exists, are these changes an inevitable consequence of age? If the answer to this question is "no", under what circumstances are there exceptions to this notion? An area of growing interest is the role of exercise in the aging CNS. Because investigations have reported that elderly subjects who exercise fail to demonstrate slowed behavior, the next section is devoted to a discussion on the relevance of exercise in CNS integrity and slowed behavior.

## POTENTIAL ROLE OF EXERCISE FOR CENTRAL NERVOUS SYSTEM INTEGRITY

### Rationale

What role does exercise play in the maintenance of CNS integrity in the older adult? Although much speculation exists, the direct experimental evidence to adequately answer this question is sparse. However, the CNS alterations may be reduced through exercise. Spirduso (1980, 1983) has reviewed some of the investigations which substantiate this hypothesis. She reported that both acute and chronic exercise increase the level of norepinepherine and serotinin, as well as some of the metabolites associated with these neurotransmitters. Furthermore, these reviews discuss the release of plasma endorphins which reflect dopamine turnover. Spirduso (1980) also addressed the increase in regional blood flow in the brain as a result of exercise and its relationship to metabolic demands. Thus, it does appear that the aging CNS can benefit from exercise. Even though more investigations are essential in understanding the effects of exercise on the aging brain, the empirical evidence to support its potential role in information processing will be considered.

All mental functions require efficient communication within the neuronal network. If an interruption in communication occurs, such as a loss of neurons, dendritic branches and spines, synapses, and reduction in neurochemical activity, a decrement in information processing is a likely consequence. Ultimately, neuronal transmission is dependent upon the synapse and synaptic activity, thus implying the importance of energy metabolism within the existing functional neurons. Because oxygen and glucose play an extremely important role in energy metabolism, consideration must be given to the ability of the older individual to adequately deliver and utilize oxygen within the CNS. Therefore, researchers have generated efforts to investigate a possible relationship between the role of aerobic exercise and information processing ability in the older adult.

Initial evidence on the role of exercise for information processing speed as measured by RT and aging has been provided by Spirduso (1975), Spirduso and Clifford (1978), and Clarkson and Kroll (1978). For excellent reviews on this information the reader is referred to Ostrow (1984) and Spirduso (1980). A review has also been written by Tomporowski and Ellis (1986) on the immediate or short-term effects of anerobic and aerobic exercise on cognitive functioning.

Since we are advocating the importance of cerebral oxygenation for information processing speed and overall cognitive functioning for the older adult, we will present recent literature that has assessed oxygen consumption as well as other physiological correlates of cardiovascular efficiency. This evidence will be integrated with measures of speed of responding and other cognitive tasks. First, we will present experiments that have investigated the relationship of $O_2$ consumption, aerobic exercise, and reaction time (RT) with exercise interventions. Secondly, those studies that investigated aerobic exercise and other indicants of cognitive functioning will be reported.

## Oxygen Consumption, Aerobic Exercise, and RT

A study by Era, Jokela, and Heikkinen (1986) examined possible performance differences between men aged 31 to 35, 51 to 55, and 71 to 75 years at different levels of complexity of psychomotor and motor tasks. They also attempted to relate psychomotor speed to living habits and physiological and psychological characteristics of health. They assessed oxygen consumption with a direct and an indirect method. The direct method was a max $\dot{V}O_2$ test, while the indirect method used three successive loads lasting four minutes and then $\dot{V}O_2$ max was estimated. Only the directly assessed maximal oxygen consumption measure correlated significantly with the psychomotor speed measures. Those correlations were $-.68$ for a visual stimulus choice reaction time (CRT) task and max $\dot{V}O_2$ for the 71-75 year olds ($p < .01$, $n = 11$), and $-.68$ for an auditory stimulus choice reaction time task and max $\dot{V}O_2$ ($p < .05$, $n = 11$). Simple reaction time (SRT) did not correlate significantly ($r = -.37$) with max $\dot{V}O_2$ for these same individuals. Unfortunately, the authors used only three practice trials and 12 actual trials of SRT and CRT in which a mean of the last five successful trials was used for analysis. Since reaction time is susceptible to practice effects (Rabbitt, 1979a), one questions whether their reaction time scores were true indicants of speed of information processing. It is likely, however, that using reaction times that were slower and/or more variable would reduce the correlation.

Another study that resulted in significant changes in SRT was conducted by VanFraechem and VanFraechem (1977). Their two month exercise program consisting of 1 hour twice a week was adapted for age and their subjects were sedentary and active females aged 70 to 80 years. Although no direct measures of oxygen utilization were administered, the sedentary group evidenced significant SRT improvement.

Dzewaltowski (1985) conducted a very commendable thesis for which he utilized 10 dependent measures to investigate $\dot{V}O_2$ and RT change with exercise. SRT and CRT were fractionated into premotor and motor components, state and trait anxiety, resting heart rate, and an estimated $\dot{V}O_2$ max (older group brought to 150 beats/min) were procured. An eight week aerobic exercise program was provided for young and old adults. Pretest $\dot{V}O_2$ max correlated significantly with SRT and CRT (SRT $= -.60$, CRT $= -.66$) across age, but none of the correlations between $\dot{V}O_2$ max change and posttest RT were significant. While this result does not appear to support a strong relationship between $O_2$ consumption and speed of responding, it is possible that the change in RT, instead of posttest RT, would need to be correlated (a positive correlation predicted) in order to achieve a meaningful relationship between the two variables. This may be true because, for example, a person with an initially high $\dot{V}O_2$max and a low (fast) RT may not change much in $\dot{V}O_2$ max and still be low in posttest RT. Many individuals like this example will weaken the predicted negative correlation between $\dot{V}O_2$ max change and posttest RT. One might also speculate that other variables that are related to $O_2$ consumption, such as heart rate, systolic blood pressure, respiratory rate, and respiratory quotient, need to be entered into a multiple regression with RT in order to account for more of the variability in RT. This might be especially so since $\dot{V}O_2$ max is a gross indicant of $O_2$ consumption for all body tissues and not just that of the CNS.

Significant changes were produced in SRT, simple premotor time, and in CRT, choice premotor time, for the older group using the multiple dependent t-tests. Since some ($n = 5$) of the older individuals experienced a mean $\dot{V}O_2$ max change of 48.99% and SRT, simple premotor time, and CRT, choice premotor time, changed for the older group as a whole (Hi and LoFit), a strong relationship between oxygen utilization and central indicants of speed of behavior is quite tenable.

Significant changes in $\dot{V}O_2$ max and RT were reported by Dustman et al. (1984) (see Chapter 3). Their 55-70 year old sedentary subjects met for three one hour sessions a week for four months. One group, the aerobic exercise group ($n = 13$), had the goal of increasing their heart rate to 70%-80% of their heart rate reserve and to maintain this for longer periods of time as their conditioning improved. Another group ($n = 15$), the exercise control group, worked on strength and flexibility exercises while the third group ($n = 15$) was the nonexercise control group. All exercise subjects experienced a true maximal $\dot{V}O_2$ test. The aerobically trained individuals improved significantly more in $\dot{V}O_2$ max than the exercise controls. The aerobic group increased by 27%, from 19.4 to 24.6 ml/kg/min, while the exercise control group increased by 9%, from 22.5 to 24.5 ml/kg/min. Results from multiple dependent t-tests, which may be questioned due to inflated type 1 error, produced significant changes in SRT for the aerobic exercise group but not for the exercise control or the nonexercise control. No improvement occured in CRT for any group. Since there was a greater increase in $\dot{V}O_2$ max for the aerobic group, and they also changed significantly more than the other groups in SRT, it may be assumed that the change in $O_2$ consumption caused the change in CNS speed.

This experiment has several commendable qualities. First, the experimental design is exactly what is needed for this type of intervention investigation. Two types of control are needed in order to clearly determine aerobic benefits; one, a nonexercise control and the other, a group that exercises but does not attempt to derive aerobic benefits. The purpose of this later group would be to determine whether strength training, for example, could affect RT via the muscular system. Another aspect of this line of investigation that appears to be essential is related to the type of $\dot{V}O_2$ max test that is given. The investigators in the Dustman et al. (1984) experiment utilized a maximal effort protocol and their RT changes were 16 msec for the aerobic exercise group and 7 msec for the exercise control group. Since only small changes in RT are being observed a precise indicant of oxygen consumption is needed. Rather than use an estimated $\dot{V}O_2$ max test, it would appear that investigators need to use maximal tests.

In summarizing the previous findings for the limited number of studies reported, it does appear that RT, especially as measured by SRT, changes with an aerobic exercise intervention for the older adult. There is also a fairly strong relationship between SRT and maximal $\dot{V}O_2$ for the older adult. The predictive nature of $\dot{V}O_2$ max change as a sole indicant of change in CNS speed is less clear. More experimentation on this relationship is certainly needed.

While research conducted in our lab (Toole, Abourezk, and Qasem, 1987) employed a different research design, it also lends support to the enhanced effects of oxygen utilization on RT speed. We sought to test McFarland's (1952, 1963) original idea concerning "oxygen want" which stated that older adults are possibly less able to utilize available oxygen or are less able to deliver available oxygen to the tissues. More recently Botwinick (1973) and Gibson and Peterson (1982) also suggested that hypoxia is a potential cause of information processing decrements. We tested ten males who ranged in age from 48 to 60 years, the majority of whom were university professors (remaining were businessmen). A bicycle ergonometer was used in order to determine their estimated $\dot{V}O_2$ max. Their scores ranged from 12.9 ml/kg/min to 36.5 ml/kg/min. Those who were active ($n = 5$) as determined by weekly jogging miles (12-30 miles/week), had maintained this level of activity for several years, and whose $\dot{V}O_2$ max values were in the "average" category using the Astrand-Rhyming (1960) classification of maximal oxygen uptake by age groups, had mean $\dot{V}O_2$ values of 34.62 ml/kg/min ($SD = 1.88$). Those who were less active ($n = 5$) by professing no regular activity and whose $\dot{V}O_2$ max values were in either the "low" or "somewhat low" category, had mean $\dot{V}O_2$ values of 24.7 ml/kg/min ($SD = 9.17$). We also measured SRT (100 trials for each $O_2$ condition) and CRT (100 trials for each $O_2$ condition) under conditions of normal $O_2$ (20.9% oxygen), 12%, and 80% oxygen (300 trials/day). All conditions were randomly assigned to subjects. In testing the "oxygen want" hypothesis, our premise was that those subjects who were less efficient in $O_2$ utilization as evidenced by low $\dot{V}O_2$ max would produce slower RTs than those who had a higher $\dot{V}O_2$

max under all $O_2$ conditions. We also speculated that the lower $\dot{V}O_2$ max subjects would benefit more from 80% $O_2$ than the higher $\dot{V}O_2$ max subjects because, possibly, they were in a state of mild hypoxia and therefore, a greater supply of $O_2$ would promote faster responses.

It can be seen from Table 2-2 that these speculations were not supported. We did not find faster RTs for the active group with normal $O_2$ nor with 12% $O_2$ or 80% $O_2$. It seems that these subjects who were classified as "average" $\dot{V}O_2$ max were not as efficient as needed to provide reaction time benefits. Both groups, however, improved significantly from the enhanced supply of $O_2$ as can be seen from Figures 2-2 and 2-3.

Figure 2-2 depicts a significant ($p < .05$) $O_2$ condition main effect for CRT while Figure 2-3 represents a significant ($p < .05$) interaction of $O_2$ condition with SRT trial blocks. For SRT and CRT for both activity groups, inhaling 80% $O_2$ produced an immediate benefit to the speed of responding.

One other investigation produced CNS improvement as manifested in behavioral response due to an enhanced $O_2$ supply (Jacobs et al., 1969). Their subjects, however, experiencing clinical manifestations of intellectual deterioration had been hospitalized, in some cases, for several years because of symptoms of senility. None experienced cardiac, metabolic, or respiratory health risks. They were provided hyperoxygenation treatment (99%-100% $O_2$), and improved significantly after $O_2$ treatment on the Wechsler Memory Scale, Bender-Gestalt Memory Phase and Tien's Organic Integrity Test. Our subjects were healthy professionals.

One other study used healthy subjects and evaluated the effect of an enhanced supply of $O_2$. Fletcher (1985) provided a 67% $O_2$ mixture for men and women ages 54 to 67 years. They were categorized as high fit ($\dot{V}O_2$ max between 32 and 47 ml/kg/min) or low fit ($\dot{V}O_2$ max between 17 and 32 ml/kg/min). Reaction time correlated ($r = .25$) low with maximal oxygen uptake, and there were no statistically significant differences between high and low fit groups for reaction time in either normoxic (20.9% $O_2$) or hyperoxic conditions (67% $O_2$), nor did either group benefit significantly from the enhanced supply of $O_2$. She concluded that possible oxygen deprivation in the central nervous system was not significantly related to psychomotor speed.

**TABLE 2.2.** *Mean (msec) Reaction Times and Standard Deviations (in parentheses) for Each of Simple (SRT) and Choice (CRT) Conditions Under Three Oxygen Conditions.*

| Oxygen Condition | SRT | | | CRT | | |
|---|---|---|---|---|---|---|
| | Normal | 12% | 80% | Normal | 12% | 80% |
| Active Group | 285(49) | 277(53) | 279(35) | 342(38) | 334(31) | 314(42) |
| Less Active Group | 276(34) | 275(54) | 254(24) | 303(28) | 320(28) | 299(16) |

*AGING AND MOTOR BEHAVIOR*

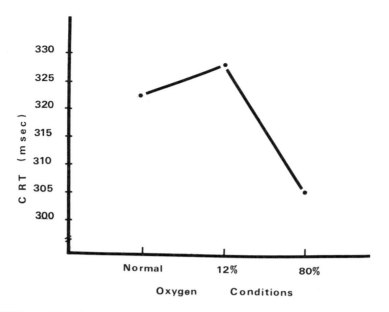

**FIGURE 2.2.** *Mean choice reaction time (CRT) in msec for each of the normal, 12%, and 80% oxygen conditions.*

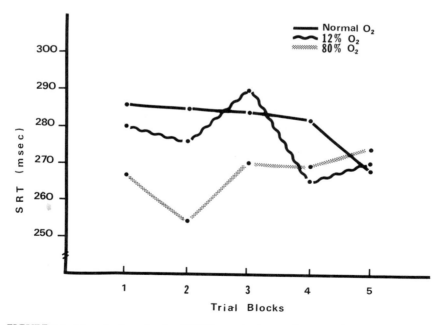

**FIGURE 2.3.** *Mean simple reaction time (SRT) in msec for the normal, 12%, and 80% oxygen conditions over each trial block.*

INFORMATION PROCESSING

55

We would prefer to speculate instead that central processing time has been confounded by the inclusion of a movement task with the reaction time task. Henry and Rogers (1960) demonstrated that simple reaction time was a function of the complexity of the task (number of subsequent movements to be performed after the reaction to the initial stimulus). It would appear that reaction time for Fletcher's subjects (normoxic $M$ = 389 msec), (average simple RT for active and inactive older adults = 195 msec, Stelmach & Diewert, 1977; 154 msec, Spirduso & Clifford, 1978) was substantially affected by the necessity of moving to another key after the stimulus light. While it is apparent that the increase in reaction time for her task is, in fact, due to central processing time (e.g., decision time to select the appropriate angle of movement to the key and programming time), a measure of reaction time without a movement component is the more conventional measure of simple and choice reaction time.

While Fletcher's results were not supportive of the effects of an $O_2$ deprived CNS for the older adult, it would seem that our results do lend support to this "oxygen want" notion as hypothesized by McFarland (1952, 1963), Botwinick (1973), and Gibson and Peterson (1982). The 80% $O_2$ could have changed the partial pressure of $O_2$ ($PO_2$) to the benefit of the tissue, the CNS. "When healthy humans with an $O_2$ saturation of 97% breathe gas mixtures containing more than 21% $O_2$, the alveolar $PO_2$ rises above 100 mm Hg" (Cherniack, Altose, & Kelsen, 1983, p. 688). Apparently, the change in alveolar $PO_2$ due to inhaling 80% $O_2$ produced immediate effects on the CNS that resulted in significant improvements in SRT and CRT. From a limited resource perspective (Salthouse, 1985), an enhanced supply of a resource essential to optimal functioning of the CNS benefitted CNS speed. This could serve to support the processing rate theory as proposed by Salthouse (1985). It would be imperative, however, to compare younger adults with older adults to determine whether 80% $O_2$ also positively affected the younger adults. If this were true, it would weaken the hypothesis that the older adult is mildly hypoxic, or experiencing a decline in utilizing or delivering this general resource of $O_2$ to the CNS.

## Physical Activity and Cognitive Function

Another aspect, that of other cognitive functions, has been examined in order to determine whether direct measures of $O_2$ consumption and overall cognitive functioning change with exercise. One such investigation, by Elsayed, Ismail, and Young (1980), utilized an exercise protocol for 70 people, age 24 to 68 years, for 3-90 minute sessions per week for four months. They conducted pre and posttests on sub-max $VO_2$, fluid and crystallized intelligence, and other physiological measures.

They used Cattell's (1963) definition of fluid intelligence as intellectual development due primarily to biological factors and crystallized intelligence as collective learning and acculturation. Then they used a regression equation with the physiological measures to determine their predictive strength for intelligence. The regression equation included submaximal exercise heart rate, percent lean body weight, max $\dot{V}O_2$ uptake for ml/kg lean body weight, submax minute volume ventilation/kg body weight, resting diastolic blood pressure, resting pulse pressure, and a constant. Fluid intelligence (using the Culture Fair Intelligence Test Scale 3, Form A, Cattell, 1957) was related to physical fitness (physiological measures) and age. Regardless of age, the high-fit group had a significantly higher total fluid intelligence score than the low-fit group.

While Powell (1974) did not measure $\dot{V}O_2$ max when he provided an exercise therapy program, he did report significant changes in two cognitive functioning tests, the Progressive Matrices Test and Wechsler Memory Scale, for geriatric mental patients after 12 weeks of exercise. Another physical activity program designed for geriatric mental patients produced changes in the Wechsler Adult Intelligence Scale (WAIS). This experiment was conducted by Stamford, Hambacher, and Fallica (1974). Those who exercised experienced significant decreases in heart rate, systolic blood pressure, and the WAIS (General Information-broad spectrum of basic facts). The WAIS digit span and Draw-A-Person Test (DAP) did not change, however. While neither of these investigations measured oxygen consumption, evidence has shown that some aspects of cognitive functioning are positively affected by aerobic exercise.

Stacey, Kozma, and Stones (1985) also reported a significant improvement in a cognitive functioning test after their six month exercise program for volunteers from a fitness club who were either new to the club or who had been active for a year or more. They used the Digit Symbol sub-test of the Wechsler Adult Intelligence Scale. $\dot{V}O_2$ max was not measured.

Other investigators who examined the effects of exercise on cognitive functioning have employed a cross-sectional design by comparing those who have been habitual exercisers with those who have had a fairly inactive lifestyle. A dissertation by Crooks (1976) is one example. He determined that level of aerobic physical activity, as professed by each individual, correlated significantly with subtest WAIS scores (Similarities, Block Design, and Digits Backward), and with the Bender-Gestalt Tests. He tested 70 adults who were 55 to 89 years old and then utilized a stepwise multiple regression technique. Systolic blood pressure and resting heart rate as well as professed level of aerobic physical activity entered into significant ($p < .01$) predictions of psychological test performance.

Powell and Pohndorf (1971) also measured cognitive functioning with a fluid intelligence indicant. The "Culture Fair" Intelligence Test, a timed test, was used for the measurement of mental ability. A group who had been running for three years was compared with a group who had not been exercising and a group who fit into neither of these groups, in that they were individuals who exercised occasionally or who had exercised regularly at one time and had since become inactive. All subjects ranged in age from 34 to 75 years ($M$ = 50.33 years). Eight tests of physiological functions, systolic and diastolic blood pressures in sitting and mild postexercise states (bench stepping), basal metabolic rate, serum cholesterol level, total peripheral resistance, and the Schneider Index, were correlated with the measures of mental ability. While fluid intelligence was inversely correlated with age ($r$ = -.57), the exercise group was not significantly better than the nonexercise group on fluid intelligence. It would be interesting to know the relationship of exercise to fluid intelligence for just the older adults who were found in this study to exhibit greater decline than the younger adults on the Culture Fair Text.

The reaction time results of Dustman et al. (1984) were reported earlier in this chapter and the reader may refer to Chapter 3 for more design detail. They also incorporated six other neuropsychological tests as indicants of cognitive functioning. Those were critical flicker fusion threshold (CFF), culture-fair intelligence, digit symbol WAIS subtest, dots estimation, digit span subtest from WAIS, and the stroop color test. It may be noted that many of these tests are timed, and therefore one could speculate that speed of responding is important for effective performance. Their aerobically trained group that completed four months of target-heart rate conditioning demonstrated significant improvement on CFF, digit symbol, dots estimation, and stroop tests. The other control groups, the strength/flexibility training group and the nonexercise group, improved significantly for only one test each; dots estimation for the exercise control and culture fair IQ for the nonexercise controls. It is clearly evident from these results that previously sedentary (as documented by $\dot{V}O_2$ max values) older adults can improve their mental functioning as well as their cardio-vascular functioning.

In a study conducted by Abourezk (1986), the effects of aerobic exercise on short-term memory function in older men was investigated. (The reader is referred to Chapter 5.) For the dichotic listening task, the active group was significantly better at short-term memory retention for the second ear ($M$ = 13.40%) than the nonactive group ($M$ = 6.70%). It was concluded that the long-term aerobic activity may have facilitated the delivery to or utilization of oxygen in the CNS which may have diminished short-term memory deficits in the older exercise trained adult.

In summary, with the exception of results reported by Powell and Pohndorf (1971), all of those reviewed have demonstrated that exercise benefits cognitive functioning for the previously sedentary older adult and, in the case of Abourezk's (1986) subjects, it appears that exercise benefitted cognitive functioning for those who had been exercising for years. One of the common elements among these cognitive functioning tests is memory. Many specific tests of memory function need to be made with the goal of understanding how memory is affected by exercise. The future directions section will address some ideas related to these issues.

## FUTURE DIRECTIONS

Many recommendations have been previously made within the text and many of those will be reviewed here as well. This section of the paper will be organized in the following way. First, suggestions will be made that relate to experimental design, procedures, and statistical analyses that test the effects of exercise on speeded tasks and tasks of cognitive function for the young and old adult. Next, tests related to Salthouse's (1985) processing rate theory will be suggested.

More intervention studies are needed with groups of younger and older adults. We need to test individuals in aerobic fitness, use a sample that possesses a large range of fitness levels, and then randomly assign them to treatment/control groups. Each of these cells then need to be sufficiently large to have adequate power. Analyses of variance should be conducted, and correlations could include $\dot{V}O_2$ max change after an aerobic exercise program with RT change.

Multiple regression could be used with RT as the criterion and $\dot{V}O_2$ max, heart rate, systolic blood pressure, respiratory rate, and respiratory quotient as predictor variables in the regression equation. This could tell us more about the strength of the relationship of many aerobic variables to speed of processing in the CNS.

Since $\dot{V}O_2$ max is a gross indicant of $O_2$ uptake, that is, all tissues that respond to an increased demand of $O_2$ with exercise stress are being measured with $\dot{V}O_2$ max, it could be suggested that researchers use a measure that more specifically reflects CNS $O_2$ consumption, that is, PET scanning. The technique utilized by Pantano et al. (1983) to determine regional blood flow could be investigated for potential use. With this technique we could start to learn more about regional cerebral blood flow, cerebral oxygen utilization, and energy metabolism as they relate to exercise.

Correlations could also be made on the relationship of age with speeded tasks for those who have a history of aerobic exercise participation and those who do not and have not participated in aerobic exercise. $\dot{V}O_2$ max could serve as the indicant of aerobic efficiency in these correlations. This would tell us more about the strength of the relationship of age, aerobic function, and speed. Subjects who range in age from youth to old age should be used. Correlations also need to be made on age, aerobic function, and cognitive function on tests such as memory and intelligence. If the correlations between age, speeded tasks, aerobic function, and cognitive function are similar, then a speed based interpretation of exercise benefits for overall cognitive function is feasible. This could be one way of testing Salthouse's (1985) processing rate theory.

Another test of Salthouse's ideas on the limited resource hypothesis involves establishing whether a critical resource, such as oxygen, does, in fact, decline or is not delivered as well or utilized as well by the CNS with increased age. These facts would help to establish whether age-related slowing of behavior is a general limited resource problem.

The limited resource interpretation might also be investigated by making a task dependent manipulation by changing the difficulty of the task, and those who possess the critical resource should not exhibit the degree of decrement in performance as those older adults who are deficient in the critical resource. This could be done, for example, by increasing the number of stimuli in a choice reaction time paradigm.

Many specific tests of memory function need to be made with the goal of understanding if and how memory is affected by exercise. Are both short-term and long-term memory affected by physical activity, is search and retrieval speed enhanced, is encoding affected, and is RT speed related to better recall? Short-term motor memory could be investigated by using the linear slide, or a force displacement task, and manipulating the retention interval. Verbal tasks could also be used; the digit symbol substitution test from the Wechsler Adult Intelligence Scale is an example. Long-term motor memory could be examined by utilizing the above motor tasks and bringing subjects back to the lab after a retention interval of days. A Sternberg paradigm (1969) would provide information about another information processing process, search speed. Dual and triple tasks could be used to investigate another central processing task, attentional regulation. Using this research strategy would shed more light on the general limited resource and specific process accounts of age-related slowing, and whether exercise affects these dimensions.

More animal experimentation coupled with human investigations are definitely needed in order to investigate the role exercise plays in neurotransmitter production, release, and resorption. PET scanning methods may be a means of determining this information for human studies. In order to study the possibility that neurochemical changes occur with aerobic training, PET measures could be taken before and after a long term exercise program. Using this technique in conjunction with measures of information processing abilities could help to further investigate the relationship between the processing rate theory and CNS integrity.

## GENERAL SUMMARY

The general phenomena of age-related slowing has been documented over decades of research. Declines have been observed in input of stimuli, attention to specific input, short-term storage, retrieval, and organization of new input just to mention a few. Salthouse's (1985) processing rate theory was reviewed due to its effectiveness in accounting for many of these age-related declines. It explains cognitive slowing by postulating a general limited resource. Salthouse assumes that the quantity of resources responsible for speed of cognitive functioning declines with age. Many types of cognitive declines such as RT slowing, encoding, attention, short-term storage, and organization could be explained by this limited resource hypothesis. An alternate view of slowing, the specific process account, was also discussed.

Next, some of the evidence concerned with age-related CNS changes was reviewed as well as explanations for psycho-motor slowing. Some of the neurophysical changes within the CNS are: neuronal, dendritic, and synaptic loss, decrease in neurotransmitter production, decrease in regional cerebral blood flow, $O_2$ consumption, and energy metabolism. Investigators have attempted to explain age-related slowing by incorporating these age-related CNS changes within their behavioral hypotheses. Those hypotheses reviewed were a neural noise explanation, loss of activation, "oxygen-want", and neuronal transmission time.

The role of exercise for CNS integrity over the age-span was discussed with importance given to the ability of the older adult to adequately deliver and utilize oxygen within the CNS, because oxygen and glucose play an extremely important role in CNS energy metabolism. Recent literature was presented that assessed information processing speed by using RT and cognitive functioning through utilizing primarily memory tasks. Many of these investigations also measure $O_2$ consumption before and after aerobic exercise interventions. The general findings were that information processing speed may change significantly from pre to posttests for the sedentary adult who participates in an aerobic exercise program. There is also a fairly strong relationship between RT and oxygen consumption for these individuals. Aerobic exercise was also found to benefit some cognitive functioning tests, namely those related to memory.

The future directions section addressed suggested experimental designs, procedures, and statistical analyses that test the effects of exercise on tasks of speed and cognitive function. Lastly, recommendations were made that related to Salthouse's (1985) processing rate theory and the role of physical activity for enhancing processing speed.

## REFERENCES

Abourezk, T. (1986). The effects of regular aerobic exercise on short-term memory efficiency in the older adult. Unpublished master's thesis, Florida State University, Tallahassee, FL.

Astrand, I. (1960). Aerobic work capacity in men and women with special reference to age. *Acta Physiologica Scandinavia, 49,* (supplement 169), 45-60.

Baron, A., Menich, S.R., & Perone, M. (1983). Reaction times of younger and older men and temporal contingencies of reinforcement. *Journal of the Experimental Analysis of Behavior, 40,* 275-287.

Birren, J.E. (1970). Toward an experimental psychology of aging. *American Psychologist, 25,* 124-135.

Birren, J.E. (1974). Translations in Gerontology—From Lab to Lib: Psychophysiology and Speed of Response. *American Psychologist, 29,* 808-815.

Birren, J.E., & Botwinick, J. (1955). Age differences in finger, jaw, and foot reaction time to auditory stimuli. *Journal of Gerontology, 10,* 429-432.

Birren, J.E., Woods, A.M., & Williams, M.V. (1979). Speed of behavior as an indicator of age changes and the integrity of the nervous system. In F. Hoffmeister & C. Miller (Eds.), *Brain function in old age* (pp. 10-44). Berlin: Springer-Verlag.

Birren, J.E., Woods, A.M., & Williams, M.V. (1980). Behavioral slowing with age: Causes, organization and consequences. In L.W. Poon (Ed.), *Aging in the 1980's* (pp. 293-308). Washington, D.C.: American Psychological Association.

Bondareff, W. (1985). The neural basis of aging. In J.E. Birren & K.W. Schair (Eds.), *Handbook of the psychology of aging (2nd ed.)* (pp. 95-111). New York: Van Nostrand Reinhold Co.

Botwinick, J. (1971). Sensory-set factors in age differences in reaction time. *Journal of Genetic Psychology, 119,* 214-249.

Botwinick, J. (1973). Processing sense information. *Aging and Behavior,* (pp. 131-153). New York: Springer Publishing Co.

Botwinick, J., Brinley, J.F., & Robbin, J.S. (1958). The effect of motivation by electric shocks on reaction in relation to age. *American Journal of Psychology, 71,* 408-411.

Botwinick, J., & Storandt, M. (1974). *Memory, related functions, and age.* Springfield, IL: Charles C. Thomas.

Brody, H. (1955). Organization of the cerebral cortex III. A study of aging in the human cerebral cortex. *Journal of Comparative Neurology, 102,* 551-556.

Caird, W.K. (1966). Aging and short-term memory. *Journal of Gerontology, 21,* 295-299.

Canestrari, R.E. (1968). Age changes in acquisition. In G.A. Talland (Ed.), *Human aging and behavior* (pp. 169-188). New York: Academic Press.

Carlson, N.R. (1986). *Physiology of Behavior* (pp. 68-77). Newton, MA: Allyn and Bacon Inc.

Cattell, R.B. (1957). The IPAT Culture fair intelligence scales. *Institute for Personality & Ability Testing,* Champaign, IL.

Cattell, R.B. (1963). Theory of fluid and crystallized intelligence: A critical experiment. *Journal of Educational Psychology, 54,* 1-22.

Cherniack, N.S., Altose, M.D., & Kelsen, S.G. (1983). The respiratory system. In R.M. Berne and M.N. Levy (Eds.), *Physiology* (pp. 639-740). St. Louis: C.V. Mosby.

Clarkson, P.M., & Kroll, W. (1978). Practice effects on fractionated response time related to age and activity level. *Journal of Motor Behavior, 10,* 275-286.

Craik, F.I.M. (1965). The nature of the age decrement in performance on dichotic listening tasks. *Quarterly Journal of Experimental Psychology, 17,* 227-240.

Craik, F.I.M. (1968). Short-term memory and the aging process. In G.A. Talland (Ed.), *Human aging and behavior* (pp. 131-168). New York: Academic Press.

Craik, F.I.M., & Byrd, M. (1982). Aging and cognitive deficits: The role of attentional resources. In F.I.M. Craik & S.E. Trehub (Eds.), *Aging and cognitive processes* (pp. 191-211). New York: Plenum.

Craik, F.I.M., & Masani, P.A. (1967). Age differences in the temporal integration of language. *British Journal of Psychology, 58,* 291-299.

Craik, F.I.M., & Masani, P.A. (1969). Age and intelligence differences in coding and retrieval of word lists. *British Journal of Psychology, 60,* 315-319.

Craik, F.I.M., & Rabinowitz, J.C. (1984). Age differences in the acquisition and use of verbal information: A tutorial review. In J. Bouma & D.G. Bouwhuis (Eds.), *Attention and performance X,* (pp. 471-499). Hillsdale, NJ: Earlbaum.

Crooks, G.M. (1976). Relationships of physical, social, and physiological variables to psychological performance in subjects 55-89 years of age. Unpublished doctoral dissertation, University of Kansas, Lawrence.

Dekoninck, W.J. (1985). Brain metabolism and aging. In M. Bergener, M. Ermini, & H.B. Stahelin (Eds.), *Thresholds in aging* (pp. 147-174). London: Academic Press Inc.

Denney, D.R. (1974). Clustering in middle and old age. *Developmental Psychology, 4*, 171-191.

Denney, D.R. & Denney, N.W. (1973). The use of classification for problem solving: A comparison of middle and old age. *Developmental Psychology, 9*, 275-278.

Dixon, R.A., Simon, E.W., Nowak, C.A., & Hultsch, D.F. (1982). Text recall in adulthood as a function of information, input modality, and delay interval. *Journal of Gerontology, 37*, 358-364.

Drachman, D.A. & Leavitt, J. (1972). Memory impairment in the aged: Storage versus retrieval deficit. *Journal of Experimental Psychology, 93*, 302-308.

Dustman, R.E., Ruhling, R.O., Russell, E.M., Shearer, D.E., Bonekat, H.W., Shigeoka, J.W., Wood, J.S., & Bradford, D.C. (1984). Aerobic exercise training and improved neuropsychological function of older individuals. *Neurobiology of Aging, 5*, 35-42.

Dzewaltowski, O.A. (1985). *The affect of aerobic exercise on information processing in older adults.* Unpublished master's thesis, West Virginia University, Morgantown.

Elsayed, M., Ismail, A.H., & Young, R.J. (1980). Intellectual differences of adult men related to age and physical fitness before and after an exercise program. *Journal of Gerontology, 35*, 383-387.

Era, P., Jokela, J., & Heikkinen, E. (1986). Reaction and movement times in men of different ages: A population study. *Perceptual and Motor Skills, 63*, 111-130.

Feldman, M.L., & Dowd, C. (1975). Loss of dendritic spines in aging cerebral cortex. *Anatomy and Embryology, 148*, 279-301.

Finch, C.E. (1973). Manoamine metabolism in the aging male mouse. In M. Rockstein (Ed.), *Development and aging in the nervous system* (pp. 199-218). New York: Academic Press

Fletcher, L.M. (1985). *The relation of maximal oxygen uptake and hyperoxia to reaction and movement times in older men and women.* Unpublished master's thesis, The Pennsylvania State University, State College, PA.

Frackowiak, R.S.J., Lenzi, G.C., Jones, T., & Heather, J.D. (1980). The quantitative measurement of regional cerebral blood flow and oxygen metabolism in normal man using oxygen-15 and positron emission tomography: Theory, procedure and normal values. *Journal of Computer Assisted Tomography, 4*, 727-736.

Frackowiak, R.S.J., Wise, R., Gibbs, J.M., & Jones, T. (1983). Oxygen extraction in the aging brain. *European Neurology, 22* (suppl. 2), 24-25.

Fraser, D.C. (1958). Decay of immediate memory with age. *Nature, 182*, 1163.

Freddari, C.B., & Giuli, C. (1980). A quantitive morphometric study of synapses of rat cerebellar glumeruli during aging. *Mechanisms of Aging and Development, 12*, 127-136.

Frolkis, V.V., & Bezrukov, V.V. (1979). Aging of the central nervous system. *Interdisciplinary Topics in Gerontology, 16*, 30-52.

Giaquito, S. & Nolfe, G. (1983). Cortical processing in the aged. *European Neurology, 22* (suppl. 2), 31.

Gibson, G.E., & Blass, J.P. (1976). Impaired synthesis of acetylcholine in brain accompanying mild hypoxia and hypoglycemia. *Journal of Neurochemistry, 27*, 37-42.

Gibson, G.E., & Peterson, C. (1982). Biochemical and behavioral parallels in aging and hypoxia. In E. Giacobini, G. Filogamo, G. Giacobini, & A. Vernadakis (Eds.), *The aging brain: Cellular and molecular mechanisms of aging in the nervous system* (pp. 107-112). New York: Raven Press.

Gibson, G.E., Peterson, C., & Sansone, J. (1981). Decreases in amino acid and acetylcholine metabolism during hypoxia. *Journal of Neurochemistry, 37* (1), 192-201.

Glick, R., & Bondareff, W. (1979). Loss of synapses in the cerebellar cortex of senescent rat. *Journal of Gerontology, 34*, 818-822.

Gordon, S.K. & Clark, W.C. (1974). Application of signal detection theory to prose recall and recognition in elderly and young adults. *Journal of Gerontology, 29*, 64-72.

Grant, E.A., Storandt, M., & Botwinick, J. (1978). Incentive and practice in the psychomotor performance of the elderly. *Journal of Gerontology, 33*, 413-415.

Hall, T.C., Miller, A.K.H., & Corsellis, J.A.N. (1979). Variations in the human Purkinje cell population according to age and sex. *Neuropathology and Applied Neurobiology, 1*, 267-292.

Hasan, M., & Glees, P. (1973). Ultrastructural age changes in hippocampal neurons, synapses and neuroglia. *Experimental Gerontology, 8*, 75-83.

Hasher, L. & Zacks, R.T. (1979). Antomatic and effortful processes in memory. *Journal of Experimental Psychology: General, 108*, 356-388.

Henderson, G., Tomlinson, B.E., & Gibson, P.H. (1980). Cell counts in human cerebral cortex in normal adults throughout life using an imaging analyzing computer. *Journal of Neurological Sciences, 46*, 113-136.

Henry, F.M., & Rogers, D.E. (1960). Increased response latency for complicated movements and a memory drum theory of neuromotor reaction. *Research Quarterly, 31*, 458-488.

Hess, T.M. & Higgins, J.N. (1983). Context utilization in young and old adults. *Journal of Gerontology, 38*, 65-71.

Huhenlucher, P.R. (1979). Synaptic density in human frontal cortex—developmental changes and effects of aging. *Brain Research, 163*, 195-205.

Hultsch, D.F. (1971). Organization and memory in adulthood. *Human Development, 14*, 16-29.

Inglis, J. & Ankus, M.N. (1965). Effects of age on short-term storage and serial rote learning. *British Journal of Psychology, 56*, 183-195.

Jacobs, E.A., Winter, P.M., Alvis, H.J., & Small, S.M. (1969). Hyperoxygenation effect on cognitive functioning in the aged. *The New England Journal of Medicine, 281,* 753-757.

Kausler, D.H. & Puckett, J.M. (1979). Effects of word frequency on adult age differences in word memory span. *Experimental Aging Research, 5,* 161-169.

Konigsmark, B.W., & Murphy, E.A. (1970). Neuronal populations in the human brain. *Nature, 228,* 1335-1336.

Ksiezak, J.J., & Gibson, G.E. (1981). Oxygen dependence of glucose and acetylcholine metabolism in slices and synaptosomes from rat brain. *Journal of Neurochemistry, 37* (2), 305-314.

Lassen, N.A., Feinberg, I., & Lane, M.H. (1960). Bilateral studies of cerebral oxygen uptake in young and aged normal subjects and in patients with organic dementia. *Journal of Clinical Investigations, 39,* 491-500.

Lassen, N.A., Ingvar, D.H., & Shihoj, E. (1978). Brain function and blood flow. *Scientific American,* (Oct), 62-71.

Lenzi, G.L., Frackowiak, R.S.J., Jones, T., Heather, J.D., Lammertsma, A.A., Rhodes, C.G., & Pozzilli, C. (1981). CMRO2 and CBF by the oxygen-inhalation technique. *European Neurology, 20,* 285-290.

Light, L.L., Zelinski, E.M., & Moore, M. (1982). Adult age differences in reasoning from new information. *Journal of Experimental Psychology: Learning, Memory, and Cognition, 8,* 435-447.

Madden, D.J. (1983). Aging and distraction by highly familiar stimuli during visual search. *Developmental Psychology, 19,* 499-507.

McFarland, R.A. (1952). Anoxia: Its effects on the physiology and biochemistry of the brain and on behavior. In P.B. Hueber (Ed.), *The biology of mental health and disease* (pp. 335-355). New York: Hueber, Inc.

McFarland, R.A. (1963). Experimental evidence of the relationship between aging and oxygen want: In search of a theory of aging. *Ergonomics, 6,* 342-365.

McGeer, E.G. (1978). Aging and neurotransmitter metabolism in the human brain. In R. Katzman, R.D. Terry, & K.L. Bick (Eds.), *Alzheimer's disease: Senile dementia and related disorders (Vol. 6)* (p. 427). New York: Raven Press.

McGeer, E.G., Fibiger, H.C., McGeer, P.L., & Wickson, W. (1971). Aging and brain enzymes. *Experimental Gerontology, 6,* 391-396.

McGeer, E.G., & McGeer, P.L. (1975). Age changes in the human for some enzymes associated with metabolism of catecholamines, GABA and acetylcholine. In Ordy & Brizzee (Eds.), *Neurobiology of aging* (pp. 287-305). New York: Plenum Publishing.

Meek, J.L., Bertilsson, L., Cheney, L., Zsilla, G., & Costa, E. (1977). Aging-induced changes in acetylcholine and serotonin content of discrete brain nuclei. *Journal of Gerontology, 32,* 129-131.

Monagle, R.D., & Brody, H. (1974). The effects of age upon the main nucleus of the inferior olive in the human. *Journal of Comparative Neurology, 155,* 61-66.

Ostrow, A.C. (1984). *Physical activity and the older adult: Psychological perspectives.* Princeton: Princeton Book Co.

Pantano, P., Baron, J.C., Lebrun-Grandie, P., Duquesnay, N., Bousser, M.G., & Comar, D. (1983). Effects of aging on regional CBF and CMRO2 in humans. *European Neurology, 22* (suppl. 2), 24-31.

Perlmutter, M. & Mitchell, D.B. (1982). The appearance and disappearance of age differences in memory. In F.I.M. Craik & S. Trehub (Eds.), *Aging and cognitive processes* (pp. 127-144). New York: Plenum.

Perry, E.K., Perry, R.H., Gibson, P.H., Blessed, G., & Tomlinson, B.E. (1977). A cholinergic connection between normal aging and senile dementia in the human hippocampus. *Neuroscience Letters, 6,* 85-89.

Ponzio, F., & Calderini, G., Lomuscio, G., Vantini, G. Toffano, G., & Algeri, S. (1982). Changes in monoamines and their metabolite levels in some brain regions in aged rats. *Neurobiology of Aging, 3,* 23-29.

Powell, R.R. (1974). Psychological effects of exercise therapy upon institutionalized geriatric mental patients. *Journal of Gerontology, 29,* 157-161.

Powell, R.R., & Pohndorf, R.H. (1971). Comparison of adult exercises and nonexercises of fluid intelligence and selected physiological variables. *Research Quarterly, 42,* 70-77

Rabbitt, P.M.A. (1979a). Current paradigms in human information processing. In V. Hamilton & D.M. Warburton (Eds.), *Human stress and cognition.* Chichester, England: Wiley (pp. 115-140).

Rabbitt, P.M.A. (1979b). Some experiments and a model for changes in attentional selectivity with old age. In F. Hoffmeister & C. Muller (Eds.), *Brain function in old age* (pp. 82-94). Berlin: Springer-Verlag.

Rabbitt, P.M.A. (1982). How do old people know what to do next? In F.I.M. Craik & S. Trehub (Eds.), *Aging and cognitive processes* (pp. 79-98). New York: Plenum.

Robinson, A.J., Niles, A., Davis, J.N., Bunney, W.E., Davis, J.M., Colburn, R.W., Bourne, H.R., Shaw, D.M., & Coppern, A.J. (1972). Aging, monamines, and monamine oxidase levels. *Lancet* (1), 290-291.

Roy, C.S., & Sherrington, C.S. (1980). On the regulation of the blood-supply of the brain. *Journal of Psychology (Lond.), 11,* 85-108.

Russell, E.M. (1982). The effects of an aerobic conditioning program on reaction times of older sedentary adults. Unpublished doctoral dissertation, The University of Utah, Salt Lake City.

Salthouse, T.A. (1980). Age differences in visual masking: A manifestation of decline in signal/noise ratio? Paper presented at the 33rd Annual Meeting of the Gerontological Society of America, San Diego, CA.

Salthouse, T.A. (1985). *A theory of cognitive aging.* Amsterdam: Elsevier Science.

Salthouse, T.A., & Lichty, W. (1985). Tests of the neural noise hypothesis of age-related cognitive change. *Journal of Gerontology, 40*, 443-450.

Samorajski, T., Rolsten, C., & Ordy, J.M. (1971). Changes in behavior, brain and neuroendocrine chemistry with age and stress in C574B410 male mice. *Journal of Gerontology, 26*, 168-175.

Scheibel, M.E., Lindsay, R.D., Tomiyasu, U., & Scheibel, A.B. (1976). Progressive dendritic changes in the aging limbic system. *Experimental Neurology, 53*, 420-430.

Schonfield, A.D. & Robertson, B. (1966). Memory storage and aging. *Canadian Journal of Psychology, 20*, 228-236.

Shaps, L.P. & Nilsson, L. (1980). Encoding and retrieval operations in relation to age. *Developmental Psychology, 16*, 636-643.

Spirduso, W.W. (1975). Reaction and movement time as a function of age and physical activity level. *Journal of Gerontology, 30*, 435-440.

Spirduso, W.W. (1980). Physical fitness, aging, and psychomotor speed: A review. *Journal of Gerontology, 35*, 850-865.

Spirduso, W.W. (1983). Exercise and the aging brain. *Research Quarterly for Exercise and Sport, 54*, 208-218.

Spirduso, W.W., & Clifford, P. (1978). Neuromuscular speed and consistency of performance as a function of age, physical activity level and type of physical activity. *Journal of Gerontology, 33*, 26-30.

Stacey, C., Kozma, A., & Stones, M.J. (1985). Simple cognitive and behavioral changes resulting from improved physical fitness in persons over 50 years of age. *Canadian Journal on Aging, 4*, 67-74.

Stamford, B.A., Hambacher, W., & Fallica, A. (1974). Effects of daily physical exercise on the psychiatric state of institutionalized geriatric mental patients. *Research Quarterly, 45*, 34-41.

Stelmach, G.E., & Diewert, G.L. (1977). Aging, information processing, and fitness. In G. Borg (Ed.), *Physical work and effort* (pp. 115-136). New York: Pergamon Press.

Sternberg, S. (1969). Memory-scanning: Mental processes revealed by reaction-time experiments. *American Scientist, 57*, 421-457.

Stones, M.J., & Kozma, A. (1985). Physical performance. In N. Charness (Ed.), *Aging and human performance* (pp. 261-291). New York: John Wiley & Sons, Ltd.

Surwillo, W.W. (1968). Timing of behavior in senescence and the role of the central nervous system. In G.A. Talland (Ed.), *Human aging and behavior* (pp. 1-35). New York: Academic Press.

Swets, J.A. (1964). *Signal detection and recognition by human observers.* New York: John Wiley & Sons, Ltd.

Talland, G.A. (1968). Age and the span of immediate recall. In G.A. Talland (Ed.), *Human aging and behavior* (pp. 93-129). New York: Academic Press.

Taub, H.A. (1979). Comprehension and memory of prose materials by young and old adults. *Experimental Aging Research, 5*, 3-13.

Till, R.E. & Walsh, D.A. (1980). Encoding and retrieval factors in adult memory for implicational sentences. *Journal of Verbal Learning and Verbal Behavior, 19*, 1-16.

Tomporowski, P.D. & Ellis, N.R. (1986). Effects of exercise on cognitive processes: A review. *Psychological Bulletin, 99*, 338-346.

Toole, T., Abourezk, T., & Qasem, F. (1987). The role of oxygen in central nervous system processing speed and short-term memory in older adults. (In preparation).

Unsworth, B.R., Fleming, L.H., & Caron, P.C. (1980). Neorotransmitter enzymes in telencepholon, brain stem and cerebellum during the entire lifespan of the mouse. *Mechanisms of Aging and Development, 13*, 205-217.

VanFraechem, J., & VanFraechem, R. (1977). Studies of the effect of a short training period on aged subjects. *Journal of Sports Medicine and Physical Fitness, 17*, 373-380.

Vijayashankar, N., & Brody, H. (1979). A quantitative study of the pigmented neurons in the nuclei locus coeruleus and subcoeruleus in man as related to aging. *Journal of Neuropathology and Experimental Neorology, 38*, 490.

Welford, A.T. (1958). *Ageing and human skill.* London: Oxford University Press.

Welford, A.T. (1977). Motor performance. In J.E. Birren & K.W. Schaie (Eds.), *Handbook of the psychology of aging* (pp. 450-496). New York: Van Nostrand Reinhold.

Welford, A.T. (1984). Between bodily changes and performance: Some possible reasons for slowing with age. *Experimental Aging Research, 10*, (2), 73-88.

Welford, A.T. (1985). Changes of performance with age: an overview. In N. Charness (Ed.), *Aging and human performance* (pp. 333-369). New York: John Wiley & Sons, Ltd.

*INFORMATION PROCESSING*                                                       **65**

# 3

## Aerobic Exercise Training and Improved Neuropsychological Function of Older Individuals[1]*

ROBERT E. DUSTMAN[2,3,4]

ROBERT O. RUHLING[5]

EVAN M. RUSSELL[6]

DONALD E. SHEARER[2]

H. WILLIAM BONEKAT[2,7]

JOHN W. SHIGEOKA[2,7]

JAMES S. WOOD[2,7]

DAVID C. BRADFORD[4]

## ABSTRACT

The effects of a four month aerobic exercise conditioning program on neuropsychological test performance, depression indices, sensory threshold, and visual acuity of 55-70 year old sedentary individuals were evaluated. Aerobically trained subjects were compared with two age-matched control groups of subjects: those who trained with strength and flexibility exercises and others who were not engaged in a supervised exercise program. The aerobically trained subjects demonstrated significantly greater improvement on the neuropsychological battery than did either control group. Depression scores, sensory thresholds, and visual acuity were not changed by aerobic exercise. The pattern of results suggests that the effect of aerobic exercise training was on central rather than on peripheral function. We

[1] This research was supported by the Veterans Administration and by funds from NIH Biomedical Research Support (Grant No. RR07092)
[2] Veterans Administration Medical Center, Salt Lake City
[3] Department of Neurology, University of Utah
[4] Department of Psychology, University of Utah
[5] College of Health, University of Utah
[6] College of Health, Wheaton College
[7] Department of Internal Medicine, University of Utah

*This chapter is reprinted with permission from the *Neurobiology of Aging*, 5, 35-42, Copyright 1984, Pergamon Journals, Ltd.

speculate that aerobic exercise promoted increased cerebral metabolic activity with a resultant improvement in neuropsychological test scores.

## INTRODUCTION

Growing old is accompanied by a gradual decline of the central nervous system (CNS). Measures of higher mental function such as intellect, memory, attention, and perception evidence decline (Botwinick, 1973), and behavior slows as demonstrated by prolonged reaction times (Botwinick, 1973), reduced brain wave (EEG) frequency (Obrist, 1976), increased latency of event related potentials (Beck, Swanson, & Dustman, 1980; Dustman & Beck, 1969), and slower nerve conduction velocities (Dorfman & Bosley, 1979).

It has been suggested that decrements in mental and electrophysiological functioning of older individuals may, in part, result from the brain being mildly hypoxic (Gibson & Peterson, 1982; McFarland, 1969). There are two factors which contribute to reduced cerebral oxygenation in old age and thus may adversely affect brain function: the increasing presence of atherosclerosis (Bierman, 1978; Mintz & Mankovsky, 1971) and an inability to efficiently transport and utilize oxygen resulting from physically inactive life-styles (deVries, 1975). The latter can be improved by aerobic exercise (deVries, 1975) and there is growing evidence suggesting that the rate of decline of physical and cognitive abilities is governed by physical conditioning level as well as by age (Bortz, 1980; Bortz, 1982; deVries, 1979; Fries & Crapo, 1980). For example, response times of older men who had maintained an active participation in physical activities such as racquet sports and running were significantly faster than those of age-matched sedentary men and little different from response times of much younger sedentry subjects (Sherwood & Selder, 1979; Spirduso & Clifford, 1978). Also, highly fit older individuals scored higher on tests of fluid intelligence than did less fit subjects (Elsayed, Ismail & Young, 1980; Powell & Pohndorf, 1971).

Results such as these raise important questions. Does the better performance of physically active older individuals reflect a predisposition for superiority in both athletic and cognitive abilities, or does exercise per se have a beneficial effect on CNS functioning? If the latter is true, can CNS functioning of older people be significantly improved by a program of physical activity even though they have maintained a sedentary life-style for many years? Is the type of exercise important? Exercise that results in increased aerobic efficiency, i.e., an improved ability to transport oxygen from the environment to consumer cells (deVries, 1979), may have more effect on brain function than physical activities that do not improve aerobic capacity.

The present study was designed to evaluate the effects of an aerobic exercise training program on brain function of sedentary older people.

## METHOD

Sedentary individuals aged 55-70 years were solicited from the community and screened for health problems which would preclude their participation in an exercise program. Those who stated that they actively engaged in physical conditioning activities were not considered further. The research was described in greater detail at a formal meeting and prospective subjects were provided an opportunity to ask questions and become familiar with a treadmill on which maximal exercise tests were to be performed. They were told they would be paid a modest sum at the end of the study for their participation and were given informed consent forms to review. The protocol for this study and consent forms were approved by the University of Utah Review of Research with Human Subjects Committee (IRB).

Individuals who elected to participate in the research were scheduled for a maximal exercise test. Immediately before this test they were examined by a physician for health problems which would exclude them from safely performing a maximal exercise test and/or engaging in an exercise program. Those selected to participate performed a modified Balke exercise test on a motor driven treadmill (Balke & Ware, 1959). During the test their electrocardiogram was continuously monitored by a physician and their blood pressure was measured every two to three minutes. The treadmill was set at a speed of 67.0 m/min and 1% slope. While the speed remained constant, the slope of the treadmill was increased 1% each succeeding minute of exercise until a maximal effort was achieved (American College of Sports Medicine, 1980). During the test a standard open-circuit indirect calorimetry system was used so that measures of minute ventilation and maximal oxygen uptake ($\dot{V}O_2$max) could be obtained. On completion of the maximal exercise test, subjects were alternately assigned to the experimental group (aerobic exercise training) or to an exercise control group. A questionnaire revealed that only three subjects smoked on a regular basis; these were in the aerobic exercise group.

Additional measures were obtained during two test sessions, each about 90 minutes in duration, from subjects in the experimental and exercise control groups and from a third group of older volunteers. The latter, nonexercise controls did not participate in an exercise program and were not tested on the treadmill. They were screened for health problems during a structured interview. Electrophysiological measures (EEG and evoked potentials), auditory, visual and somatosensory thresholds, and a measure of visual acuity were obtained during one test session. During the other, measures were obtained for several neuropsychological tests and two depression inventories, the Beck Depression Index (Beck, Ward, Mendelson, Mock & Erbaugh, 1961) and the Self-Rating Depression Scale (Zung, 1967). The EEG and evoked potential results will be reported elsewhere. All subjects reported they were right-handed.

## Sensory Thresholds and Visual Acuity

As part of the procedures for recording auditory brain stem potentials, an auditory threshold was measured. Both ears were tested; the best ear was reported. Clicks were generated by a Grass Auditory Stimulus Control Module (S10ASCM) and delivered monaurally to subjects via earphones. Somatosensory thresholds were established for 0.5 msec shocks generated by a Grass S10SCM stimulator and delivered to the median nerve of the dominant hand. Flashes, generated by a Grass PS22 Photostimulator, backlighted a narrow black diagonal line placed in a viewing box towards which the subject's gaze was oriented. Neutral density filters were used to change stimulus intensity. Visual threshold was defined as the lowest intensity at which subjects could correctly report the orientation, left or right, of the line (Dustman, Snyder & Schlehuber, 1981). Visual acuity was measured with a Bausch and Lomb Vision Tester (Model 712241). Vision of a number of subjects was corrected by glasses which were worn during testing procedures.

## Neuropsychological Tests

(1) *Critical Flicker Fusion Threshold* (CFF) was measured with a Lafayette Instrument Flicker Fusion Control Unit (Model 12025) with attached viewing chamber (Model 12026) which presented a flashing light to the dominant eye. The light/dark ratio of the stimuli was 1:1. CFF threshold was the frequency (Hz) at which the flashes appeared to fuse into a continuous light. (2) *Culture-Fair Intelligence*, scale 3, Form A, consisting of four timed paper and pencil tests was used as a measure of intellectual performance (*Measuring Intelligence with the Culture Fair Tests*, 1973). (3) *Digit Span*, a subtest from the Wechsler Adult Intelligence Scale (WAIS) (Wechsler, 1981), provided a measure of recent memory. The subject's score was the number of digits in the longest series of numbers he/she could correctly repeat plus the number in the longest series which he/she could correcly report in reverse order. (4) *Digit Symbol WAIS subtest* (Wechsler, 1981). Subjects were asked to match numbers with appropriate symbols to be drawn below the numbers. A key illustrating number-symbol matches was provided. Their score was the number of matches correctly made in 90 sec. (5) *Dots Estimation*. Sixteen slides, each containing from 1 to 16 opaque dots, were presented tachistoscopically on a screen for 200 msec. Subjects were asked to estimate the number of dots displayed with the score being the number of errors (difference between

his/her estimate and the actual number of dots) averaged over two repetitions. (6) *Reaction Time.* Measures of simple and choice reaction time were obtained. Subjects sat facing a video screen while holding a response switch in each hand and were instructed to respond to appropriate stimuli as quickly as possible. For simple reaction time the imperative stimulus was an X. During choice reaction time trials an X and an O were presented simultaneously, one on the left and the other on the right of the screen. Subjects responded with their left switch when the X appeared to their left and with the right switch when the X was displayed to their right. Imperative stimuli were preceded by a warning stimulus, a small rectangle. The interval between warning and imperative stimuli was randomly varied among 0.50, 0.75, 1.00 and 1.25 sec. Inter-trial intervals were 1 sec. Fifty valid simple and choice reaction time trials were obtained from each subject. Invalid trials were those for which reaction times were less than 100 msec (anticipation), longer than 500 msec, or a wrong switch was depressed. The fastest and slowest five trials were discarded and mean reaction time was computed from the remaining 40 trials. (7) *Stroop Color Test.* Three 35.5×10 cm cards were used as stimulus materials. Card 1 consisted of 17 color names printed in black ink. Card 2 consisted of 17 colored bars. On card 3 were 17 color names printed in a different color of ink (e.g., the work "red" was printed in blue ink). Word and color bars, each about 2-3 cm in length, were ordered vertically on the cards. Subjects completed four tasks, in order, as follows. They were asked to read the color words on card 1 (Task I), name the colors on card 2 (Task II), read the color words on card 3 (Task III), and to name the color of the ink used for each color word on card 3 (Task IV). The latter, an "interference" task, provides a measure of a subject's ability to "shift his perceptual set to conform to changing demands" (Lezak, 1983, p. 523), and is particularly sensitive to the effects of adult aging (Cohn, Dustman & Bradford, 1984). Each task was timed and subjects were asked to work as rapidly as possible.

## Exercise Protocol

The exercise groups met for three one hour sessions a week over a four month period; each was supervised by a graduate student trained in exercise physiology. Every two weeks the instructors alternated groups. Subjects in the experimental group, following a few minutes of "warm up" exercises, then concentrated on aerobic exercise, consisting mostly of fast walking with occasional slow jogging. Their goal was to increase their heart rate to 70-80% of the heart rate reserve and to maintain it at this rate for longer periods of time as their conditioning improved (American College of Sports Medicine, 1980). The exercise control group participated in strength and flexibility exercises. They also monitored their heart rates but were encouraged to keep them below a level reported to improve aerobic efficiency. On conclusion of the four month exercise program, subjects in the exercise groups again performed the maximal exercise test; the remaining tests were administered to all subjects.

The aerobic exercise, exercise control and nonexercise control groups included, respectively, 13 subjects aged 55-68 years (mean = 60.6), 15 subjects aged 55-70 years (mean = 62.3) and 15 subjects aged 51-70 years (mean = 57.4). Nine of the subjects in each group were males. The groups were equivalent in terms of number of years of education (15-16 years), scores on the Culture Fair Test of Intelligence, and mean number of days between pre- and posttreatment tests (about 140 days). The groups were not equal, however, with respect to age as subjects in the nonexercise control group were younger than those in the exercise control group ($p < .05$).

## RESULTS

Subjects in the two exercise groups were compared with respect to six physiological measures which are indicative of physical health condition: resting systolic and diastolic blood pressure, resting heart rate, maximum heart rate, maximum minute ventilation and maximum oxygen uptake ($\dot{V}O_2$max). The latter three measures were obtained while subjects were performing the initial treadmill test; the other measures were obtained just before they walked on the treadmill. As shown in Table 3-1, the exercise groups did not differ on any of these measures. Nor, with the exception of age, did the experimental and control groups differ on any of the other measures obtained during pre-exercise testing ($p > 0.10$).

To determine if our subjects had made a maximal effort on the treadmill exercise test, we compared mean $O_2$ uptake for the minute

**TABLE 3.1.** *Physiological measures obtained from the aerobic and exercise control subjects while at rest immediately before their initial treadmill test (blood pressure and heart rate) and while they walked on the treadmill (maximum heart rate and maximum minute ventilation ($V_E$).*

|  | Aerobic | | Exercise Control | |  |
|---|---|---|---|---|---|
|  | Mean | S.D. | Mean | S.D. | t-Value |
| Blood Pressure (mm Hg) |  |  |  |  |  |
| Systolic | 140.1 | 15.3 | 135.8 | 9.2 | 0.882 |
| Diastolic | 90.7 | 6.1 | 85.9 | 9.1 | 1.651 |
| Heart Rate (BPM) |  |  |  |  |  |
| At Rest | 82.4 | 16.3 | 79.9 | 12.5 | 0.450 |
| Maximum | 148.0 | 12.8 | 147.5 | 12.6 | 0.110 |
| Maximum $V_E$ (L/min) | 64.9 | 22.1 | 65.2 | 18.8 | 0.025 |
| $VO_2$max (ml/kg/min) | 19.4 | 5.7 | 22.5 | 5.1 | 1.507 |

The probability for each t-value was > 0.10 (26 *df*).

*AGING AND MOTOR BEHAVIOR*

preceding the final minute of effort (22.1 ml/kg/min) with that for the final minute (22.9 ml/kg/min), a 0.8 ml/kg/min difference. Means were based on pre- and posttest evaluations of all of the exercise subjects. Maximum oxygen uptake is reportedly achieved if the difference between consecutive $\dot{V}O_2$ readings, with increasing work loads, is less than 2.1 ml/kg/min (Taylor, Buskirk & Henschel, 1955). Our data suggest that this criterion was met.

A Group × Session ANOVA was computed on pre- and posttreatment $\dot{V}O_2$max values for the two exercise groups. A significant treatment effect was found with $\dot{V}O_2$max means being larger at the conclusion of the exercise programs, $F(1,26)=23.6$, $p<0.001$. While the groups were not different for combined pre- and posttreatment values ($p>0.10$), a significant interaction, $F(1,26)=4.89$, $p=0.036$, indicated a differential effect of type of training on $\dot{V}O_2$max improvement. $\dot{V}O_2$max increase for the experimental group was significantly greater than that for the exercise control subjects as determined by a $t$-test of $\dot{V}O_2$max change, $t(26)=2.153$, $p=0.04$. $\dot{V}O_2$max for the aerobically trained group increased by 27% from 19.4 to 24.6 ml/kg/min, $t(12)=4.08$, $p<0.002$, and 9%, 22.5 to 24.5 ml/kg/min, for the exercise control subjects, $t(14)=2.40$, $p=0.04$. The greater improvement for the aerobic subjects was not the result of more training hours since, on the average, individuals in the exercise control group attended 3.9 more training sessions than did the aerobically trained subjects.

Analyses of variance on scores from pretest and posttest sessions (Group × Sessions ANOVAs) revealed that sensory thresholds and indices of depression were not significantly changed from initial values after the four month experimental period. Visual acuity, however, improved significantly, from 20/23 to 20/21 ($p<0.05$). A nonsignificant Group × Session interaction indicated that the improvement was common to all groups suggesting a learning effect for this particular test.

Aerobic exercise training, however, was associated with a significant improvement on most neuropsychological measures. The aerobically trained group demonstrated significant improvement on Critical Flicker Fusion, Digit Symbol, Dots Estimation, Simple Reaction Time, and Stroop tests (Table 3-2). Their improvement on Digit Span approached significance ($p=0.08$). Digit span forward and backward each improved by 0.5 digits. Performance of the control groups significantly improved for only one test each: Dots Estimation for the exercise controls and Culture Fair IQ for the nonexercise controls. No improvement in Choice Reaction Time occurred, either for groups combined or for individual groups ($p>0.10$).

An evaluation was made of overall neuropsychological test improvement. Pre- and posttest scores of the 43 subjects for each of the eight measures listed in Table 3-2 were converted to standard scores with

**TABLE 3.2.** *Pre- and Posttreatment values for eight neuropsychological tests and for the eight tests combined.*

| | Aerobic | | | Exercise Control | | | Nonexercise Control | | |
|---|---|---|---|---|---|---|---|---|---|
| | Pre | Post | p | Pre | Post | p | Pre | Post | p |
| CFF (Hz) | 38.2 | 39.4 | =0.002 | 38.5 | 38.8 | ns* | 38.8 | 38.8 | ns |
| Culture Fair IQ | 97.6 | 100.1 | ns | 94.4 | 99.3 | ns | 85.5 | 92.1 | =0.014 |
| Digit Span | 12.6 | 13.6 | =0.080 | 11.9 | 12.3 | ns | 11.7 | 11.5 | ns |
| Digit Symbol | 54.8 | 61.0 | <0.001 | 54.1 | 56.0 | ns | 55.1 | 55.4 | ns |
| Dots (errors) | 40.8 | 34.9 | =0.020 | 42.3 | 33.1 | =0.005 | 38.0 | 35.7 | ns |
| Simple Reaction Time (msec) | 199.2 | 182.6 | =0.020 | 196.0 | 189.0 | ns | 188.7 | 185.1 | ns |
| Stroop (sec) Interference | 18.1 | 15.2 | <0.001 | 18.7 | 18.2 | ns | 17.2 | 16.9 | ns |
| Total | 41.6 | 36.1 | <0.001 | 41.0 | 40.2 | ns | 38.1 | 38.0 | ns |
| Combined Tests (Std scores) | 97.3 | 106.1 | <0.001 | 96.5 | 100.6 | =0.011 | 99.7 | 100.6 | ns |

Pre-and posttests, separated by a four month interval, were administered to older individuals who received aerobic or strength and flexibility training (exercise control) or did not participate in an exercise program (nonexercise control).

Probability values were based on $t$-tests for correlated means.

*Not significant.

a mean of 100 and a standard deviation of 15. Scores were inverted about the mean when necessary so that for all tests a higher score represented better performance. A mean of the pre- and posttest standard scores was calculated for each subject and a Group × Session ANOVA was computed on these means. Mean standard scores of the three groups (combined across sessions) were not different. Posttest means, for groups combined, were significantly larger than pretest means, $F(1,40)=43.7$, $p<0.001$. The Group × Session interaction was also highly significant, $F(2,40)=8.23$, $p=0.001$, indicating a differential pre- and posttest change in performance among the three groups. Evaluation of change for each group by $t$-test documented significant cognitive improvement for both the aerobic ($t=5.66$, $p<0.001$) and the exercise control ($t=3.52$, $p<0.001$) groups. Cognitive performance of the nonexercise control subjects did not reliably improve ($p>0.10$). Mean pre- and posttest standard score values are illustrated in Figure 3-1.

A single factor ANOVA was computed on post- minus pretest differences in mean standard scores to determine if the improvement evidenced by the aerobically trained individuals was significantly greater than that of the control groups. A significant Group effect was obtained, $F(2,40)=7.95$, $p<0.002$. *Post-hoc* comparisons of differences among group means indicated that test performance of the aerobically trained subjects improved more than the performance of the exercise control ($p<0.05$) and the nonexercise control ($p<0.01$) groups. The control groups did not reliably differ from each other with respect to amount of pre- posttest change.

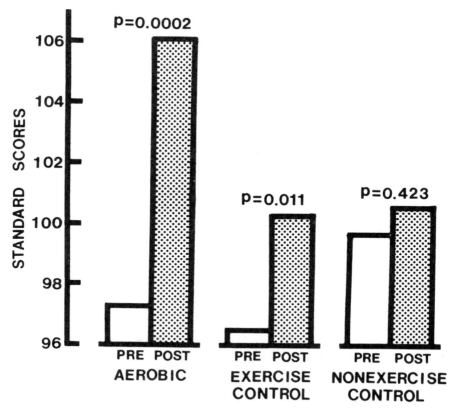

**FIGURE 3.1.** *Standard scores, averaged across the eight tests listed in Table 3-2 (see text), for three groups of older individuals: those who participated in an aerobic conditioning program (AEROBIC), in a program of strength and flexibility exercises (EXERCISE CONTROL), or who did not participate in an organized exercise program (NONEXERCISE CONTROL). Pre- and posttests were separated by four months. p (probability) values indicate significance of pre- posttest differences.*

Additional analyses were performed to increase our understanding regarding the significant time savings demonstrated by our aerobically trained subjects on the Stroop Interference Test (Task IV, see Table 3-2). First, a Group × Sessions ANOVA was computed on Stroop Task I scores, speed of reading color words printed in black. Two significant effects were obtained (Table 3-3). Reading times for groups combined were faster for the postexercise than for the preexercise session ($p < 0.02$). A significant interaction ($p < 0.001$) indicated that the time saving was not equal across groups. Analyses by $t$-test showed that reading speed was increased only for the aerobically trained individuals; mean reading time for Task I declined from 6.2 to 5.7 sec ($p = 0.004$; $p > 0.10$ for the two control groups). Second, to determine if the time savings at posttesting for the aerobic subjects on Stroop Task IV was a result of improved speed of reading rather than a reduction of an interference effect, Task I pretest values were subtracted from Task IV pretest values; similar data were derived from posttest scores. The results of an ANOVA computed on these data are listed in Table 3-3. Again pre-posttest differences were evaluated by $t$-test. A significant reduction in interference effect was observed for the aerobically trained individuals ($p < 0.002$) but not for the two control groups ($p > 0.10$) (see Figure 3-2).

The three subjects in the aerobic group who smoked were compared with the remaining ten who did not smoke on pre-treatment $\dot{V}O_2$max and neuropsychological test values and on amount of improvement in $\dot{V}O_2$max and neuropsychological function at posttreatment testing. Scores of the two groups did not differ appreciably.

## DISCUSSION

Following a four month program of exercise training, physical fitness level and neuropsychological test performance of previously sedentary elderly individuals were clearly improved. That the subjects had been sedentary was documented by their level of physical fitness prior to the start of the exercise activities. On the basis of their $\dot{V}O_2$max values, 70% were rated as being in poor or very poor physical condition (Cooper, 1977); the remaining 30% were in fair condition. Our results strongly support the concepts that physically unfit elderly people can participate in a program of regular exercise at an intensity sufficient to significantly

**TABLE 3.3.** *Means and standard deviations (in parentheses) and F and p values from group x session ANOVAs computer on Stroop Color Test Task I scores (time and seconds to read a column of color words) and on Task IV (Interference test) scores after Task I scores had been subtracted.*

|  | Task I | Task IV-Task I |
|---|---|---|
| Group |  |  |
| Aerobic | 5.92 (0.88) | 10.76 (3.86) |
| Exer Cont | 5.83 (0.69) | 12.59 (4.40) |
| Nonexer Cont | 5.77 (0.58) | 11.31 (2.56) |
| F (2/40 df) | 0.18 | 1.00 |
| p | $>0.10$ | $>0.10$ |
| Session |  |  |
| Pre | 5.90 (0.74) | 12.10 (3.48) |
| Post | 5.77 (0.68) | 11.07 (3.91) |
| F (1/40 df) | 6.09 | 13.07 |
| p | $<0.02$ | $<0.001$ |
| Group × Session |  |  |
| F (2/40 df) | 8.87 | 4.62 |
| p | $<0.001$ | $<0.02$ |

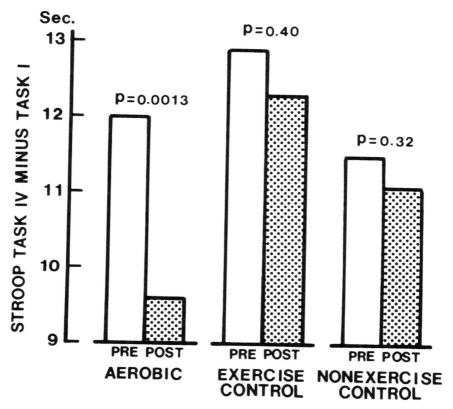

**FIGURE 3.2.** *The time to read a list of color names (Stroop Task I) was subtracted from the time required to name the colors in which color names were printed (Stroop Task IV, Interference test). This was done to determine if the improved scores at posttesting on the Interference test for the aerobically trained subjects were the result of improved motor ability. As illustrated, after Task I times were subtracted the aerobically trained subjects still demonstrated a significant pre- posttest time savings for Task IV. Note that this was not true for the control groups.*

improve their physical fitness level (deVries, 1975) and that exercise can improve their mental as well as physical functioning.

Two complementary findings merit comment. The first is that on the average, both exercise groups improved on the neuropsychological tests, while the nonexercise control group did not. Moreover, the type of exercise was strongly related to the magnitude of test improvement. Subjects participating in aerobic activities, fast walking and some slow jogging, improved significantly more than those who did strength and flexibility exercises even though the latter subjects participated in slightly more exercise sessions. Differences in performance cannot be attributed to pre-existing differences between groups, as subjects were randomly assigned to the two types of exercise programs (resulting in equivalence between groups on all of the relevant measures) and training for both was administered by the same people.

The second relevant finding is that while groups differed in their mean scores, thus demonstrating an overall relationship between type of exercise and degree of cognitive improvement, that relationship did not hold up in analysis of individual scores. There was no correlation between posttreatment residual scores on the cognitive tests and posttreatment $\dot{V}O_2$max residuals for either exercise group, where residuals were formed by partialling the pretreatment scores from the posttreatment scores. This finding is not surprising since our $\dot{V}O_2$max measure, used to document exercise training effects, is not a measurement of regional oxygen consumption; rather it measures overall body oxygen consumption and is weighted more toward muscle than brain, e.g., the brain requires only about 20% of total body oxygen (Ordy & Kaack, 1975). Since $\dot{V}O_2$max is not specific for brain oxygen consumption and since there is no reason to expect that exercise related increases in oxygen to the brain would closely parallel increases to muscle, a direct relationship between $\dot{V}O_2$max and neuropsychological measures would not be predicted.

The pattern of results, i.e., improved neuropsychological function with no change in sensory threshold following aerobic conditioning, suggests that the effects of aerobic exercise were primarily on central rather than on peripheral mechanisms. The effects appeared to be widespread since improvement was observed for a variety of areas including the recall and reproduction of verbal and auditory materials, visuo-motor speed, critical flicker fusion threshold, and "mental flexibility," the ability to shift perceptual set as measured by Task IV of the Stroop Interference test (Lezak, 1983).

As we were unable to monitor physiological changes that may have occurred in the brain as a consequence of our treatment procedures, we can only speculate that improved neuropsychological performance of our aerobically trained subjects occurred because of enhanced cerebral metabolic activity. There is reasonably good evidence that for average elderly people, those who do not experience unusually good health, brain perfusion and oxygen levels are reduced (Frackowiak, Lenzi, Jones & Heather, 1980; Kuhl, Metter, Riege & Phelps, 1982; Sokoloff, 1975). Oxygen is not only necessary for glucose metabolism at the cellular level but is an important substrate for turnover of neurotransmitters that are essential for cognitive and motor activities (Bartus, Dean, Beer & Lippa, 1982; Gibson & Peterson, 1982; Simon, Scatton & Le Moal, 1980). Neuropsychological test performance has proven to be sensitive to reduced levels of oxygen as demonstrated by impaired performance of young adults at altitude (McFarland, 1969) and adverse altitude effects have been shown for some of the tasks used in the present study: critical flicker fusion threshold (Sen Gupta, Mathew & Gopenath, 1979), digit symbol (Evans, Carson & Shields, 1969), memory (McFarland, 1969), and response time (Cahoon, 1972; Kobrick, 1972; Ledwith, 1970). The administration of oxygen to elderly subjects and to patients with chronic obstructive pulmonary disease has resulted in improved cognitive performance (Block, Castle & Keitt, 1974; Jacobs, Winter, Alvis & Small, 1969; Krop, Block & Cohen, 1973; Krop, Block, Cohen, Croucher & Shuster, 1977), in the absence of recent memory loss (Raskin, Gershon, Crook, Sathananthan & Ferris, 1978) or other evidence of a dementing process (Ben-Yishay, Diller & Reich, 1979; Levin & Peters, 1977; Thompson, 1975).

As a result of the aerobic conditioning program $\dot{V}O_2$max levels for our experimental group increased by 27%. The increase was 9% for the exercise control subjects who also demonstrated a reliable, although much smaller, increase in performance for combined neuropsychological tests. We suggest that the improved transport and utilization of oxygen was realized in brain as well as in other body tissues. An increase in cerebral oxygen might result in improved neuropsychological function because of increased turnover of neurotransmitters which are dependent upon oxygen for their metabolism. Hypoxia has been shown to cause a decline in acetylcholine metabolism (Gibson & Peterson, 1982) and oxygen is utilized directly for the synthesis and degradation of dopamine, norepinephrine (NE), and serotonin (5-HT) (Gibson & Peterson, 1982; Gibson, Pulsinelli, Blass & Duffy, 1981). Each of these neurotransmitters has been implicated in human behavior and the functioning of each declines with approaching senescence (Beck, 1978).

Spirduso (1983), reporting that the ability of rats to initiate fast movements was clearly related to nigrostriatal dopaminergic efficiency, suggested that chronic exercise can influence neurotransmitter systems. Direct evidence of this was provided by Brown and his colleagues (Brown et al., 1979; Brown & Van Huss, 1973). They found an increase in whole brain levels of NE and 5-HT for rats which had participated in a running program designed to simulate middle distance running by humans.

It should not be surprising that mental function of older individuals can be improved since in recent years studies have documented that the "old" brain can be modified. For elderly rats housed in environments which provided for increased sensory and motor stimulation, the size and complexity of neuronal structures were increased, forebrains were larger and heavier, and cholinergic activity was enhanced (Connor & Diamond, 1982; Connor, Wang & Diamond, 1982; Cummins, Walsh, Budtz-Olsen, Konstantinos & Horsfall, 1973; Riege, 1971; Uylings, Kuypers, Diamond & Veltman, 1978). These changes may have occured because of increased perfusion and oxygenation of brain tissue. There is substantial evidence that movement, sensory stimulation, and even ideation results in an immediate increase of cerebral blood flow in activated cortical areas (Engel, Kuhl, & Phelps, 1982; Gross, Marcus, & Heistad, 1980; Larsen, Skinhoj & Lassen, 1979; Mazziotta, Phelps, Carson & Kuhl, 1982; Phelps, Kuhl & Mazziotta, 1981), with a concomitant flow increase in frontal association areas (Ingvar, 1980). The physical activities associated with our exercise programs, in addition to improving aerobic efficiency, may have provided sufficient cortical stimulation to promote structural and functional change.

The fact that aerobic conditioning resulted in improvement for a variety of neuropsychological tests may indicate that this type of exercise affects processes underlying attention and concentration which in turn determine level of performance. Attention wanes during periods of hypoxia (Petajan, 1973), perhaps due to a release of cortical inhibitory influence on the ascending reticular activating system (Dell, Hugelin & Bonvallet, 1961; Petajan, 1973). On the basis of event related potential data, we have reported evidence of reduced inhibitory control in healthy elderly people which we speculated might be related to reductions in certain populations of cortical cells and to less efficient neurotransmitter systems (Dustman & Snyder, 1981; Dustman, Snyder & Schlehuber, 1981; Podlesny & Dustman, 1982).

The two depression scales were included in our battery of tests since it is known that there is a greater incidence of depression in the elderly (Zung, 1967) and that aerobic exercise may reduce level of depression (Morgan, Roberts, Brand & Feinerman, 1970). For our subjects there was no change in scores of depression following four months of physical conditioning with aerobic or with strength and flexibility training, possibly because of their relatively good mental health. For example, none had scores on the Beck Depression Inventory which were as high as the mean score for a group of 127 patients rated by Beck et al. (1961) as being mildly depressed. Morgan et al. (1970) stated that while regular physical exercise reduces depression scores of depressed individuals, scores do not change for those who are not initially depressed. A correlation of Beck Depression Inventory with Self-rating Depression scale scores of our 43 subjects was 0.72 ($p < 0.001$).

In summary, we report that following a four month protocol of aerobic exercise training, performance of previously sedentary older individuals on a variety of neuropsychological tasks was significantly improved. These tasks purportedly measured response time, visual organization, memory, and mental flexibility. We suggest that improved neuropsychological performance of the aerobically trained group occurred as a result of enhanced cerebral metabolic activity. However, validation of our hypothesis must await research which employs modern noninvasive techniques to measure cerebral metabolism before and after an aerobic exercise training program.

## ACKNOWLEDGEMENTS

Thanks are extended to D. Heinig, MD, A. Kralios, MD, H. Kuida, MD, R. Latin, PhD, P. Matlin, MS, L. Steinhaus, MS, D. Thurman, MD, and J. Wagner, MD for their assistance.

## REFERENCES

ACSM-America College of Sports Medicine (1980). *Guidelines for graded exercise testing and exercise prescription.* Philadelphia: Lea & Febiger.

Balke, B., & Ware, R.W. (1959). An experimental study of "physical fitness" of Air Force personnel. *United States Armed Forces Medical Journal, 10,* 675-688.

Bartus, R.T., Dean, R.L., Beer, B., & Lippa, A.S. (1982). The cholinergic hypothesis of geriatric memory dysfunction. *Science, 217,* 408-417.

Beck, A.T., Ward, C.H., Mendelson, M., Mock, J., & Erbaugh, J. (1961). An inventory for measuring depression. *Archives of General Psychiatry, 4,* 561-571.

Beck, C.H.M. (1978). Functional implications of changes in the senescent brain: A review. *Canadian Journal of Neurological Sciences, 5,* 417-424.

Beck, E.C., Swanson, C., & Dustman, R.E. (1980). Long latency components of the visually evoked potential in man: Effects of aging. *Experimental Aging Research, 6,* 523-545.

Ben-Yishay, Y., Diller, L., & Reich, T. (1979). Oxygen therapy fails to reverse senility. *Geriatrics, 34,* 116-117.

Bierman, E.L. (1978). Atherosclerosis and aging. *Federation Proceedings, 37,* 2832-2836.

Block, A.J., Castle, J.R., & Keitt, A.S. (1974). Chronic oxygen therapy: Treatment of chronic obstructive pulmonary disease at sea level. *Chest, 65,* 279-288.

Bortz, W.M. (1980). Effect on exercise on aging-effect of aging on exercise. *Journal of American Geriatrics Society, 28,* 49-51.

Bortz, W.M. (1982). Disuse and aging. *Journal of American Medical Association, 248,* 1203-1208.

Botwinick, J. (1973). *Aging and behavior.* New York: Springer.

Brown, B.S., Payne, T., Kim, C., Moore, G., Krebs, P., & Martin, W. (1979). Chronic response of rat brain norepinephrine and serotonin levels to endurance training. *Journal of Applied Physiology, 46,* 19-23.

Brown, B.S., & Van Huss, W.D. (1973). Exercise and rat brain catecholamines. *Journal of Applied Physiology, 34,* 664-669.

Cahoon, R.L. (1972). Simple decision making at high altitude. *Ergonomics, 15,* 157-164.

Cohn, N.B., Dustman, R.E., & Bradford, D.C. (1984). Age-related decrements in Stroop Color Test performance. *Journal of Clinical Psychology, 40,* 1244-1250.

Connor, J.R., & Diamond, M.C. (1982). A comparison of dendritic spine number on pyramidal neurons of the visual cortex of old adult rats from social or isolated environments. *Journal of Comparative Neurology, 210,* 99-106.

Connor, J.R., Wang, E.C., & Diamond, M.C. (1982). Increased length of terminal dendritic segments in old adult rats' somatosensory cortex: An environmentally induced response. *Experimental Neurology, 78,* 466-470.

Cooper, K.H. (1977). *The aerobics way.* New York: Bantam Books.

Cummins, R.A., Walsh, R.N., Budtz-Olsen, O.E., Konstantinos, T., & Horsfall, C.R. (1973). Environmentally-induced changes in the brains of elderly rats. *Nature, 243,* 516-518.

Dell, P., Hugelin, A., & Bonvallet, M. (1961). Effects of hypoxia on the reticular and cortical diffuse systems. In H. Gastaut & J.S. Meyer (Eds.), *Cerebral anoxia and the electroencephalogram* (pp. 46-58). Springfield: Thomas.

deVries, H.A. (1975). Physiology of exercise and aging. In D.S. Woodruff & J.E. Biren (Eds.), *Aging* (pp. 257-276). New York: Van Nostrand.

deVries, H.A. (1979). Tips on prescribing exercise regimes for your older patients. *Geriatrics, 34,* 75-81.

Dorfman, L.J., & Bosley, T.M. (1979). Age-related changes in peripheral and central nerve conduction in man. *Neurology, 29,* 38-44.

Dustman, R.E., & Beck, E.C. (1969). The effects of maturation and aging on the waveform of visually evoked potentials. *Electroencephalography and Clinical Neurphysiology, 26,* 2-11.

Dustman, R.E., & Snyder, E.W. (1981). Life-span changes in visually evoked potentials at central scalp. *Neurobiology of Aging, 2,* 303-308.

Dustman, R.E., Snyder, E.W., & Schlehuber, C.J. (1981). Life-span alterations in visually evoked potentials and inhibitory function. *Neurobiology of Aging, 2,* 187-192.

Elsayed, M., Ismail, A.H., & Young, R.J. (1980). Intellectual differences of adult men related to age and physical fitness before and after an exercise program. *Journal of Gerontology, 35,* 383-387.

Engel, J., Kuhl, D.E., & Phelps, M.E. (1982). Patterns of human local cerebral glucose metabolism during epileptic seizures. *Science, 218,* 64-66.

*AEROBIC EXERCISE TRAINING*

Evans, W.O., Carson, R.P., & Shields, J.L. (1969). The effect of high terrestrial environment on two different types of intellectual functioning. In A.H. Hegnauer (Ed.), *Biomedicine of high terrestrial elevations* (pp. 291-294). Washington, D.C.: U.S. Army Research Institute of Environmental Medicine.

Frackowiak, R.S.J., Lenzi, G-L, Jones, T., & Heather, J.D. (1980). Quantitative measurement of regional cerebral blood flow and oxygen metabolism in man using $^{15}0$ and positron emission tomography: Theory, procedure, and normal values. *Journal of Computer Assisted Tomography, 4*, 727-736.

Fries, J.F., & Crapo, L.M. (1980). *Vitality and aging.* San Francisco: Freeman.

Gibson, G.E., & Peterson, C. (1982). Biochemical and behavioral parallels in aging and hypoxia. In E. Giacobini, G. Filogamo, G. Giacobini & A. Vernadakis (Eds.), *The aging brain: Cellular and molecular mechanisms of aging in the nervous system* (pp. 107-122). New York: Raven Press.

Gibson, G.E., Pulsinelli, W., Blass, J.P., & Duffy, T.E. (1981). Brain dysfunction in mild to moderate hypoxia. *American Journal of Medicine, 70*, 1247-1254.

Gross, P.M., Marcus, M.L., & Heistad, D.D. (1980). Regional distribution of cerebral blood flow during exercise in dogs. *Journal of Applied Physiology, 48*, 213-217.

Ingvar, D.H. (1980). Regional cerebral blood flow and psychopathology. In J.O. Cole & J.E. Barrett (Eds.), *Psychopathology in the aged* (pp. 73-78). New York: Raven Press.

Jacobs, E.A., Winter, P.M., Alvis, H.J., & SMall, S.M. (1969). Hyperoxygenation effects on cognitive functioning in the aged. *New England Journal of Medicine, 281*, 753-757.

Kobrick, J.L. (1972). Effects of hypoxia on voluntary response time to peripheral stimuli during central target monitoring. *Ergonomics, 15*, 147-156.

Krop, H.D., BLock, A.J., & Cohen, E. (1973). Neuropsychologic effects of continuous oxygen therapy in chronic obstructive pulmonary disease. *Chest, 64*, 317-322.

Krop, H.D., Block, A.J., Cohen, E., Croucher, R., & Shuster, J. (1977). Neuropsychologic effects of continuous oxygen therapy in the aged. *Chest, 72*, 737-743.

Kuhl, D.E., Metter, E.J., Riege, W.H., & Phelps, M.E. (1982). Effects of human aging on patterns of local cerebral glucose utilization determined by the [$^{18}$F] fluorodeoxyglucose method. *Journal of Cerebral Blood Flow and Metabolism, 2*, 163-171.

Larsen, B., Skinhoj, E., & Lassen, N.A. (1979). Cortical activity of left and right hemisphere provoked by reading and visual naming. A rCBF study. *ACTA Neurologica Scandinavia, 60*, Supplement 72, 6-7.

Ledwith, F. (1970). The effects of hypoxia on choice reaction time and movement time. *Ergonomics, 13*, 465-482.

Levin, H.S., & Peters, B.H. (1977). Hyperbaric oxygenation in the treatment of postencephalitic amnesic syndrome. *Aviation, Space, and Environmental Medicine, 48*, 668-671.

Lezak, M.D. (1983). *Neuropsychological assessment,* 2nd edition. New York: Oxford University Press.

Mazziotta, J.C., Phelps, M.E., Carson, R.E., & Kuhl, D.E. (1982). Tomographic mapping of human cerebral metabolism: Sensory deprivation. *Annals of Neurology, 12*, 435-444.

McFarland, R.A. (1969). Review of experimental findings in sensory and mental functions. In A.H. Hegnauer (Ed.), *Biomedicine of high terrestrial elevations* (pp. 250-265). Washington, D.C.: U.S. Army Research Institute of Environmental Medicine.

*Measuring Intelligence with the Culture Fair Tests, Manual for Scales 2 and 3* (1973). Los Angeles: Western Psychological Services.

Mintz, A.Y., & Mankovsky, N.B. (1971). Changes in the nervous system during cerebral atherosclerosis and aging. *Geriatrics, 26*, 134-144.

Morgan, W.P., Roberts, J.A., Brand, F.R., & Feinerman, A.D. (1970). Psychological effects of chronic physical activity. *Medicine and Science in Sports and Exercise, 2*, 213-217.

Obrist, W.D. (1976). Problems of aging. In G.E. Chatrian & G.C. Lairy (Eds.), *Handbook of electroencephalography and clinical neurophysiology* (Vol. 6, Part A, pp. 275-292). Amsterdam: Elsevier.

Ordy, J.M., & Kaack, B. (1975). Neurochemical changes in composition, metabolism, and neurotransmitters in the human brain with age. In J.M. Ordy & K.R. Brizzee (Eds.). *Neurobiology of aging* (pp. 253-285). New York: Plenum.

Petajan, J.H. (1973). Neuropsychological acclimatization to high altitude. *Journal of Human Evolution, 2*, 105-115.

Phelps, M.E., Kuhl, D.E., & Mazziotta, J.C. (1981). Metabolic mapping of the brain's response to visual stimulation: Studies in humans. *Science, 211*, 1445-1448.

Podlesny, J.P., & Dustman, R.E. (1982). Age effects on heart rate, sustained potential, and P3 responses during reaction-time tasks. *Neurobiology of Aging, 3*, 1-9.

Powell, R.R., & Pohndorf, R.H. (1971). Comparison of adult exercisers and nonexercisers on fluid intelligence and selected physiological variables. *Research Quarterly for Exercise and Sport, 42*, 70-77.

Raskin, A., Gershon, S., Crook, T.H., Sathananthan, G., & Ferris, S. (1978). The effects of hyperbaric and normobaric oxygen on cognitive impairment in the elderly. *Achives of General Psychiatry, 35*, 50-56.

Riege, W.H. (1971). Environmental influences on brain and behavior of year old rats. *Developmental Psychobiology, 4*, 157-167.

Sen Gupta, J., Mathew, L., & Gopenath, P.M. (1979). Effect of physical training at moderate altitude (1950m) on hypoxic tolerance. *Aviation, Space, and Environmental Medicine, 50*, 714-716.

Sherwood, D.E., & Selder, D.J. (1979). Cardiorespiratory health, reaction time, and aging. *Medicine and Science in Sports, 11*, 186-189.

Simon, H., Scatton, B., & Le Moal, M. (1980). Dopaminergic A10 neurons are involved in cognitive functions. *Nature, 286,* 150-151.

Sokoloff, L. (1975). Cerebral circulation and metabolism in the aged. In S. Gershon & A. Raskin (Eds.), *Aging,* (pp. 45-54). New York: Raven Press.

Spirduso, W.W. (in press). Nigrostriatal dopaminergic function in aging, exercise, and movement initiation. In K. Bohrer & T. White (Eds.), *Frontiers in exercise biology.*

Spirduso, W.W., & Clifford, P. (1978). Replication of age and physical activity effects on reaction and movement time. *Journal of Gerontology, 33,* 26-30.

Taylor, H.L., Buskirk, E., & Henschel, A. (1955). Maximal oxygen intake as an objective measure of cardio-respiratory performance. *Journal of Applied Physiology, 8,* 73-80.

Thompson, L.W. (1975). Effects of hyperbaric oxygen on behavioral functioning in elderly persons with intellectual impairment. In S. Gershon & A. Raskin (Eds.), *Aging,* Volume 2, (pp. 169-177). New York: Raven Press.

Uylings, H.B.M., Kuypers, K., Diamond, M.C., & Veltman, W.A.M. (1978). Effects of differential environments on plasticity of dendrites of cortical pyramidal neurons in adult rats. *Experimental Neurology, 62,* 658-677.

Wechsler, D. (1981). *WAIS-R Manual.* New York: Psychological Corporation.

Zung, W.W.K. (1967). Depression in the normal aged. *Psychosomatics, 8,* 287-292.

# Part III
# Aging and Motor Memory

## INTRODUCTION

One of the more popular and systematic approaches to studying the sensory-motor system in relation to aging has been to conceptualize human skillful performance in terms of an information-processing model. The execution of a motor response is thought to invoke a series of stages that involve the acceptance, storage, and processing of information before effector mechanisms are activated. An information-processing model provides a framework for identifying what stages during motor performance are most affected by aging processes. This viewpoint is not new and has found much support, particularly in papers by Welford (1965), Birren (1974), Stelmach and Diewert (1977), and Birren, Woods, and Williams (1980).

A dynamic perspective on information processing during movement assumes that information is retained or stored for future use during the various stages of processing. The framework or systems involved in this storage have been labeled memory. Schmidt (1987) defined memory as "the persistence of the acquired capability for responding" (p. 493). He noted, however, that memory should be viewed as the *capability* for responding, rather than a site where that capability is stored.

Within this information-processing framework, it is hypothesized that there are at least three separate memory systems labeled *short-term sensory store*, *short-term memory*, and *long-term memory*. These three systems differ in terms of the amount and type of information that is stored and the rate of loss of information (Schmidt, 1987). Research evidence (e.g., Birren et al., 1980) exists indicating that the efficiency of all three systems decline with advancing age. For example, in terms of long-term memory, reviews of research literature by Botwinick (1978) and Stelmach and Diewert (1977) suggest that age-related declines in long-term memory, at least in terms of new learning, center more on declines in *recall* (the searching and retrieval of stored information), than on declines in *recognition* (the matching of stored information without retrieval). However, there may be little decline with age in the retrieval of very old, basic information.

In the chapter that follows, Benham and Heston examine memory retrieval and motor behavior in the aged. The authors first examine what is known about age-related differences in recall and recognition in verbal memory. After concluding that age-related deficits are greater for verbal recall than verbal recognition, the authors contrast these findings with what is known about motor memory and aging. Based on limited research, Benham and Heston speculate that explanations for deficits in motor memory with advancing age may parallel findings in the verbal memory literature.

In Chapter Five, Abourezk examines the relationship of aerobic activity to short-term memory efficiency in older adult males. Retrospective analyses of active older runners compared to inactive older subjects revealed that the active group was able to remember more information than the inactive group on a dichotic listening task. In the discussion that follows, Abourezk explores possible mechanisms that may explain why the active group was significantly better at short-term memory retention.

### REFERENCES

Birren, J.E. (1974). Translations in gerontology-from lab to life. Psychophysiology and speed of response. *American Psychologist, 29*, 808-815.
Birren, J.E., Woods, A.M., & Williams, M.V. (1980). Behavioral slowing with age: Courses, organization,

and consequences. In L.W. Poon (Ed.), *Aging in the 1980s* (pp. 293-308). Washington, D.C., American Psychological Association.

Botwinick, J. (1978). *Aging and behavior* (2nd edition). New York: Springer.

Schmidt, R.A. (1987). *Motor control and learning* (2nd edition). Champaign, IL: Human Kinetics.

Stelmach, G.E., & Diewert, G.L. (1977). Aging, information processing and fitness. In G. Borg (Ed.), *Physical work and effort* (pp. 115-136). New York: Pergamon Press.

Welford, A.T. (1965). Performance, biological mechanisms and age: A theoretical sketch. In A.T. Welford & J.E. Birren (Eds.), *Behavior, aging, and the nervous system* (pp. 3-20). Springfield, IL: Charles C. Thomas.

# 4

## Memory Retrieval in the Adult Population

TAMI BENHAM

MELISSA HESTON

### ABSTRACT

A deficiency in retrieval operations has been postulated as an underlying factor in observable age differences in the performance of memory tasks. The purpose of this chapter is to examine the literature pertaining to memory retrieval in the aged. Findings of age-related differences in recall and recognition in both the verbal memory and the motor memory literature are examined. The use of verbal recall for retrieving information appears to place greater demands upon the information processing system demands which the aged are often unable to meet under standard laboratory conditions. The aged seem to be able to meet the processing demand of verbal recognition more readily. These retrieval processes may be influenced by factors such as the familiarity of information, task difficulty, encoding ability, and rehearsal strategies. Limited data on motor memory in the aged indicate that older adults do display patterns of retrieval deficits similar to those found for verbal memory. At this time, a considerable number and variety of questions about motor memory retrieval in the aged remain to be answered.

### INTRODUCTION

According to the information processing paradigm, in order to perform a previously learned movement skill, it is first necessary to recall from memory the information needed to perform the movement correctly and efficiently. If retrieval problems prevent the effective "calling up" of a movement skill from long-term memory, then difficulties in producing efficient movement should result (Ostrow, 1984). The purpose of this chapter is to examine the literature pertaining to memory retrieval in the aged and to address the following question: Is a deficiency in retrieval operations an underlying factor in observable age differences in the performance of memory tasks?

Unfortunately, the motor learning literature focusing on the aging population is limited. Literature regarding motor memory retrieval in elderly adults is almost nonexistent. Thus, this chapter will initially focus on age differences in retrieval, as measured by cognitive tasks requiring the use of recall and recognition memory. These research findings may then lend themselves to the field of motor learning and indicate appropriate lines of study. The second section of this chapter will review literature concerning recognition and recall in motor memory in general, and then consider in detail the few studies in which motor memory in the aged has been examined. In the final section of this chapter, possible relationships between verbal and motor recall and recognition will be discussed. In addition, questions that could be addressed in future research will be posed.

## MEMORY RETRIEVAL: RECALL AND RECOGNITION

The memory process has often been described as consisting of two stages: the retention (or storage) of information, and the retrieval (or accessing) of information. Memory retrieval is generally measured using cognitive tasks which require the recognition and/or recall of previously learned information. Recall memory is believed to involve a search for and subsequent retrieval of the desired information (Botwinick, 1973). Recognition memory, however, is held to require only a single matching of information in the environment with information in long-term storage (Stelach, 1982).

During recognition tasks, the intensity of the retrieval load is considered to be lighter since the correct alternative is always present (Botwinick, 1984). During a recall task, however, the retrieval load increases because no clues or correct alternatives are provided. Information must be retrieved solely by calling it up from long-term storage. In both types of tasks, there is an assumption that age-related differences may tentatively imply retrieval deficiencies. If memory retrieval problems do increase with age, and memory recall tasks do make greater processing demands than memory recognition tasks, then one might hypothesize that: (1) recognition memory would be superior to recall memory in the aged population and in the non-aged population, and (2) greater performance differences between the aged and non-aged populations would be found for recall versus recognition tasks.

### Age Differences in Recall and Recognition Memory

In an early study, Schonfield and Robertson (1966) investigated the hypothesis that performance differences between older and younger adults would be smaller on a recognition task than on a recall task. These researchers also predicted that there would be greater differences between the recognition and recall scores of older adults than between the scores of younger adults. The subjects were 134 adults between the ages of 20 and 75. Subjects were given untimed recall and recognition tests in which they responded to two 24 word lists. Results indicated that there was little difference in the performances of the two age groups on the recognition test. On the recall test, however, a steady decline with age was found. Schonfield and Robertson concluded that while there was no apparent decline with age in recognition memory, there was "a loss of almost 50% between the scores of this group of younger and older people" (p. 233) in recall. Additionally, older adults displayed greater differences between recognition and recall scores than younger adults. The authors concluded that aging was causal factor in the retrieval difficulties of older individuals.

More recently, Rankin and Hyland (1983) found age-related differences in recall and recognition as a function of an orienting task. Three groups of subjects (young, M age = 18.44 years; middle age, M age = 47.11 years; older, M age = 69.55 years) were asked to recall a list of words based on varied initial instructions. More specifically, subjects were asked if the word to be recalled rhymed with another word, or if the word was a synonym of another word, or were simply instructed to learn the word. Subjects were then given a recall task. Findings indicated a performance difference between the age groups when the instructions involved simply telling the subjects to learn the word. Under this condition, younger subjects recalled more words than middle-aged or elderly subjects. However, no age-related differences in recognition memory were found. The authors posited that the ability of younger subjects to recall more information may be due to age-related differences in either memory trace strength or accessibility. This pattern of age-related differences in recall memory, in which younger adults recall more than older adults, has been demonstrated in several other studies (Erber, 1974; Howard, Heisey & Shaw, 1986; Rabinowitz, 1984; Shaps & Nilsson, 1980).

Age differences in recognition memory have been found less frequently than age differences in recall memory. Neither Schonfield and Robertson (1966) nor Rankin and Hyland (1983) found performance differences between younger and older subjects on tasks requiring the use of recognition memory. This absence of significant age-related differences in recognition memory has been documented in other studies (Shaps & Nilsson, 1980; West & Boatwright, 1983). However, some researchers have found age-related differences in recognition memory.

Based on the hypothesis that older adults would show declining performances in recognition memory as task difficulty increased, Erber (1974) tested 80 subjects aged 19-75 years, divided into two age groups, on more recognition difficult tasks. Task difficulty was manipulated by increasing the number of words to be learned, and by using a five alternative forced-choice test. In earlier research, forced-choice recognition tests typically had four alternatives from which to chose. Under these conditions, a strong main effect for age was found, with younger subjects scoring better than older subjects. List length was found to affect the performances of subjects in both age groups, with most subjects performing better on the shorter lists.

Erber (1974) concluded that previous examinations of recognition memory may not have produced age-related differences due to insufficient task difficulty. Further support for Erber's conclusion has been provided by Burke and Yee (1984). These researchers found an age difference in recognition memory favoring younger (M age = 25.3 years) over older (M age = 68.5 years) subjects on a task requiring semantic processing of sentences.

Thus the literature on age-related differences in recall seems to support the notion that the aged population, as compared to the younger population, is less capable of this form of information retrieval. Findings of age-related differences in recognition memory seem less clear. Under standard experimental conditions, elderly adults perform as well as younger adults. However, with increases in task difficulty, which presumably would make the processing demands of recognition more similar to those of recall, age-related differences in recognition become evident. These findings lead one to wonder if reducing the processing demands of recall and recognition might reduce performance differences between young and aged individuals. One method for manipulating task difficulty, and thus processing demands, is to vary the familiarity of the information to be retrieved. This procedure has been used in several studies.

## Familiarity and Age Differences

Hanley-Dunn and McIntosh (1984) investigated the influence of information familiarity on the recall performance of two age groups (young, M age = 20.3 years, and old, M age = 71.9 years). Subjects were asked to recall names from four lists: (1) national politicians (presumably meaningful to both cohorts), (2) big band musicians (presumably more meaningful to the older cohort), (3) contemporary singers (presumably more meaningful to the younger subjects), and (4) nonmeaningful names (unfamiliar to both cohorts). Significant differences were found in the lists that were best recalled. Politicians' names were recalled best, followed by singers and nonmeaningful names. Under these conditions, older subjects recalled slightly more items in total than younger subjects, and in particular, were better at recalling the names of national politicians and big band musicians. Younger subjects outperformed older subjects in their recall of singers' names. Overall, older subjects performed as well as, if not better than, younger subjects.

Worden and Sherman-Brown (1983) demonstrated similar effects on recall memory for information meaningfulness and cohort after testing young (M age = 20.76 years) and older (M age = 73.65 years) adults. Four types of word lists were used in this study: (1) "popular" words (words which were used with high frequency by both cohorts), (2) "dated" words (words that were used with high frequency by older subjects), (3) contemporary words (words which were used with high frequency by the younger cohort), and (4) "rare" words (words which were used infrequently by both cohorts). A significant age group by task interaction was found. The older subjects performed significantly better on the recall of the popular and dated lists than on the contemporary and rare lists. For the younger subjects, the only significant difference in recall performance was between the popular and rare lists. The authors explained their findings by suggesting that "high-frequency words from one's youth are particularly memorable, especially for elderly individuals" (p. 521).

Similar findings of a task by age interaction have been reported by Poon and Fozard (1978). These researchers found that older subjects had shorter naming latencies when asked to identify dated unique objects. These objects were deemed relatively more familiar to older subjects than to younger subjects. However, when asked to name common contemporary objects, younger subjects had shorter latencies. Thus, the familiarity, or meaningfulness, of information seems to be an important influencer of recall memory performance, particularly among aged populations.

Finally, Rabinowitz (1984) examined recognition memory in younger ($M$ age = 20 years) and older ($M$ age = 70 years) adults, and found age differences in the performance of a series of paired-association tests. Based on the belief that recognition involves both retrieval and familiarity, the author analyzed each characteristic for differences. Younger adults recognized more words and committed fewer errors, suggesting a difference in retrieval processes. However, after adjusting for age-related differences in familiarity, no differences between the two age groups were found. Rabinowitz suggested that the familiarity of information may well determine whether or not age-related differences in recognition will be observed. In summary, familiarity seems to play an influential role in both memory recall and recognition, regardless of age.

## Deficiencies in Retrieval, or Something Else?

When age-related differences in memory retrieval have been found, it has generally been assumed that these differences are the result of deficiencies in retrieval processes. However, a variety of other executive control processes are used during the initial processing and storage of information. Is it possible that deficits in these other control processes are at least partially responsible for the poorer recall and sometimes poorer recognition performances of the elderly? This question has been addressed.

**Encoding deficiencies:** West and Boatwright (1983) posited that encoding and retrieval processes might not be independent, and thus difficulties in encoding could be at least partially responsible for the retrieval deficits found in aged populations. To investigate this possibility, these researchers examined recall and recognition in three groups of adults (20-39 years of age, 40-59 years of age, and 60-79 years of age). Initially, subjects were given either an acoustic or semantic orienting task, followed by a distracting task. Acoustic word pairs included two words that were considered to rhyme when the vowel and final consonants of the words matched. For the semantic word pairs, subjects attempted to generate a precisely specified relationship between the two words. Then, each encoding group was divided in half and given either a self-paced recognition or cued recall test. The recognition and recall tests were either semantic or acoustic in nature.

West and Boatwright's (1983) data displayed the typical pattern of age differences in recall performance, with older subjects performing more poorly than either middle-age or younger subjects. No group differences were found in recognition performance. Additionally, recognition scores were generally higher than cued recall scores. Interestingly, all subjects performed better when encoding instructions and retrieval requirements were similar. Semantic-orienting instructions combined with a semantic test produced the best scores. Thus the role of encoding as an influential factor in memory retrieval should not be discounted. Perhaps better encoding would reduce or eliminate age-related differences in retrieval.

**Ineffective use of rehearsal strategies:** The ability of older adults to utilize appropriate memory rehearsal strategies may also be a factor in age-related differences in recall and recognition performance. It has been suggested that the aged often display ineffective use of cues and associations on cued recall tests, and thus tend to score lower than young individuals (Howard et al., 1986; Perlmutter, 1979). Mitchell and Perlmutter (1986) investigated this hypothesis by comparing the performances of younger (M age = 23 years) and older (M age = 65 years) adults on incidental and expected tests of recall and recognition. The largest age difference, which favored the younger group, was seen in the intentional memory task. The authors suggested their data might indicate a more effective use of mnemonic strategies by younger subjects. Overall, however, Mitchell and Perlmutter concluded that both the younger and the older subjects employed similar retrieval strategies.

Sanders et al. (1980) also proposed that ineffective rehearsal strategy use by older adults would result in age-related differences in memory retrieval. In this study, the rehearsal strategies of young (M age = 23.9 years) and older (M age = 73.9 years) adults in a free recall task were compared. Younger adults performed better than older adults, and this difference in performance was associated with age-related differences in rehearsal strategies. Younger subjects employed active, serial, and categorically-organized rehearsal, while older adults used inactive, nonstrategic rehearsal. Among older subjects, the probability of recall rose as the number of rehearsals increased.

Drawing upon the findings of Sanders et al. (1980), Schmitt, Murphy, and Sanders (1981) hypothesized that age differences in recall could be due to greater inactivity among older adults. They also proposed that older adults may simply lack available rehearsal strategies. To test these notions, three groups of older adults ($M$ age = 72.1 years) were given different instructions concerning rehearsal strategies and tested on a free recall task over four categorizable word lists. One group received direct instruction on the importance of active rehearsal. The second group was also given these instructions, plus additional instructions on the use of an efficient category rehearsal strategy. The third group served as a control group, receiving no instructions on either rehearsal or categorization. Prior to exposure to the experimental conditions, all groups were given a practice task and received identical instructions. There were no performance differences between the groups on this practice task. However, following the presentation of differential instruction, differences between the groups were found.

The group which received instruction concerning both active rehearsal and categorization had a higher overall mean score for recall, recalled more items per category, and displayed more organization at recall than either the active rehearsal only group or the control group. Interestingly, the active rehearsal and categorization group correctly recalled an average of 78% of the items. College-aged subjects in the Sanders et al. (1980) study averaged only 79% correct. Moreover, the rehearsal patterns of both groups appeared to be similar in nature. Schmitt et al. (1981) concluded that "it is clear that older adults' potential substantially exceeds their spontaneous performance" (p. 336), at least in free recall tasks.

## CONCLUSION

Age differences have been observed quite readily in performances requiring the use of recall; results from studies of recognition memory have been less conclusive. This difference in findings for recall versus recognition seems to be a function of a difference in the processing demands which each process poses. Retrieval of information using recall apparently places greater demands upon the information processing system, demands which the elderly seem less able to meet under typical laboratory conditions. The demands of recognition retrieval do not appear to be as difficult for the aged to meet under some circumstances, thus the inconsistent findings concerning this process. In addition, factors such as familiarity of information, task difficulty, encoding ability, and rehearsal strategies may strongly influence the recall and recognition performances of the aged. In particular, if effective encoding and rehearsal techniques can be taught to older adults, then it may be possible to decrease, if not eliminate completely, the age-related retrieval differences often found in laboratory studies.

## RECALL AND RECOGNITION IN MOTOR SKILLS

Motor memory, defined as "the persistence of the acquired capability for responding" (Schmidt, 1982, p. 606), has been the focus of much research, particularly since the mid to late 1960s. For the most part, this work has been done within the general box model of information processing in which long-term memory and short-term memory are basic hypothetical constructs. Investigators have pursued questions on a variety of topics, including the retention of continuous (Fleishman and Parker, 1962; Meyers, 1967; Ryan, 1962, 1965) and discrete motor skills (Neumann and Ammons, 1957) in long term memory, the nature of encoding of movement information in short-term motor memory (Diewart, 1975; Gundry, 1975; Roy, 1977; Walsh, Russell, and Crassini, 1981; Wrisberg and Winter, 1985), and the effects of interpolated tasks on movement reproduction (Dickinson and Higgins, 1977; Laabs, 1974; Norrie and Henry, 1978).

In most of these studies, however, motor memory recall was the primary dependent variable. Only a modest body of literature has developed concerning motor memory recall *and* motor memory recognition as separate processes. Studies in this area were conducted in response to the theoretical proposals of Adams (1971), and Schmidt (1975). Both of these classic works centered on motor learning, and in both proposals, motor memory recall and recognition were treated as essential and independent processes.

According to Adams (1971, 1976), learning a motor skill results from the development of two independent memory structures. The first structure, termed a memory trace, is used to select and initiate the desired movement. Memory traces are relatively simple motor programs and are responsible for movement recall. The second memory structure, the perceptual trace, is used to evaluate the correctness of the movement response initiated by the memory trace. Perceptual traces consist of sensory feedback and knowledge of results (KR), information from previous performances, and are used by the learner to recognize errors in the performance of motor skills. During slow movements, these errors can be recognized and corrected while the movement is in progress. During fast movements, however, errors cannot be recognized in time to properly correct the movement, and thus correction must occur on the next performance.

Schmidt's (1975, 1976; Shapiro and Schmidt, 1982) schema theory of motor learning also emphasized the role of recall and recognition in the acquisition and performance of motor skills. This theory consists of three major components: (1) generalized motor programs (GMP), (2) recall schemata, and (3) recognition schemata. The GMP is an abstract memory structure which controls a particular class of movements. The defining feature of the movements in a given class is a common motor pattern. This motor pattern is contained in the GMP and is modified via a recall schema to meet the specific demands of the eliciting motor task situation. That is, the recall schema is a rule representing the relationship between the motor commands a learner sends to the musculature, and the results of those commands in terms of actual limb movement and/or the movement's effect on the environment. The recall schema is analogous to Adams' (1971) memory trace.

The recognition schema is used to evaluate the correctness of a movement response, and thus is analogous to Adams' (1971) perceptual trace. This schema is a rule based on the relationship between the actual outcome of a response and the sensory feedback from that response. When a movement response is evaluated, actual sensory consequences are compared with the sensory consequences predicted by the recognition schema associated with the GMP being used. Discrepancies between the two sets of consequences are identified as errors. As was the case with Adams' (1971) model, errors can be detected and corrected promptly during slow movements, and on the next trial in fast movements.

Three reasons have been posited for the independence of memory traces and perceptual traces, or of recall and recognition schemata. First, if the mechanism responsible for movement initiation were also the mechanism used to determine movement correctness, then the movement would have to be judged correct. With a single mechanism, there could be no discrepancies between the motor commands being sent out and the sensory feedback from the executed movement unless external forces intervened unexpectedly. Second, development of the perceptual trace used to recognize errors and make corrections can only occur after the response has been initiated and sensory feedback and KR have become available. Thus, some other mechanism is needed to initiate the movement. Finally, use of a memory trace or recall schema is an instance of motor recall, while use of a perceptual trace or recognition schema is an instance of motor recognition. Recall and recognition processes have been purported to be independent in verbal memory tasks, and might reasonably be expected to be independent in motor tasks as well. A number of research studies have been conducted in order to test the independence of these two memory processes.

*MEMORY RETRIEVAL*

# Independence of Recall and Recognition

Newell and Chew (1974) had subjects perform a rapid linear positioning task under varying conditions of sensory feedback: (1) with both visual and auditory feedback, (2) with visual, but no auditory feedback, and (3) with auditory, but no visual feedback, and (4) with no visual or auditory feedback. The task required subjects to learn to move a slide 24.03 cm in 150 msec. Subjects were given 70 learning trials with experimenter-provided KR, followed by 40 retention trials without KR. Recall memory strength was measured in absolute error in movement time, and recognition memory strength was measured by having subjects estimate the correctness of their performance on each trial. Withdrawal of KR was followed by an immediate decrement in recognition memory. However, recall memory did not decay with KR withdrawal. The finding of differential decay in recall and recognition memory was interpreted as evidence of the independence of these two memory structures. However, these authors also noted that it may ultimately be possible to manipulate recall and recognition separately for only a limited period of time, since changes in recognition memory should lead to changes in the nature of the errors being detected. This latter change should in turn lead to an updating of the recall memory for the movement to be performed.

Williams (1978) reported two experiments in which additional evidence was found to support the independence of recognition and recall memory for movement. In the first experiment, one group of subjects practiced a linear positioning task in which they moved the slide various distances with endpoints marked by stops. A second group of subjects was trained to allow the experimenter to make the movement for them. It was hypothesized that this passive movement group would develop recognition memory since sensory feedback was available. However, it also was predicted that passive subjects would not develop recall memory because they did not actually structure or initiate the movement. After 36 trials with KR, four recognition test trials were given in which subjects were asked if the particular stop had been practiced. For two of the test trials, subjects did move to stops that had been practiced. For the other two trials, the stops were novel. Subjects were also asked to estimate how much a particular test stop differed from the practice stops. Results on both of these recognition measures supported the hypothesis that movement recognition memory could develop in the absence of a movement recall memory, when sensory feedback and KR were available.

In the second experiment (Williams, 1978), the role of active versus passive movement in the establishment of recall memory was investigated. One group of subjects experienced passive movement while the other group performed active movement. Subjects in both groups were given four movement trials on each of five different lengths, followed by

*AGING AND MOTOR BEHAVIOR*

four recall test trials. In two of the trials, subjects were asked to reproduce movements that had been practiced. In the other two trials, subjects were asked to produce movements of novel lengths. The active movement group proved to be clearly superior. Williams concluded that although his findings did support Schmidt's (1975) proposal for the existence of different roles for recall and recognition schemata in motor skill performance, the data did not provide much substantial support for the theoretical independence of these two memory structures. Rather, it was deemed possible that some form of interaction could occur between the recall and recognition schemata for a particular movement skill.

Kelso (1978) also used an active versus passive movement paradigm with a slow linear positioning task to test the independence of recall and recognition schemata. Knowledge of results were provided during 17 acquisition trials, followed by 20 trials without KR. No differences were found in the ability of the two groups to acquire the response. However, the performance of the active group declined when KR was removed, while the passive group's performance remained stable. If slow movements were actually controlled by recognition alone, then no differences between the active and passive movement groups should have appeared upon withdrawal of KR. Thus, Kelso proposed that slow movements may not be controlled by recognition alone, rather some other "additional (perhaps separate) process" (p. 73) seemed to be involved.

Kelso also suggested that the active group, which had acquired both a recall and a recognition memory for the movement, may actually have been utilizing recall memory to control the movement. The passive movement group, however, was limited to use of a recognition schema. Drawing on findings from the verbal memory literature, Kelso noted that recognition memory performance was typically found to be superior to recall memory performance. One explanation of this recognition-recall memory difference emphasized the notion that an actual memory search is not required with recognition because the needed information is available in the environment. Thus, the recognition process may be relatively robust against possible deficits in search and retrieval strategies, while recall memory may not. In addition, recall memory may take longer to develop than recognition memory. Thus, if subjects in the active group were utilizing recall memory to control movement, this memory may have been relatively weak compared to the recognition memory which subjects in the passive group had to use.

In two related experiments, Wallace and McGhee (1979) also tested the hypothesis that recall and recognition motor memory were independent structures. In the first experiment, subjects performed a linear positioning task under one of two conditions. One group of subjects actually moved the slide to a criterion position. The second group of subjects had to locate the slide handle and grasp it after the experimenters had positioned the slide at the criterion position. Subjects in both conditions were given 15 practice trials, 50 acquisition trials with KR on the criterion movement, followed by 10 test trials without KR. During these no KR trials, all subjects made active movements. Absolute error was used to measure recall performance, while the difference between actual error and subjects' estimates of error were used to measure recognition performance.

Results indicated that subjects in the actual slide movement condition developed strong recall memories, while subjects in the other condition did not. Unfortunately, this conclusion has to be considered tentative since two other inequalities existed between the groups. First, the actual slide movement group could select the end point for their movements while the other group could not. Recall of criterion movements has been found to be better when subjects select the end locations of their movements as compared to recall of criterion movements in which experimenters select the end locations (Schmidt, 1982). Second, the non-slide movement group did not experience the same sensory feedback associated with the criterion movement, because their movements were not along the slide track. It has been established that sensory feedback about both the end location for movement and the extent of the movement are important for movement reproduction (Schmidt, 1982). The non-slide movement group experienced only relevant sensory feedback about end location, and thus were at a disadvantage in terms of the sensory information. An attempt was made to eliminate the two inequalities in a second experiment.

The second study also utilized the active movement versus passive movement paradigm, which allowed both groups to experience similar sensory information about both end location and movement extent. In addition, subjects in both conditions were allowed to select the end point for each movement. Subjects received 25 acquisition trials with KR, followed by 10 test trials without KR. Absolute error and differences between objective and subject-estimated error again served as measures of recall and recognition, respectively.

Findings indicated that both groups developed strong recognition memories during acquisition. Furthermore, the active movement group demonstrated superior recall performance on the first test trial. However, passive subjects displayed improvement in performance during the remaining test trials. This finding indicated that passive subjects were able to use their strong recognition memories to develop increasingly accurate recall memories for the criterion movement. Another interesting finding, similar to a pattern found in Kelso's (1978) data, was that the recall performance of active subjects declined in the absence of KR. However, in the first experiment by Wallace and McGhee (1979), active movement subjects showed no such decline. This inconsistency may have arisen because subjects in the second experiment performed only half the number of acquisition trials as subjects in the first experiment. Thus, these data support Kelso's notion that recall memory may take longer to develop than recognition memory.

Based on their findings, Wallace and McGhee concluded that recognition memory development can indeed occur independent of recall memory development. However, recall memory can be developed in the absence of previous practice when recognition memory is well developed. This relationship has been documented in other studies (Zelaznik, Shapiro & Newell, 1978; Zelaznik & Spring, 1976). Thus, it appears that while recall and recognition memory can develop independently, under normal circumstances, there may be some dependency between these two processes.

## Movement Recall and Recognition in the Aged

Unfortunately, very little work has been done on movement recall and recognition in the aged population. In an early study, Jordan (1978) compared the performances of 30 young (*M* age = 20.6 years) and 30 elderly (*M* age = 70.2 years) adults on a linear-positioning task. Subjects were given eight trials on each of five different movement distances, with retention intervals of 5, 10, 20 or 50 seconds between the criterion movement and the reproduction movement. In addition, subjects were assigned to one of five treatment groups which experienced different conditions during the retention interval, and were tested under sighted and blindfolded conditions.

Under the blindfolded condition, no age differences were found in performance; younger subjects, however, performed better than elderly subjects under the sighted condition. Furthermore, younger subjects' performances showed larger decrements in response to interpolated tasks than did elderly subjects. Both findings were attributed to a possible difference in sensitivity to sensory feedback between the two groups. More specifically, it was proposed that older subjects failed to make use of much of the sensory information available. Thus, they performed more poorly than younger subjects under the sighted condition because they were unable to make full use of the visual feedback present in the task. On the other hand, older subjects may have been less sensitive to the potentially disruptive sensory feedback of the interpolated tasks, and as a result, showed smaller performance decrements than younger subjects.

More recently, Toole, Pyne, and McTarsney (1984) examined recall memory for series of consecutive movements of varying numbers. Subjects in four age groups (18-32 years, 33-47 years, 48-62 years, and 63-77 years) participated. Task series having up to 12 consecutive movements were performed. No performance differences were found between younger and older subjects on shorter movement series. However, the performance of older subjects was significantly poorer on longer movement series (series with 9 to 12 consecutive movements). These data parallel findings for verbal memory in that age-related differences are few when the demands on memory are relatively light. However, as processing demands rise, such age differences increase in magnitude and are found more frequently.

In a second experiment by Toole, Pyne, and McTarsney (1984), the effect of experimenter-imposed organizational schemes was investigated using linear positioning tasks. Subjects were undergraduate and graduate students, and older adults 60-70 years of age. On tasks which made relatively low demands on memory, older subjects displayed improved recall when using the organizational schemes. However, as the demands on memory were increased, age differences in recall did appear.

Finally, Marshall, Elias and Wright (1985) used a simple motor task to study the ability of young (18-21 year olds), middle-aged (40-52 year olds), and older (60-79 year olds) adults to detect and correct movement errors. Error detection was tested by having subjects identify which of two movements had been previously presented. In the error correction task, subjects were required to correct a movement so that it matched a previously performed criterion movement. The performances of both the middle-aged and older subjects were inferior to the performance of the young subjects on the error detection task. Older subjects also performed more poorly than young subjects on the error correction task.

Based on the limited research available, it appears that older adults do demonstrate some deficits in motor memory recall and recognition, and that these deficits may be similar to those demonstrated in verbal memory. Generally, age-related decrements in motor memory seem to increase in magnitude as the demands on memory grow, although the data are not fully consistent. Jordan (1978), for example, found no significant age differences in recall under a blindfolded condition. Reasons for age-related differences in motor memory are unknown at this time. However, it is possible that the same factors responsible for age-related deficits in verbal memory are also responsible for such differences in motor memory. For example, it may be that older adults are less efficient encoders of movement information. If this is the case, one could expect that older adults, as compared to younger adults, would require more practice on a given motor skill in order to develop recall and recognition memories that result in effective movement and efficient error detection, respectively. Furthermore, if motor memory recall is harder to establish than motor memory recognition, then age-related differences in motor memory recall may be particularly pronounced. At this point, the available data are so limited that one can only speculate.

# DIRECTIONS FOR FUTURE RESEARCH

An appropriate starting point for future research in age-related differences in motor memory recall and recognition would be the full identification and description of any such differences. In connection to this research, a variety of questions could be asked. What is the role of encoding in accounting for any motor memory recall and recognition deficits associated with age? Can techniques be identified and tested which might facilitate the development of both types of motor memory in the aged? How does motor memory for novel skills relate to motor memory for skills learned much earlier in life? Anecdotal data, for example, indicates that some continuous motor skills such as swimming and bicycle riding are never lost to healthy elderly people, even though they may not have used those skills in years. Is motor memory for discrete skills that were learned years before as "good" as motor memory for continuous skills seems to be?

Are there developmental changes in the way people encode information about movement? For example, it has been well established that young adults tend to use both location cues and movement extent cues when reproducing simple movements, with location cues being used more for long movements and distance cues for short movements (Schmidt, 1982; Wrisberg and Winter, 1985). Is there a shift with age in the type of cues used to reproduce certain kinds of movements? More importantly, given that most motor memory studies use very simple motor tasks which do not reflect accurately the complexities of movements used everyday by young and old alike, what is the relationship between motor memory for these artificial tasks, and motor skills which are ecologically valid?

Finally, how similar are recall and recognition processes for verbal and motor memory, and could these similarities change with age? While there do appear to be some tentative similarities, such as changes in the frequency and magnitude of age-differences as a function of task processing demands, there also may be some dissimilarities; for example, recall and recognition seem to be more interdependent in motor memory than in verbal memory. It would, of course, be parsimonious if the same principles and mechanisms could explain both motor and verbal memory. However, substantially more research is needed to answer this and other questions.

# SUMMARY

The purpose of this chapter was to review the literature on memory retrieval in the aging population, and to address the hypothesis that an underlying factor in age-related differences found in the performance of memory tasks may be a deficiency in retrieval operations. Retrieval, the accessing of information from long-term memory, is often assessed via a cognitive task which requires recall and/or recognition of previously learned information. Recall memory involves a search and retrieval process, whereas recognition is simply the matching of environmentally produced information to that which is stored in memory. It has been suggested that recognition involves a lighter retrieval load since the correct alternative is always present.

Based on the assumption that age-related differences may tentatively imply retrieval deficiencies, two hypotheses were generated. First, recognition memory should be superior in both aged and younger populations due to lesser processing loads, and second, greater age differences would be displayed in recall and recognition. The literature review did reveal apparent age-related differences in recall. Although appearing less frequently, age-related differences in recognition were also found. When processing demands were reduced through increased familiarity, recall and recognition were enhanced regardless of age. Encoding deficiencies, as well as ineffective rehearsal strategies, were also purported to influence age-related differences in memory retrieval.

Interest in motor memory recall and recognition developed in response to the motor learning theories of Adams (1971), and Schmidt (1975). Both theorists posited these two memory processes to be independent of each other. Research evidence generally has indicated that these two processes can develop and operate independently under certain experimental conditions. However, the independence of recall and recognition in the acquisition and performance of motor skills in the natural environment has not been established. Rather, it seems likely that in the "real world" motor task situations, recall and recognition are to some undetermined degree, interdependent.

Relatively little research has been conducted on age-related differences in motor memory recall and recognition. Limited data have indicated that age-related differences in motor memory do occur. Furthermore, these differences have paralleled similar differences reported in the verbal memory literature. The finding that age-related differences in motor memory recall and recognition increase as processing demands increase is an example of this similarity. The origin of apparent age-related deficits in motor memory is unknown at present. It is possible that these deficits are due to age-related declines in motor memory recall and recognition per se. However, it is also possible that age-related declines in processes such as encoding and rehearsal are important factors as well. Currently, a definitive conclusion does not seem possible. Clearly, there is a need for substantially more research into the nature and source of age-related differences in motor memory recall and recognition.

# REFERENCES

Adams, J.A. (1971). A closed-loop theory of motor learning. *Journal of motor behavior, 3,* 111-149.

Adams, J.A. (1976). Issues for a closed-loop theory of motor learning. In G.E. Stelmach (Ed.), *Motor control: Issues and trends* (pp. 87-107). New York: Academic Press.

Botwinick, J. (1973). *Aging and behavior.* New York: Springer Publishing Comapny.

Botwinick, J. (1984). *Aging and Behavior* (3rd edition). New York: Springer Publishing Company.

Burke, D.M. and Yee, P.L. (1984). Semantic priming during sentence processing by young and older adults. *Developmental Psychology, 20,* 930-910.

Dickinson J. and Higgins, N. (1977). Release from proactive and retroactive interference in motor short-term memory. *Journal of Motor Behavior, 9,* 61-66. Diewert, G.L.

————. (1975). Retention and coding in motor short-term memory: A comparison of storage codes for distance and location information. *Journal of Motor Behavior, 7,* 183-190.

Erber, J.T. (1974). Age differences in recognition memory. *Journal of Gerontology, 29,* 177-181.

Fleishman, E.A. and Parker, J.F. (1962). Factors in the retention and relearning of perceptual motor skill. *Journal of Experimental Psychology, 64,* 215-226.

Gundry, J. (1975). The use of location and distance in reproducing different amplitudes of movement. *Journal of Motor Behavior, 7,* 91-100.

Hanley-Dunn, P. and McIntosh, J.L. (1984). Meaningfulness and recall of names by young and old adults. *Journal of Gerontology, 39,* 583-585.

Howard, D.V., Heisey, J.G. and Shaw, R.J. (1986). Aging and the priming of newly learned associations. *Developmental Psychology, 22,* 78-85.

Jordan, T. (1978). Age differences in visual and kinesthetic short-term memory. *Perceptual and Motor Skills, 46,* 667-674.

Kelso, J.A.S. (1978) Recognition and recall in slow movements: separate memory states? *Journal of Motor Behavior, 10,* 69-76.

Laabs, G.J. (1974). The effect of interpolated motor activity on the short-term retention of movement distance and end-location. *Journal of Motor Behavior, 6,* 279-288.

Marshall, P.H., Elias, J.W. and Wright, J. (1985) Age related factors in motor error detection and correction. *Experimental Aging Research, 11,* 201-206.

Meyers, J. (1967). Retention of balance coordination learning as influenced by extended lay-offs. *Research Quarterly, 38,* 72-78.

Mitchell, D.B. and Perlmutter, M. (1986). Semantic activation and episodic memory: Age similarities and differences. *Developmental Psychology, 22,* 86-94.

Neumann, E. and Ammons, R.B. (1957). Acquisition and long term retention of simple serial perception motor skill. *Journal of Experimental Psychology, 53,* 158-161.

Newell, K.M. and Chew, R.A. (1974). Recall and recognition in motor learning. *Journal of Motor Behavior, 6,* 245-253.

Norrie, M.L. and Henry, F.M. (1978). Influence of an interpolated non-related motor task on short- and long-term memory learning and retention of a gross motor skill. *Perceptual and Motor Skills, 46,* 987-994.

Ostrow, A.C. (1984). *Physical activity and the older adult: Psychological perspectives.* Princeton, N.J.: Princeton Book Company.

Perlmutter, M. (1979). Age differences in adults' free recall, cued recall and recognition. *Journal of Gerontology, 34,* 533-539.

Poon, L.W. and Fozard, J.L. (1978). Speed of retrieval from long-term memory in relation to age, familiarity and datedness of information. *Journal of Gerontology, 33,* 711-717.

Rabinowitz, J.C. (1984). Aging and recognition failure. *Journal of Gerontology, 39,* 65-71.

Rankin, J.L. and Hyland, T.P. (1983). The effects of orienting tasks on adult age differences in recall and recognition. *Experimental Aging Research, 98,* 159-164.

Roy, E.A. (1977). Spatial cues in memory for movement. *Journal of Motor Behavior, 9,* 151-156.

Ryan, E.D. (1962). Retention of stabilometer and pursuit rotor skills. *Research Quarterly, 33,* 592-598.

Ryan, E.D. (1965). Retention of stabilometer performance over extended periods of time. *Research Quarterly, 36,* 46-51.

Sanders, R.E., Murphy, M.D., Schmitt, F.A. and Walsh, K.K. (1980). Age differences in free recall rehearsal strategies. *Journal of Gerontology, 35,* 550-558.

Schmidt, R.A. (1975). A schema theory of discrete motor skill learning. *Psychological review, 82,* 225-260.

Schmidt, R.A. (1976). The schema as a solution to some persistent problems in motor learning theory. In G.E. Stelmach (Ed.), *Motor control: Issues and trends* (pp. 41-65). New York: Academic Press.

Schmidt, R.A. (1982). *Motor control and learning.* Champaign, IL: Human Kinetics Publishers.

Schmitt, F.A., Murphy, M.D. and Sanders, R.E. (1981). Training older adult free recall rehearsal strategies. *Journal of Gerontology, 36,* 329-337.

Schonfield, D. and Robertson, B.A. (1966). Memory storage and aging. *Canadian Journal of Pyschology, 20,* 228-236.

Shapiro, D.C. and Schmidt, R.A. (1982). The schema theory: Recent evidence and developmental implications. In J.A.S. Kelso and J.E. Clark (Eds.), *The development of movement control and co-ordination* (pp. 113-150). Chichester, Great Britain: John Wiley and Sons.

Shaps, L.P. and Nilsson, L.G. (1980). Encoding and retrieval operations in relation to age. *Developmental Psychology, 16,* 636-643.

Stelmach, G.E. (1982). Information-processing framework for understanding human motor behavior. In J.A.S. Kelso (ed.), *Human motor behavior: An introduction* (pp. 63-91). Hillsdale, NJ: Lawrence Erlbaum.

Toole, T., Pyne, A., and McTarsney, P.A. (1984). Age differences in memory for movement. *Experimental Aging Research, 10,* 205-210.

Wallace, S.A. and McGhee, R.C. (1979). The independence of recall and recognition in motor learning. *Journal of Motor Behavior, 11,* 141-151.

Walsh, W.D., Russell, D.G. and Crassini, B. (1981) Interference effects in recalling movements. *British Journal of Psychology, 72,* 287-298.

West, R.L. and Boatwright, L.K. (1983). Age differences in cued recall and recognition under varying encoding and retrieval conditions. *Experimental Aging Research, 9,* 185-189.

Williams, I.D. (1978). Evidence for recognition and recall schematas. *Journal of Motor Behavior, 10,* 45-52.

Worden, P.E., and Sherman-Brown, S. (1983). A word-frequency cohort effect in young versus elderly adults' memory for words. *Developmental Psychology, 19,* 521-530.

Wrisberg, C.A. and Winter, T.P. (1985). Reproducing the end location of a positioning movement: The long and short of it. *Journal of Motor Behavior, 17,* 242-254.

Zelaznik, H.N., Shapiro, D.C. and Newell, K.M. (1978). On the structure of motor recognition memory. *Journal of Motor Behavior, 10,* 313-323.

Zelaznik, H. and Spring, H. (1976). Feedback in response recognition and production. *Journal of Motor Behavior, 8,* 309-312.

**104**          *AGING AND MOTOR BEHAVIOR*

# 5

## The Effects of Regular Aerobic Exercise on Short-Term Memory Efficiency in the Older Adult

Tami Abourezk

### ABSTRACT

The purpose of this chapter is to investigate the effects of aerobic activity on short-term memory efficiency in the older adult. Twenty males aged 50 to 70 years subdivided into two groups (active and nonactive) were tested on a dichotic listening task. The active group ran an average of 25 miles a week for the past five years, while the nonactive group did not exercise aerobically on a regular basis. Subjects from both groups were equally able to report a high percentage of digits during monaural presentation. Thus it was assumed that the subjects could hear and understand the presented digits. Likewise, when subjects were asked to selectively attend to one ear, both groups were not significantly different in the percentage of digits recalled. During dichotic presentation in which the subjects reported one ear and then the other ear, no significant difference existed for the first ear (active first ear $M$ = 23.10 and nonactive first ear $M$ = 22.20). However, the active group ($M$ = 13.40) reproduced more digits from the second ear than the nonactive group ($M$ = 6.70).

These findings demonstrate that under relatively simple conditions, there is no exercise related difference in memory capacity for physically active and inactive older adults. In contrast, when memory capacity was stressed, physically active older adults remembered more information than their inactive counterparts. This latter result supports the notion that a regular regimen of exercise can benefit cognitive functioning in the aged.

### INTRODUCTION

Birren (1974) proposed that advancement in age leads to a slowing down of the central nervous system (CNS) which is exhibited as a decrement in information processing time. This decrement is evident in the time it takes an older individual to respond to a single stimulus (simple reaction time) or multiple stimuli (choice reaction time). It has been repeatedly demonstrated that both simple reaction time (SRT) and choice reaction time (CRT) are slower with an increase in age (Birren, 1964; Borkan & Norris, 1980; Hodgkins, 1963). In addition to a lengthening in decision making time, the effect of age on other mental abilities has also been demonstrated. For example, many studies report a deterioration in memory (see Craik, 1977; Erber, 1981; Salthouse, 1982 for detailed reviews). These decrements are also evident in the short-term memory of the older adult, especially when the individual must divide his/her attention (Craik, 1977).

In a dichotic listening task, subjects must divide their attention between lists of digits presented simultaneously in both ears. Similar to a reaction time task, time is also an important variable in dichotic listening performance. Because the digits held in the second ear decay over time, it is critical that the subject retrieve the first ear digits rapidly in order to prevent this decay. Utilizing a dichotic listening task, investigations have repeatedly demonstrated the diminished capacity of short-term memory in subjects between the ages of approximately 50 and 70 years (Clark & Knowles, 1973; Inglis & Caird, 1968; Parkinson, Lindholm, & Urell, 1980).

Although it would seem, based on these studies, that a decrease in information processing abilities are an inevitable consequence of age, studies have indicated exceptions to this view. For example, research conducted by Spirduso (1975) and Spirduso and Clifford (1978) suggest that one's cardiovascular fitness level, rather than age per se may be responsible for the slowing down of the CNS. Spirduso (1975) reported that men (50-70 years of age) who participated regularly (three times a week over the past 30 years) in racquet sports or handball were significantly faster in SRT, discrimination reaction time (DRT), and movement time (MT) than their inactive counterparts. These findings were replicated in a study which included runners (Spirduso & Clifford, 1978). Older men who maintained an active lifestyle, either racquet sports or running, reacted and moved significantly faster than their sedentary peers. Additional studies which have also resulted in faster SRT's in older adults, have done so by means of aerobic training programs (Stacey, Kozma, & Stones, 1985; Van Fraecham & Van Fraecham, 1977).

Physical activity may also enhance cognitive function in older adults. Subjects placed in an exercise therapy program significantly improved their scores on the Wechsler Memory Scale and the Progressive Matrices Test (Powell, 1974). Elsayed, Ismail, and Young (1980) reported that a four month exercise program resulted in higher fluid intelligence (i.e., Culture Fair Intelligence Test Scale) for the high-fit group. Studies conducted by Crooks (1976) and Dustman et al. (1984) also seem to suggest a positive relationship between one's cardiovascular fitness level and cognitive functioning in the aged.

In light of the foregoing research, the purpose of this experiment was to investigate a specific deficiency in short-term memory and its relationship to aerobic exercise in the older adult. It was predicted that the active group would exhibit less short-term memory deficiency, utilizing a dichotic listening task, as compared to the nonactive group.

# METHOD

## Subjects

A total of 20 older adult males (nine university professors, eight state employees, and three self-employed) volunteered for participation in this experiment. The subjects were divided into two groups, active and nonactive, ranging in age from 50 to 70 years. The 10 subjects in the active group (M age = 57.00 years, SD = 7.01) reported they ran an average of 25 miles per week for the past five years. These subjects were recruited from a local running club. The nonactive group (M age = 59.40 years, SD = 7.95) consisted of 10 subjects who did not and had never participated in aerobic exercise on a regular basis.

In order to determine the homogeneity of the two groups, all subjects completed a questionnaire concerning demographic and health information. Each subject was: 1) from a socioeconomic status of middle to upper middle class (as determined by annual income), 2) at least a high school graduate, and 3) a nonsmoker and free from cardiovascular diseases (as determined by the response given by the subject). Because the task utilized in this study had an auditory component, all subjects were given a pure-tone audiometer examination. All subjects had normal hearing threshold levels (American National Standards Institute, 1969). Furthermore, each subject's resting heart rate and blood pressure were determined.

## Task

A dichotic listening task was utilized which consisted of listening through stereophonic headphones to digit pairs presented simultaneously to both ears. The subject's task was to verbalize the digits presented to one or both ears. All digits were recorded on audio tape by a male native speaker of American English.[1] The digits were randomly selected from the digits 1 through 10 with the restriction that no digit appear more than once in a single trial. Each trial was comprised of three-digit pairs and there were 100 trials. Based on the study conducted by Parkinson, Lindholm, and Urell (1980), the duration of the digits was set at 300 msec with a 200 msec interstimulus off-time between adjacent pairs within a trial. Thus, the rate of presentation was two pairs of digits per sec. There was also a 10 sec interval between consecutive trials.

---

[1] The dichotic tape used in the present study was prepared by Haskins laboratory with assistance from NICHD contract No 1-HD-5-2910.

## Procedure

The following test procedure was adopted from research conducted by Parkinson, Lindholm, and Urell (1980). The procedure for this experiment was subdivided into three phases. In the first phase, 20 trials were presented monaurally. The subject heard 10 trials in the right ear and then 10 trials in the left ear. The purpose of this phase was to determine if subjects could hear and understand the spoken digits.

The second phase consisted of 30 trials presented dichotically. Each subject was told to attend to one ear while ignoring the other ear. The subject verbally recalled the digits from the attended ear, 15 trials per ear. The intention of this phase was to determine if the subject could selectively attend to one ear.

In the third phase, the remaining 50 trials were presented dichotically. After hearing three pairs of digits, the subjects attempted to verbally recall, in order of presentation, all six digits (three from one ear and three from the other ear). Furthermore, the experimenter specified, prior to digit presentation, which ear to recall first, the "right" ear or "left" ear. Ear order recall was random and equal across all trials. If the subject was unable to recall a digit(s), he was instructed to respond "blank" for the omitted digit(s). Serial recall scoring was used in which digits were counted as correct only if they were reported in the correct order and from the correct ear.

## RESULTS

### Descriptive Data

Prior to the actual dichotic test, each subject's resting heart rate and blood pressure were determined. These measures were taken as further indicants of the individuals cardiovascular fitness level. The subjects in the active group had a mean heart rate of 53.20 beats/min while the mean heart rate for the nonactive group was 72.20 beats/min. Average blood pressures for the active and nonactive groups were 107-70 and 122-76, respectively.

### Digit Comprehension

A 2 x 2 (Active/Nonactive x Right/Left Ear) ANOVA with repeated measures on the last factor was conducted for phase one and two. The analysis performed on phase one revealed that the group main effect, $F (1,18) = .14, p > .05$, was not significant statistically, with the active group ($M = 99.70$) and the nonactive group ($M = 99.50$) recalling a similar percentage of digits. All subjects correctly reported at least 95% of the total number of digits presented to either the left or the right ear. It was concluded from this result that the digits were intelligible for all subjects in both groups. Furthermore, the number of digits recalled from the right ear ($M$ = 99.35) was not significantly different from the number of digits recalled from the left ear ($M$ = 99.85). The analysis for this later main effect yielded an $F (1,18)$ = .83, $p > .05$. Finally, the interaction effect, $F (1,18)$ = .84, $p > .05$, was not significant statistically.

## Selection Attention

The second phase analysis demonstrated that all subjects from both groups were able to selectively attend to one ear. The group main effect, $F (1,18)$ = .10, $p > .05$, failed to show a statistically significant difference between the active group ($M$ = 92.65) and the nonactive group ($M$ = 91.25). In addition, the right ear ($M$ = 90.80) was not significantly different, $F (1,18)$ = 2.30, $p > .05$, from the left ear ($M$= 93.10). The interaction effect, $F (1,18)$ = 1.00, $p > .05$ also lacked statistical significance.

## Short-Term Memory

A 2 x 2 (Active/Nonactive x 1st/2nd Ear) factorial analysis of variance with repeated measures on the second factor was conducted on the third phase data. This phase was necessary to test the hypothesis that the active group would recall more digits from the second ear as compared to the nonactive group. The dependent measure was the "percent correct recalled" for the 50 trials in this phase. The analysis of variance revealed a significant group by ear interaction, $F (1,18)$ = 6.12, $p < .05$. Figure 5-1 illustrates the means from the interaction effect (active group first ear $M$ = 23.10; second ear $M$ = 13.40; nonactive group first ear $M$ = 22.20; second ear $M$ = 6.70). Although a Tukey Analysis revealed that a significant difference did not exist between the first ear for the active and nonactive groups, the active group did report significantly more digits than the nonactive group from the second ear (C.Diff = 4.69).

## DISCUSSION

Based on the results reported in the first two phases of this investigation, both the active and nonactive subjects were capable of receiving (hearing and understanding) and translating or selectively attending to (distinguishing left ear digits from right ear digits) the presented digits. Difficulty in hearing or understanding the monaurally presented digits would have resulted in significant differences between the two groups. However, both groups recalled the digits presented in the first phase with 95% accuracy for both the right and left ears. Furthermore, when subjects were instructed to deliberately ignore the digits presented to one ear while attending with the other ear (phase 2), both groups were equally capable of selectively attending to either ear.

The data obtained from the third phase indicate that the active group

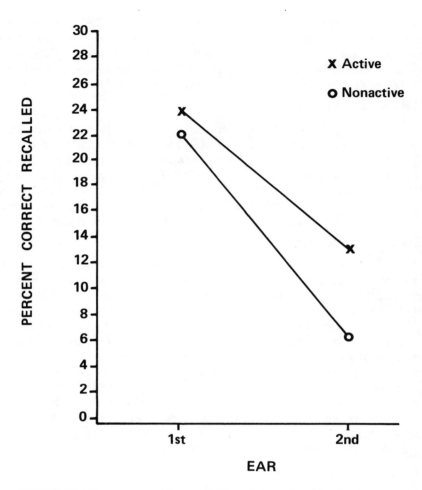

**FIGURE 5.1.** *Mean percentage of digits recalled from the first and second ear based on exercise.*

was more efficient than the nonactive group at storing and retrieving the digits presented to the second ear. During the third phase the digits were presented simultaneously. As expected both groups recalled fewer digits from the second ear. Apparently the digits from the second ear were held in storage for a period of time and were vulnerable to decay (Inglis & Ankus, 1965). However, the interaction effect (group by ear) revealed that the active group was significantly better at short-term memory retention for the second ear than the nonactive group.

Because this study was an indirect measure of the possible link between aerobic activity and age-related decrements in short-term memory, the actual underlying mechanism(s) responsible for the results obtained have not been explained. However, several researchers have speculated on the possible reasons why older individuals who maintain an active lifestyle do not exhibit information processing deficits such as an increase in decision making time, or increase in memory loss to the degree that their inactive cohorts do. One explanation for this consistent finding is the notion that regular exercise may facilitate an increase in the oxygen supply to the brain (Birren, Woods, & Williams, 1980; Spirduso, 1975). McFarland (1963) suggested that with increased age there is either less oxygen available to the CNS due to ineffective transport, or available oxygen is less adequately utilized. He amplified this view by exposing young subjects to altitudes of 10,000 feet and above. This hypoxic condition resulted in decrements in short-term memory, attention, and processing time. He suggested that these behavioral deficits are similar to the deficits observed with older adults. Thus, for whatever reason, as an individual ages the brain receives less and less oxygen, resulting in a decline of processes. Other experiments (Patel, 1977; Smith & Sokoloff, 1982) have reported in both man and animal that with age there is a decrease in energy metabolism. They suggested a link between a diminished supply of oxygen and a decrease in energy metabolism in the CNS.

Another rationale is that exercise may also increase the production of certain neurotransmitters such as serotonin, norepinepherine, and dopamine (see Spirduso, 1980; 1983 for detailed reviews). Communication among neurons is directly related to neurotransmitters and their function. Therefore, any breakdown in communication may manifest itself in decrements in information processing abilities often observed in the aging individual.

The present investigation did not attempt to directly measure the effect of oxygen on the aging CNS. However, according to the research previously discussed, it is possible that for the present study, the active group's fitness level may have had a positive effect on their ability to accurately report the second ear digits. The notion of increased oxygen to the aging CNS is an attractive hypothesis which warrants further and more direct investigations.

Although the results of this study are interesting, there are some limitations which must be addressed for future research. First, the inclusion of younger subjects, active and nonactive, could provide more information concerning the role of aerobic activity in the maintenance of a healthy CNS. If the short-term memory performance of the older active group was superior to the young nonactive group, support for the relationship between cardiovascular fitness and cognitive function would be provided. Although heart rate and blood pressure provided a measure of comparison between the active and nonactive groups for the present study, testing the subject's $\dot{V}O_2$max would be more insightful. A

$\dot{V}O_2$max indicates the greatest volume of oxygen used by the cells of the body per unit of time (Lamb, 1984). $\dot{V}O_2$max would be a more precise measure of determining one's ability to deliver oxygen to the CNS.

Furthermore, future researchers should attempt to use a group of subjects acting as their own control. Pre and post dichotic listening performance could be established before and after subjects have improved their fitness level after a six month aerobic training program. Because a long-term aerobic conditioning program would parallel the aging process per se, it could be established how enhanced $\dot{V}O_2$max levels affect processing efficiency of the aging CNS. Considerations should also be given to direct measures of processing time, the time from the presentation of the last pair of digits to the verbalization of the first digit, as well as total verbalization time. This dependent variable would measure the time aspect of the dichotic listening task. Finally, future researchers should attempt to use more direct measures of oxygen supply to the CNS (i.e., indicants of cerebral blood flow). This will help determine if the aging CNS is in a state of hypoxia and how exercise may improve it.

## SUMMARY

The primary purpose of this experiment was to investigate the effects of regular aerobic exercise on short-term memory in older adults 50-70 years of age. The analysis on the third phase supported the notion that fewer digits are recalled from the second ear on a dichotic listening task due to decay. Additionally, the active group reproduced a higher percentage of digits from the ear reported second. The differences in the third phase could not be explained in terms of the subject's lack of ability to understand, hear or selectively attend to the digits. Rather, the significant differences for phase 3 may have resulted due to the active group's fitness level. Several physiological hypotheses have been presented as possible rationales for this finding. Although the findings for the present study are important, at best they have provided indirect support for the role of aerobic exercise in the aging CNS. Therefore, future research should attempt to answer important questions about this relationship by means of more direct measures.

### REFERENCES

American National Standards Institute (1969). *Specifications for audiometers* (Report No. 53.6 - 1969). New York: ANSI Inc.

Birren, J.E. (Ed.). (1964). *The psychology of aging* (pp. 274-279). Englewood Cliffs, New Jersey: Prentice Hall.

Birren, J.E. (1974). Translation in gerontology from lab to life: Psychophysiology and speed of response. *American Psychologist, 29,* 808-815.

Birren. J.E., Woods, A.M., & Williams, M.V. (1980). Behavioral slowing with age: Causes, organization and consequences. In L.W. Poon ( Ed.), *Aging in the 1980's* (pp. 293-308). Washington D.C.: American Psychological Association.

Borkan, G.A., and Norris, A.H. (1980). Assessment of biological age using a profile of physical parameters. *Journal of Gerontology, 35,* 177-184.

Clark, L.E., & Knowles, J.B. (1973). Age differences in dichotic listening performance. *Journal of Gerontology, 28*, 173-178.

Craik, F.I.M. (1977). Age differences in human memory. In J.E. Birren & K.W. Schaie (Eds.), *Handbook of the psychology of aging* (pp. 384-420). New York: Van Nostrand Reinhold.

Crooks, G.M. (1976). Relations of physical, social, and physiological variables to psychological performance in subjects 55-89 years of age. Unpublished doctoral dissertation, University of Kansas, Lawrence.

Dustman, R.E., Ruhling, R.O., Russell, E.M., Shearer, D.E., Bonekat, H.W., Shigeoka, J.W., Wood, J.S., & Bradford, D.C. (1984). Aerobic training and improved function in older individuals. *Neurobiology of Aging, 5*, 35-42.

Elsayed, M., Ismail, A.H., & Young, R.J. (1980). Intellectual differences of adult men related to age and physical fitness before and after an exercise program. *Journal of Gerontology, 35*, 383-387.

Erber, J.T. (1981). Remote memory and age: A review, *Experimental Aging Research, 1*, 189-199.

Hodgkins, J. (1963). Reaction time and speed of movement in males and females of various ages. *Research Quarterly, 34*, 335-343.

Inglis, J., & Ankus, M.N. (1965). Effects of age on short-term storage and serial rote learning. *British Journal of Psychology, 56*, 183-195.

Inglis, J. & Caird, W.K. (1963). Age differences in successive responses to simultaneous stimulation. *Canadian Journal of Psychology, 17*, 98-105.

McFarland, R.A. (1963). Experimental evidence of the relationship between aging and oxygen want. In search of a theory of aging. *Ergonomics, 6*, 339-366.

Lamb. D.R. (1984). *Physiology of exercise: Responses and adaptations.* New York: Macmillan.

Parkinson, S.T., Lindholm J.M., & Urell, R. (1980). Aging, dichotic memory and digit span. *Journal of Gerontology, 35*, 87-95.

Patel, M.S. (1977). Age-dependent changes in the oxidative metabolism in rat brain. *Journal of Gerontology, 32* (6), 643-646.

Powell, R.R. (1974). Psychological effects of exercise therapy upon institutionalized geriatric mental patients. *Journal of Gerontology, 29*, 157-161.

Salthouse, T.A. (1982). *Adult cognition: An experimental psychology of human aging.* New York: Springer Verlag.

Smith, C.B., & Sokoloff, L. (1982). Age-related changes in local glucose utilization in the brain. In S. Hoyer (Ed.), *Experimental brain research suppl. 5: The aging brain: Physiological and pathophysiological aspects* (pp. 76-85). New York: Springer Verlag.

Spirduso, W.W. (1975). Reaction and movement time as a function of age and physical activity level. *Journal of Gerontology, 30*, 435-440.

Spirduso, W.W. (1980). Physical fitness, aging, and psycho-motor speed: A review. *Journal of Gerontology, 35*, 850-865.

Spirduso, W.W. (1983). Exercise and the aging brain. *Research Quarterly for Exercise and Sport, 54*, 208-218.

Spirduso, W.W., & Clifford, P. (1978). Replication of age and physical activity effects on reaction and movement time. *Journal of Gerontology, 33*, 26-30.

Stacey, C., Kozma, A., & Stones, M.J. (1985). Simple cognitive and behavioral changes resulting from improved physical fitness in persons over 50 years of age. *Canadian Journal on Aging, 4*, 67-74.

Van Fraecham, J., & Van Fraecham, R. (1977). Studies of the effect of a short training period on aged subjects. *Journal of Sports Medicine and Physical Fitness, 17*, 373-380.

# Part IV
# Aging, Mental Health, and Exercise

## INTRODUCTION

In my earlier book, *Physical Activity and the Older Adult: Psychological Perspectives* (Ostrow, 1984), I noted that the physical and mental health benefits of exercise are not circumscribed by age. It has only been in the last two decades, however, that we have come to realize that older people are trainable, and that in spite of years of inactivity, we can restore some of the vigor associated with youth. Exercise physiology investigations indicate that improvements in vital capacity, oxygen uptake, systolic and diastolic blood pressure, working heart rate, blood volume, percentage of body fat, and blood lactate concentrations can be expected among individuals, young or old, who participate in regular and vigorous programs of physical activity (see the excellent reviews by Hodgson & Buskirk, 1977; Shephard & Sidney, 1979; and Sidney, 1981). Similarly, as the reader will note from the chapters by Berger and Hecht and by Hird and Williams that follow, there is encouraging evidence that exercise is beneficial to the mental health of older people.

However, the results of studies on the effects of exercise on mental health are more equivocal. The difficulty of documenting the role of exercise in ameliorating the mental health of older people becomes apparent after reading the empirical investigations by Richardson and Rosenberg and by Blankfort-Doyle and her colleagues that follow. While Richardson and Rosenberg found some reductions in (somatic) anxiety after middle-aged women participated in a 7-week walk/jog program, Blankfort et al. were unable to verify that an extended 15-month program of ergometry exercise improved the psychological or functional status of a sample of nursing home residents. However, Chapter Nine by Blankfort et al. is excellent in terms of addressing the unique concerns of implementing a data-based exercise program for nursing home residents.

Numerous conceptual and methodological issues must be resolved before we can have a better understanding of the psychological effects of exercise among people as they age. For example, are there unique personality and behavioral changes that occur as people grow older, that interact with the forms of psychological change that can be expected to occur through exercise? Given the increased heterogeneity of people as they grow older on many measures of human performance, are the research designs, assessment strategies, and statistical models currently in vogue most appropriate for investigating, from a developmental perspective, the psychological effects of exercise? What are the optimum exercise regimens in terms of frequency, intensity, duration, and type for producing positive psychological change among older people? To what extent is a training effect a precursor for demonstrating psychological change in the elderly? What psychological principles govern the programming of exercise so that older adults derive maximal physical and psychological benefits? These and other issues form the basis for the chapters that follow in this section of the book.

#### References

Hodgson, J.L., & Buskirk, E.R. (1977). Physical fitness and age, with emphasis on cardiovascular function in the elderly. *Journal of the American Geriatrics Society, 25*, 385-392.
Ostrow, A.C. (1984). *Physical activity and the older adult: Psychological perspectives.* Princeton: Princeton Book Co.

Shephard, R.J., & Sidney, K.H. (1979). Exercise and aging. In R. Hutton (Ed.), *Exercise and sport science reviews* (Vol. 6) (pp. 1-57). Philadelphia: Franklin Institute Press.

Sidney, K.H. (1981). Cardiovascular benefits of physical activity in the exercising aged. In E.L. Smith & R.C. Serfass (Eds.), *Exercise and aging* (pp. 36-58). Hillside, NJ: Enslow.

# 6

# Exercise, Aging, and Psychological Well-Being: The Mind-Body Question[1]

BONNIE G. BERGER

LILLIAN MUSHABAC HECHT

## ABSTRACT

Psychological, social, and physiological benefits of exercise are examined in this chapter because the three concerns are inextricably related to the aging process. "As one ages, exercise becomes unimportant, or even superfluous" is a socially accepted truism. This chapter examines experimental evidence that suggests the reverse—that exercise becomes increasingly important throughout one's life. With exercise, the biological signposts of aging can be noticeably reduced. The psychological benefits associated with exercise as reported by the elderly are particularly pronounced. Older people who are physically active tend to be happier and score higher in self-esteem and in life quality than do the sedentary. In addition, elderly exercisers also report less anxiety, depression, and muscular tension. Because of the importance of exercise for the elderly, tentative guidelines for enhancing the psychological benefits of exercise are suggested. The exercise should be enjoyable. It also should induce deep abdominal breathing, be noncompetitive and predictable, and be frequent enough to facilitate ease of participation. In addition, exercise should be of moderate intensity and extend for at least 20 to 30 minutes.

## INTRODUCTION

There has been a slow, evolving shift in the age structure of the American population. Although the length of life may be fixed, life expectancy has increased and the population has aged (Fries, 1980; Jette & Branch, 1981). The average life expectancy in the United States was 47 years in 1900; by 1980, it had jumped to 73 years (Fries, 1980). Elimination of premature death, decreases in acute disease such as smallpox, and the postponement of chronic illness have contributed to the huge increase in life expectancy and to the rectangularization of the survival curve (Comfort, 1979; Fries, 1980) (see Figure 6-1).

The statistics have become familiar. The 65 and older population grew twice as fast as the rest of the population during the past two decades (Collins, 1987). Nine percent of the population is now over 65 years

[1] Supported in part by a Professional Staff Congress-Board of Higher Education Research Awards from the City University of New York, Nos. 6-64167, 6-63202, and 6-61055 to the first author.

**117**

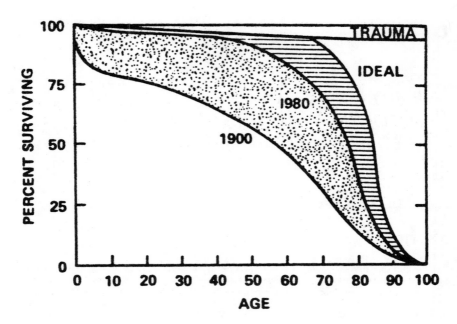

**FIGURE 6.1.** *The increasingly rectangular survival curve. Approximately 80 percent (stippled area) of the difference between the 1900 curve and the ideal curve (stippled area plus hatched area) had been eliminated by 1980. Trauma is now the dominant cause of death in early life. (From Fries, 1980, p. 131). Reprinted by permission.*

of age. By the year 2000, it is estimated that the statistic will be 12%. The figure will increase to 15 or 17% between the years 2010 and 2020 when the "baby boom" generation reaches the age of 65 (McPherson, 1986). By 2030, one fifth of all Americans will be over 65 (Collins, 1987). Since the age range of people over 65 is so large, the elderly often are separated into two categories: the young-old (65 to 75 years) and the-old old (75 to 85 and older), (Schaie & Geiwitz, 1982). This graying of the population, the greater visibility of old people and changing role models have attracted the attention of researchers and the public who wish to explore the role of exercise in delaying the "normal" aging process.

Aging does not begin suddenly at age 60 or 65. It actually begins at birth. An inherent linear decline in organ reserve (and a concomitant decrease in the ability to restore homeostasis as a result of illness or injury) begins at approximately 30 years of age (Jette & Branch, 1981). Fortunately, the decline in functional capacity can be modified substantially by exercise, weight control and diet. This chapter focuses specifically on the role of exercise in enhancing the quality of life. In addition to improving life quality, exercise, along with dietary and healthful living habits,

*AGING AND MOTOR BEHAVIOR*

increases the likelihood of living to one's full life expectancy (85 ± 5 years), (Spirduso, 1986).

Psychological, social, and physiological benefits of exercise are examined in this chapter because the three are inextricably interrelated to the aging process. Emphasizing the importance of psychological factors in aging, Pelletier (1981, p. 170) stressed in his book on aging, "Psychological factors have been demonstrated to be the *single most significant predictor of both optimum health and longevity* [italics added]."

Mark Twain once commented, "Age is a case of mind over matter; if you don't mind it, it doesn't matter." Unfortunately, not many people have adopted Twain's philosophy. "Age grading," or the inappropriateness of various types of physical activity for people in older age groups, tends to be learned by the age of 20 (Ostrow, Jones, & Spiker, 1981). In fact, preschool children have already learned that exercise is less appropriate with advancing age (Ostrow, Keener, & Perry, 1986-87). Since age-role stereotypes in regard to exercise are learned so early in life, it is not surprising that adults aged 60 and older viewed physical activity as increasingly inappropriate as the exerciser advances in age from 20 to 40 to 60 and to 80 years (Ostrow & Dzewaltowski, 1986).

The age-grading of exercise, a socially based concept, is a great detriment to regular participation in physical activity. Many people, especially women with young children, become sedentary as they leave school and enter the work-a-day world. People in their 30's and 40's do not exercise regularly because of a multitude of reasons: ageism, work and family responsibilities, low valuation of exercise, a false belief that they exercise enough, absence of role models, and lack of motor skills and facilities (e.g., McPherson, 1986; Rosenberg, 1986). By the time people reach their 60's and 70's, many have not exercised for several decades! Only 7% of the people between 65 and 69 years of age who were tested in a Canadian fitness survey demonstrated a recommended level of cardiovascular fitness (Canada Fitness Survey, 1982).

The interrelationship between exercise and aging is complex. For example, it is almost impossible to distinguish between decreases in physical abilities resulting from physical inactivity, or hypokinetic disease, and those resulting from the aging process itself. With the accumulated years of insufficient physical activity, people in their 30's, 40's and 50's began to notice a lack of physical endurance, decreased strength, increased body fat, and sagging muscles. As a result, they incorporate the feeling of "being old" in their self concepts and participate even less in physical activity for fear of a heart attack or exercise-related injury. A self-fulfilling prophecy has begun. The decrease in physical activity produces even greater changes in body composition, more noticeable deficits in physical ability, and the cycle continues as the individual exercises even less. (See Figure 6-2 for the exercise-aging cycle.)

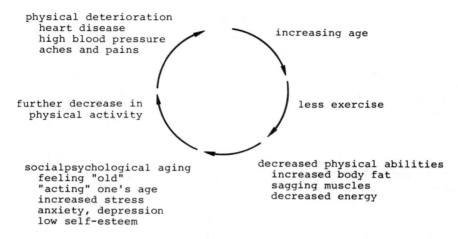

physical deterioration
  heart disease
  high blood pressure
  aches and pains

increasing age

further decrease in
  physical activity

less exercise

socialpsychological aging
  feeling "old"
  "acting" one's age
  increased stress
  anxiety, depression
  low self-esteem

decreased physical abilities
  increased body fat
  sagging muscles
  decreased energy

**FIGURE 6.2.** *The exercise-aging cycle.*

To understand the mind-body-aging relationship, it is important to critically examine the physiological and socio-psychological processes of aging. Then, the exercise specialist can knowledgeably explore the role of exercise in slowing and interrupting the "normal" aging processes.

## BIOLOGICAL AGING: MAJOR SIGNPOSTS

### Cardiovascular Changes

Aging is accompanied by both functional and structural changes in the cardiovascular system. It is difficult, however, to disassociate the effects of disease and a sedentary life style from the actual physiological deterioration of aging (Spirduso, 1986). The following changes probably reflect a *combination of aging and disuse.* The average decrease in maximum oxygen consumption ($\dot{V}O_2$max) of about 10% per decade beginning in adulthood reflects a decline in one's ability to transport oxygen to the body (Bortz, 1982). Maximal heart rate is also reduced, but cardiac output seems to be maintained in the healthy aging adult (Rodeheffer et al., 1984).

Left ventricular function can be described by preload measurements, afterload or impedance measurements, and inotropic or contractile parameters. In the aged adult, end-diastolic volume (EDV) is similar to that of younger individuals.[1] However, the rate of filling during diastole is 50% slower in the 65 to 80 year olds than in 25 to 44 year old individuals. In healthy older people, however, the EDV is the same and most probably is associated with a prolonged relaxation phase of contraction (Weisfeldt, 1985).

Impedance to ejection of blood is increased at rest in the healthy aged and is manifested by an increase in systolic blood pressure. Systolic blood pressure tends to increase in the aged as a result of a stiffening of the aorta and arterial tree, which occurs even in the absence of atherosclerosis. This is compensated, in part, by an age-related ventricular hypertrophy.

The contractile state of the heart is very difficult to measure directly. Most of the research has come from isolated hearts or intact hearts in animal experiments. Therefore, extrapolation of data from these studies to a human model must be done with careful consideration. The myocardium of aged animals has the same capacity to develop force as that of young animals. However, the duration of contraction is prolonged in the aged. This is due to both an increase in time to peak force development and relaxation time (Lakatta & Yin, 1982).

## Respiratory Signposts

With increasing age, the respiratory system is characterized by an increase in dead space, a decrease in lung weight, and a decrease in surface area for gas exchange (Krumpe et al., 1985). Oxygen tension in the arterial blood decreases, causing respiration rate to increase (Shephard & Sidney, 1979). In addition, the recoil ability of the lungs tends to decrease as lung cartilage calcifies. However, the respiratory changes that occur with aging in healthy individuals are very gradual. Respiration still remains effortless and relatively little change is perceived.

## Demineralization

Decalcification, or osteoporosis, often has been defined by bone fractures which occur as the result of mild trauma, or even spontaneously (Smith, Sempos, & Purvis, 1981). Osteroporosis is prominent in the long bones of the body, especially the radius, ulna, femoral neck, and vertebral column. The process of demineralization affects women to a much greater degree than it does men and is related to low estrogen production, prolonged calcium insufficiency, and low levels of physical activity (Smith, Sempos, Purvis, 1981; Stillman et al., 1986). Since women have less initial bone mass than men, they have less they can afford to lose. In

---

[1] This differs from individual to individual. In college students, it might be at 90% of age-adjusted heart rate. In the elderly, maximal preferred intensity of exercise might be at 70 to 80% of age adjusted heart rate.

addition, onset of osteoporosis is at a much earlier age (30 to 35 years of age) in women than in men (50 to 55 years of age). Once demineralization begins, it continues at a rate of 1 to 3% per decade in both men and women. However, superimposed on this percentage for women is a hormone-related loss of bone tissue after menopause of an additional 6% per decade (Smith & Gilligan, 1986; Stillman et al., 1986). Actual rate of bone loss reported varies from researcher to researcher (e.g., Mazess, 1982, Stillman et al., 1986). Approximately 25 to 40% of all post-menopausal women develop osteoporosis (Nordin, 1979).

## Changes in Strength, Endurance, Body Composition, and Metabolism

The aging body changes in many ways. The most noticeable changes include

1) atrophy of skeletal musculature, and

2) increase in total body fat (Bortz, 1982; Kavanagh & Shephard, 1977; Wells, 1985, pp. 181-182). Abdominal girth in women often increases 25 to 35% (Shephard, 1978).

Additional changes with age include a decline in physical stature, decreases in muscular strength and endurance, metabolic changes and decreased flexibility. Physical stature tends to decline as an individual ages due to compression of the vertebral column, a weakening of the back muscles, and osteoporosis. Physical strength decreases, because there is less muscle tissue available to perform work. Muscular endurance also declines with age, but does so to a lesser extent than does strength. As noted by Spirduso (1986), it is difficult to determine whether decreased muscular activity causes the decline, whether the decline leads to less activity, or a combination of the two explanations. Metabolic changes include a general decline in enzymatic activity and a resulting decrease in the ability to process lipids and a glucose intolerance (Shephard, 1978). Flexibility, as measured by the sit-and-reach test, decreased 23% in men and 18% in women by the age of 65. Collagen cross-linkage, joint ankylosis, and arthritis cause the major flexibility decrements (Shephard, 1986b).

Despite the decreases in physical ability with age, regular aerobic exercise enables individuals to function at much higher levels than those who are inactive (Costill, 1986). See Figure 6-3 for the U.S. records in the 10-kilometer race that remain fairly stable between ages 20 to 60. Running 6.8 miles in 40 minutes or less is an admirable accomplishment at any age. As indicated in Figure 6-3, the very best performances occur between 20 and 30 years of age. Aging does take its toll even in world class athletes. However, as illustrated in Figure 6-4, there are large differences—at every age—in the maximum oxygen uptake of highly trained runners, joggers, inactive men, and inactive women. It is encouraging to

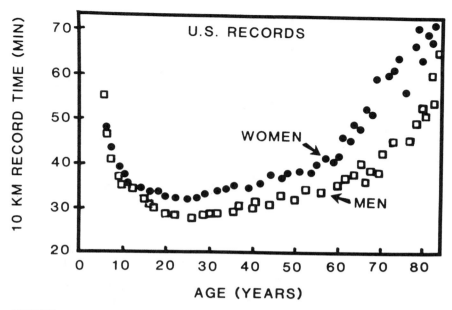

FIGURE 6.3. *U.S. records for 10 kilometers for male and female runners ranging in age from five to 83 years. (From Costill, 1986, p. 166). Reprinted by permission.*

note that the $\dot{V}O_2$max at age 70 of trained runners and joggers surpassed the $\dot{V}O_2$max of 30-year-old sedentary men and women as illustrated in Figure 6-4.

## Nervous System

There is a blunting of the abilities to see, hear and taste as the peripheral and central nervous systems age (Bortz, 1982). Interestingly, similar decreases in central nervous system function are observed with inactivity and sensory deprivation. Central nervous system changes include decreases in the rapid eye movement stage of sleep, catecholamines, hippocampal neurons, dopamine uptake, and receptor binding and turnover (e.g. Sapolsky, Krey, & McEwen, 1985). Because of these changes, the elderly do not perform as well on tests of motor performance as do younger individuals. Simple and choice reaction times are prolonged in the elderly although the exact mechanism(s) for this is not yet understood. It is known, however, that premotor latency accounts for 75% of the decline in reaction time. Motor latency accounts for the remaining 25%. With age, white muscle fibers are gradually replaced by red muscle fiber in the sedentary, possibly explaining the reduction in motor speed. Reaction time, however, can be modified with practice and can approximate, but not quite equal, that of younger individuals. Perhaps practice

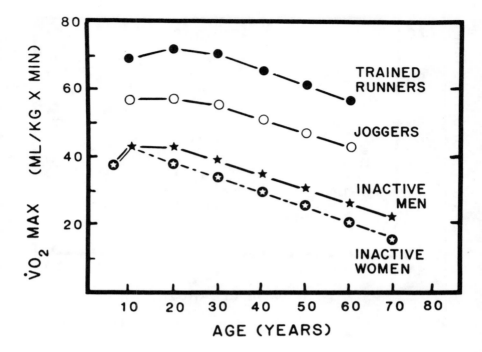

**FIGURE 6.4.** *Relationship between aging and maximal oxygen uptake ($\dot{V}O_2$ max) for inactive men and women, joggers, and highly trained runners. These cross-sectional data suggest that after the age of 20 to 25 years $\dot{V}O_2$ max declines at a steady rate for all adults, regardless of their activity level (From Costill, 1986, p. 173). Reprinted by permission.*

reduces the effect of memory deficit that older adults manifest. (Spirduso, 1985, 1986). Increases in the amplitude of movement at the center of gravity may indicate a balance disturbance with aging (Era and Heikkinen, 1984).

## PSYCHOLOGICAL HEALTH IN THE ELDERLY: MAJOR SIGNPOSTS

Despite the common perception that old people are cantankerous and crotchety, there is considerable evidence that mental health tends to improve as one ages. Anxiety in particular tends to decrease with age. Contrary to popular thought, there also is evidence that depression tends to be slightly less in people who are over 50 than in those who are between the ages of 19 and 49 (Lin, Ensel, & Dean, 1986). Although the elderly are no more depressed than other age groups, depression still is the most common psychiatric complaint among the elderly.

In examining psychological characteristics of the very old (individuals between 90 to 100 years of age), it seems that adaptability, or a *moderate and flexible attitude toward life*, is the most common characteristic (Schaie & Geiwitz, 1982, pp. 341-342). In addition to being very adaptable, very old people exercise frequently, are neither junk-food gluttons nor health-food fanatics, enjoy alcoholic drinks in moderation, but lead very different lives from one another in terms of stress and pressure (Schaie & Geiwitz, 1982).

Supporting the importance of psychosocial characteristics in the aging process, Pelletier (1981, pp. 281-318) selected five characteristics that are common in centenarian communities throughout the world such as those in the Ecuadorian Andes, Pakistan's Himalayan Karakoram range, and the Caucasus Mountains in the Soviet Union. Although it is not certain that these people live as long as claimed, they do live a long time, and it is interesting to focus on the commonalities across the communities. A century of life often has been associated with the following (Pelletier, 1981; Rosenfeld, 1978).

1) *Social environment*
   *The single most important* and frequently overlooked factor in longevity is the social dimension (Pelletier, 1981, p. 306). Included in the social environment are
   • psychological dimensions,
   • prolonged and productive involvement in community and family affairs,
   • an enduring sense of meaning in life,
   • the association of aging with wisdom and dignity, and
   • personal growth and change throughout the later years of life.
2) *Exercise*
   "Physical activity is . . . perhaps most important factor in the longevity and optimum health exhibited in these centenarian communities" (Pelletier, 1981, p. 299).
3) *Physical environment*
   This longevity factor includes such influences as the quality of water, mountainous terrain that encourages exercise, and environmental stimulation.
4) *Genetic factors*
   This influence is probably cited more often than any other, and may reflect a tendency to ascribe any unknown influence to genetic endowment.
5) *Nutrition*
   Vegetarian diets as well as a low caloric intake seem to be related to long lifespans.
6) *Sexual activity*
   Anecdotal evidence in centenarian communities include reports of women in their late 50's bearing children and of healthy sperm

specimens for 119-year-old men. Colloquialisms such as "dirty old man" and "out to pasture" reveal a negative attitude toward sexuality in the elderly (Pelletier, 1981; Rosenfeld, 1978, p. 57). Sexist thinking, as well as ageism, is prevalent in regard to sexuality. For example, there is a more positive reaction to an older man with a younger woman rather than to an older woman with a younger man, although there is no rational reason for the preference.

## Developmental Tasks of the Elderly

For many years, children, adolescents, and young adults were thought to pass through developmental stages. It is now clear that adults in their 30's, 40's, 50's, 60's, 70's, 80's are adjusting to very different issues (Helson & Moane, 1987; Levinson et al., 1978; Sheehey, 1976). Nearly 20 years ago, Havighurst (as indicated by Schaie & Geiwitz, 1982), described six developmental tasks of the elderly. Some of the following tasks are most applicable to the young-old; others, to the old-old. In addition to the six tasks listed below, Schaie & Geiwitz (1982) noted that the task of facing one's own death becomes increasingly important, the longer one lives.

Havighurst's [see Schaie and Geiwitz (1982)] developmental tasks for the elderly included the following.

1) *Adjusting to decreasing strength and health*
   Exercise is especially useful in maintaining and in developing physical ability and skills to offset those that are diminished.
2) *Adopting and adapting social roles in a flexible way*
   By adopting new activities (including exercise) to replace the role of worker and by participating in social-recreational groups, the elderly can expand their horizons. Social withdrawal or disengagement from the community is negatively correlated with life satisfaction in both the young-old and the old-old.
3) *Adjusting to retirement and reduced income*
   The importance of one's job and income to self-concept and feelings of worth influence the ease with which the elderly navigate the hurdle of retirement. Careful planning of post retirement activities and choice of where to live geographically can ease the difficulty of this developmental task.
4) *Adjusting to death of a spouse*
   Losing one's life companion drains emotional resources and requires considerable adjustment.
5) *Establishing an explicit association with one's age group*
   Community organizations such as churches, neighborhoods, and clubs provide greatly needed opportunities to establish ties with other members of one's age group.

6) *Establishing satisfactory physical living arrangements*
The elderly need to have easy access to shopping, medical care, friends, and recreational activities that is not a burden to their adult children. Dependency (physical, financial, emotional, and total) is a major fear in old age.

## Depression

Depression is the most common psychiatric complaint among the elderly and accounts for as much as 50% of all mental disorders in the aged (Gatz, Smyer, & Lawton, 1980; Rosenfeld, 1978). A high suicide rate among older adults, especially white males, emphasizes the importance of treating depressive symptoms. Helplessness, pessimism, feelings of worthlessness, and despair are common symptoms (Gallagher, Thompson, & Levy, 1980). Depression in the elderly is difficult to treat because often there are real reasons for feeling depressed: failing health; loss of friends, spouses, and relatives; financial problems.

Intensifying the difficulty of treating depression in the older adult, is the likelihood that family and friends do not enjoy being around a depressed person who tends to be dependent and demanding. Depressed older adults need interventions that recognize their concerns as valid and that help them to mobilize their resources (Gatz, Smyer, & Lawton, 1980). Although the causes of depression in the elderly may differ from those in younger populations, there seems to be no relationship between age and outcome of psychotherapy and/or medication in treating depression (Rosenfeld, 1978, p. 133). Exercise also has been an effective treatment mode for older adults (Bennett, Carmack, & Gardner, 1982; Martinsen, Medhus, & Sandvik, 1985; Morgan et al., 1970; Uson & Larrosa, 1982; Valliant & Asu, 1985). Its efficacy will be reviewed later in this chapter.

## RETARDING THE AGING PROCESS WITH EXERCISE: THE RESEARCH

The aging process as just described sounds ominous and leaves one with a bleak picture of the future. However, there is emerging evidence that exercise can abate the severity of these changes. After years of conducting research in the area of exercise and aging, Shephard (1986a) concluded,

A well-designed training program not only increases life satisfaction, but also augments maximum oxygen intake by at least 20%, with associated increases of muscle strength and joint flexibility, dispersal of accumulated fat, and halting of bone mineral loss. The subsequent rate of aging is unchanged, but it takes many more years to reach the situation where working capacity is insufficient to meet the demands of either occupation or personal care (p. 41).

Older people who are physically active can be productive and strong throughout most of their lives. Many age-related changes in body composition, and in the cardiovascular and pulmonary systems can be ascribed to a sedentary lifestyle (Bortz, 1982). In fact, the results of a classic study indicate that the long-term consequences of inactivity are comparable to the incapacitating results of 20 days of complete bed rest (Saltin et al., 1968). As noted by Smith (1981), "Some of the current research suggests that *50% of the decline frequently attributed to physiological aging is, in reality, disuse atrophy* [italics added] resulting from inactivity in an industrialized world" (p. 16).

## Research Designs: A Note of Caution

The relationship between exercise and the aging process is difficult to investigate. For example, many fitness and training programs designed for the elderly attract only a select portion of older adults—those who are physically healthy and who see themselves as physically competent. Such volunteers, however, have been estimated to represent only 10% of a given population (Brown, & Shephard, 1967). This small number responding to exercise program opportunities may reflect the low status assigned to exercise by many Americans who matured before the current wave of exercise consciousness. Throughout the life cycle of many older adults, exercise was not valued, and its benefits were unknown. Today, older individuals who volunteer for exercise programs generally are more health conscious than those who do not volunteer, better educated, and tend to be from middle and upper socioeconomic groups (Conrad, 1976).

Because of the inherent differences between older people who exercise and those who do not, results of research studies using only exercise volunteers are difficult to interpret. For example, Lobstein, Mosbacher, & Ismail (1983) compared habitual joggers between the ages of 40 and 60 who had jogged at least 20 minutes three to six times a week for a minimum of three years with sedentary controls. The major difference between the two groups were the joggers' low depression scores as measured by the Minnesota Multiphasic Personality Inventory (Dahlstrom, Welsh, & Dahlstrom, 1979). Joggers also were significantly higher in extroversion than the non-exercisers. In a study like this, it is impossible to determine whether the exercise caused these changes, or whether the exercisers initially were different from the controls.

## Training Effects in the Elderly

Despite the design problems, it seems that physically active older women and men manifest training effects similar to those of younger

*AGING AND MOTOR BEHAVIOR*

individuals (e.g., Haber et al, 1984; Johannessen et al., 1986; Larsson, et al., 1984; Shephard, 1986b). For example in one study, men between the ages of 60 to 76 years trained three to four times a week for 30 to 60 minutes by running cross-country (Larsson et al., 1984). The runners had been physically active throughout their lives. They significantly decreased their resting heart rate, blood pressure, and body weight and also increased lean body mass. Similar results have been reported by Haber and colleagues (1984). Men and women between the ages of 67 and 76 who rode bicycle ergometers for three months decreased their submaximal exercise heart rates, increased their maximal workload, and increased in maximal $\dot{V}O_2$.

With intense training (80% of maximum predicted heart rate), $\dot{V}O_2$max has been shown to improve by 25%. Arteriovenous $O_2$ difference (the amount of oxygen extracted by the working muscles) increased by 14%, and submaximal heart rate decreased about 15% (Seals et al., 1984). As in younger populations, the training response is similar in men and women and is dependent on the intensity and duration of the program (Sidney & Shephard, 1978; Wells, 1985, p. 181). Although the absolute gains decrease with aging, many of the training effects seem likely to increase the quality and possibly the quantity of the residual lifespan (Shephard, 1986b).

## Specific Age-Retarding Effects of Exercise

Aging processes proceed more slowly in physically active individuals than in the general population. Dramatic changes can be made in the age-related deterioration curves of cardiovascular functioning, endurance, strength and psychomotor functioning (Spirduso, 1986). Exercise seems to reduce many of the ravages of age, resulting in a younger appearance, an increase in energy, and enhanced physical capabilities. More specifically, the older peson who is physically active

- can decrease the loss of physical stature until age 70 or possibly 90
- has less body fat
- can preserve lean body mass until the age of 80
- has fewer ECG abnormalities
- can increase his/her cardiorespiratory fitness
- experiences a smaller decrease in aerobic power
- can reduce the rate of bone demineralization
- may delay the onset of menopause (in women) and reduce the severity of its symptoms (Kavanagh & Shephard, 1977; Wells, 1986)

## Reaction Time and Exercise

Physically active individuals also have faster simple and choice reaction times than aged-matched sedentary controls. Physically active men and women have demonstrated a greater initiating motor response to visual and auditory stimuli (Spirduso, 1980, 1985, 1986). Physically active individuals regularly participated in athletic events including racquetball, squash, and handball at least three times a week for the previous six months (Spirduso & Clifford, 1978). As noted by Spirduso (1985),

> while exercise may certainly postpone some deterioration in reaction time to the extent that older exercisers sometimes have faster reaction time than young sedentary individuals, older exercisers as a group never have reaction times that are as fast as younger exercisers as a group. Nevertheless, the degree to which age-related deterioration can be postponed in both gross motor performance and psychomotor behavior with consistent practice . . . is quite remarkable. (Spirduso, 1985, p. 66).

It is unclear exactly how physical training of the whole body affects the performance of untrained single digit reaction time. Peripheral factors such as changes in morphology or in the electrical properties of motor units cannot account for the magnitude of the change in the elderly (Spirduso, 1980). The search for mechanisms which prolong the integrity of the motor system is just beginning. Spirduso (1982, 1986), however, has described a few possibilities. These include (1) enhanced blood flow to the brain, (2) neuroendocrine adaptations to exercise stress, (3) morphological brain changes that accompany motor activity, and (4) increased whole brain catecholamine levels resulting from exercise.

Studies of exercise-trained aged rats support the widespread physiological benefits of exercise. Trained rats have increased mitochondrial enzymes and coronary flow and develop greater peak systolic pressures in comparison to sedentary, age-matched controls (Starnes, Beyer, & Edington, 1983). Training also reduced the contraction duration and stiffness coefficient of heart muscle fibers to levels seen in young rats. This suggests that aspects of the contractile mechanism in the heart that decline with age are not fixed but can be modified (Spurgeon, Steinbach, & Lakatta, 1983). After a swimming-training program, an increase in the enzyme that is responsible for the regulation of contraction (Myosin ATPase) was observed in older rats. This represents a delay in the usual decline seen with aging (Rockstein, Chesky, & Lopez, 1981).

## Exercise May Increase Life Expectancy

The effect of exercise on longevity is a complex issue and has been widely debated. Current evidence supports the likelihood that regular physical activity increases *life expectancy*, but that it has a less dramatic effect on extending the actual *life span*. Fries and Crapo (1981) noted that the human life span is generally considered to be about 85 + 5 years. Of course, numerous moderating variables such as genetic influences, diet, and an inability to assign people randomly to exercise conditions complicate research projects using human subjects.

Animal studies allow control of such moderating variables and are a useful approach in gaining insight into the relationship between exercise and longevity even though the results are not directly applicable to human beings. In one study of male and female rats, "lifelong voluntary exercise" resulted in an 11.5% and 19.3% respective increases in *life expectancy* (Goodrick, 1980). In another study of rats (males only), wheel running led to a significantly longer *life span* than either sedentary free-eating or sedentary pair-weighted controls. The exercising rats, however, did not live as long as sedentary food-restricted rats (Holloszy et al., 1985). Thus, one value of exercise on longevity might be in its weight control benefits. As previously noted, data from animal studies is encouraging. It is impossible, however, to make predictions regarding longevity between species.

Life expectancy also seems to be sex-related with females outliving males in most species. Several hypotheses that might explain this include

1) decreased metabolic rate of women
2) decreased rate of atherogenesis in women
3) the presence of an extra X chromosome acting as a DNA reserve against sex chromosome damage,
4) hormonal differences between genders (Andres, Bierman, & Hazzard, 1985), and
5) lifestyle influences (Pelletier, 1981, p. 171).

Recent population studies support the likelihood that sufficient exercise can increase life expectancy (e.g., Paffenbarger et al., 1986; Paffenbarger, Wing, & Hyde, 1978). Harvard alumni ($N$ = 16,936) who exercised less than 2000 kcal a week had a 64% greater risk for myocardial infarction than those who exercised more (Paffenbarger, Wing, & Hyde, 1978). (See Figure 6-5 for the relationship between increased caloric expenditure and incidence of heart attack in specific age groups.)

More recently, it was reported that Harvard alumni who expended 2000 kcal or more per week had a mortality rate that was 24 to 33% lower than those who exercised less (Paffenbarger et al., 1986). Men who exercised more than 2000 kcal per week lived one to two years longer than those who exercised less, even when the influences of cigarette smoking, body weight, hypertension, and early parental death were controlled. Further substantiating the benefits of exercise was the consistent trend toward a lower death rate as energy expenditure increased from 500 to 2000 kcal per week. The maximal life span seems to be constant, or very slowly evolving (Fries, 1980; Jette & Branch, 1981). However, physical exercise can abate the age-related decline in organ performance.

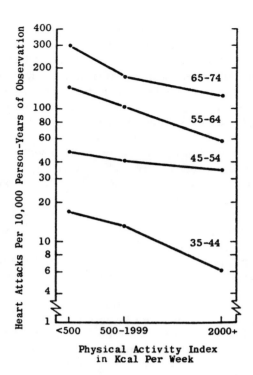

**FIGURE 6.5.** *Age-specific first heart attack rates, and physical activity index in a 6 to 10 year follow-up of Harvard male alumni. (From Paffenbarger et al., 1978, p. 166). Reprinted by permission.*

## PROGRAMS FOR THE ELDERLY DESIGNED TO ENHANCE PHYSICAL BENEFITS

In addition to the age-grading of exercise, two *fallacies* contribute to the small percentages of older people who are regular exercisers. The fallacies promoted by the age stratification of exercise activities need to be dispelled through educational programs before many elderly will consider a vigorous exercise program! These fallacies that prevent more extensive exercise participation by the elderly include the beliefs that:

1) a person needs less exercise as she or he ages (i.e., exercise is primarily for children), and
2) exercise is hazardous to the health of many older people either by
   a) precipitating a heart attack, or elevating blood pressure, or by
   b) exacerbating pre-existing medical conditions such as arthritis or Parkinsons disease.

One way to help elderly participants dispel such fallacies is to provide an exercise program that is initially closely supervised by a team of ex-

*AGING AND MOTOR BEHAVIOR*

perts such as a cardiologist, an exercise physiologist, and a sport psychologist. This has been done in an exercise study at Brooklyn College in which participants ranged in age from 65 to 80 years (Berger, Michielli, & Cohen, 1988). Psychological and physiological responses were monitored closely throughout a 12 week program. The participants grew more confident about their physical abilities, reported mood enhancement, and improved on a variety of fitness indices. They also recognized their need for exercise as illustrated by their actual hiring of the exercise leader to continue the exercise program as a group activity upon completion of the study.

As previously noted, nearly fifty percent of the functional decline in the elderly can be attributed to disuse (Smith, 1981). Thus, exercise training produces noticeable benefits for older adults who participate in a suitable program. Exercise programs of even moderate intensity can result in increased endurance, strength, flexibility and balance in older individuals who have been sedentary (Shephard, 1986b). With individualized planning, the same training principles regarding exercise intensity, duration, and frequency in younger individuals apply to older adults.

## Medical Clearance: A First Step

To participate in an exercise program, medical clearance by a physician is necessary for apparently healthy individuals over the age of 45 who previously have been sedentary (American College of Sports Medicine, 1986, p. 2). A maximal exercise test is desirable, but a submaximal test is useful in some circumstances to eliminate the possibility of exacerbating pre-existing medical problems. Even for people with medical problems, exercise often is desirable. Because of the benefits of exercise, Shephard (1986b) concluded that abnormal exercise electrocardiograms are no reason to prohibit physical activity in otherwise asymptomatic senior citizens. People with cardiovascular disease and other disabilities can exercise (Naughton, 1985). However, the guidelines for these individuals are beyond the scope of this chapter.

## Aerobic Component

After medical approval for a training program is obtained, the exercise prescription should be individualized. A stress test is useful in determining either maximal heart rate or oxygen uptake as target goals for the participant. Older adults with a mean age of 65 years who trained at 60% of their maximal $\dot{V}O_2$, three times a week (high frequency, high intensity), showed the greatest improvement in cardiovascular response from the sedentary state in comparison to individuals who exercised at lower intensity and frequency (Sidney & Shephard, 1978). (See Figure 6-6 for the considerably greater benefits of high frequency (HF), high intensity (HI) exercise in an elderly population.) If lower intensity (LI) exercise is

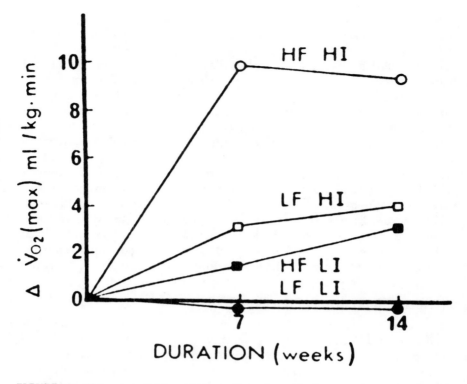

**FIGURE 6.6.** *Changes in predicted aerobic power with 7 and 14 weeks of training. Effects of frequency and intensity of effort. (From Sidney & Shephard, 1978, p. 127). Reprinted by permission*

employed, the duration and frequency of the training sessions should be increased to compensate. No training effect was seen when exercise was performed two days a week or less (LF) at a heart rate of 120 beats per minute (LI). When exercising at a heart rate of 120 beats per minute, three to four sessions per week were needed to achieve a significant but minimal training effect (Sidney & Shephard, 1978).

To further individualize exercise programs, the participants should be taught to monitor their own exercise heart rates, fatigue, and discomfort levels. Type of exercise also should be individualized. For example, people with joint pain should walk or swim rather than ride a bicycle for aerobic training. The aerobic benefits of fast walking are becoming increasingly accepted—especially in the elderly. For example, Pocari et al. (1987) found that 91% of the women and 83% of the men age 50 or older reached a training heart rate (70% of maximal heart rate) when they walked a mile as fast as possible.

*AGING AND MOTOR BEHAVIOR*

## Flexibility, Strength, and Balance Components

For a rounded fitness program, exercise sessions should include flexibility, strength building, and balance segments. These abilities, just like cardiorespiratory capabilities, decline with disuse and age (Bortz, 1982; Shephard, 1986b). Lack of flexibility, strength, and balance greatly diminishes the quality of life and may lead to even less physical activity (see Figure 6-1) and increased possibility of injury. Stretching exercises and Hatha yoga are recommended to promote flexibility which is important in reaching and twisting without pain. Working with free weights and weight machines such as the Universal or Nautilus equipment is an effective way to improve strength, increase lean muscle mass, tone muscles, and decrease osteoporosis. Dance and racquet sports help to improve balance and coordination, two factors which are important in avoiding falls.

## Conclusion: A Need for Organized Exercise Programs

How society as a whole should deal with exercise for the increasing proportion of the elderly is a complex issue. Despite the difficulties, however, systematic, well planned programs designed to improve the quality of life for older people are greatly needed.

Psychosocial considerations determine exercise compliance. On the basis of the emerging research, health care needs of older adults can be markedly reduced with balanced programs of exericse. To encourage the elderly to exercise, however, the "age-grading" that society has structured must change. Codes of "appropriate" behavior of the aging population generally have excluded exercise (Ostrow & Dzewaltowski, 1986; Ostrow, Jones, & Spiker, 1981; Ostrow, Keener, & Perry, 1986-87). Age-grading has created long term damage to how older people see themselves and to their perceived usefulness. It clearly has detracted from their active participation in society.

Enjoyment of the activity is of great importance in encouraging exercise compliance (Wankel & Kreisel, 1985). Psychological factors and the type of exercise selected are important determinants of lifelong participation. If an exerciser is bored, frustrated, or overburdened by the regimen, attrition will increase and the possible benefits are of no value. In conclusion, a personally tailored exercise program can do much to improve physical well being and to retard the functional decline of the aging adult. However, a variety of psychological factors must be considered when designing exercise programs for the elderly—or for anyone.

## PSYCHOLOGICAL BENEFITS OF EXERCISE FOR OLDER ADULTS

The popular press has publicized the exciting possibilities that exercise is accompanied by reductions in undesirable mood states such as anxiety, depression, anger, and fatigue. However until recently, Morgan and associates (Bahrke & Morgan, 1978; Greist et al., 1979; Morgan, 1979, 1980, 1987) were the few researchers conducting sequential research in the area. In these studies, differences in methodological procedures such as mood measures, types of exercise, and the exercise parameters of intensity and duration make it difficult to ascertain the types of exercise programs that maximize the mood benefits. The exciting aspect within this diversity, however, is the general conclusion that people do "feel better" after exercising (Berger, 1984a, 1984b; Berger & Owen, 1983, in press, 1988; Morgan & Goldston, 1987; Sachs & Buffone, 1984). Although relatively few studies in the massive exercise and mental health literature have focused specifically on elderly exercisers, the elderly who have been tested did report a variety of psychological benefits (Blumenthal et al., 1982; deVries & Adams, 1972; Hogan & Santomier, 1984; Olson, 1975; Sidney & Shephard, 1976).

## Need to Investigate Activities Other Than Jogging— Especially for the Elderly

Many mood and exercise studies have been confined to running programs. This narrow focus reflects the large number of researchers who jog (e.g., Sachs & Buffone, 1984) and the widespread interest in running as a vehicle for establishing cardiovascular health (e.g., Kavanagh & Shephard, 1977; Kavanagh et al., 1977). The research on jogging, however, is of little value to a large portion of the aging population. As noted by Berger and Owen (1983, 1988), there is a great need to investigate the psychological benefits of exercise other than jogging. Such information would be of particular value to the elderly, overweight, individuals with overuse injuries or other disabilities, and people who simply do not enjoy the activity.

## Methodological Considerations

It is encouraging to note that highly disparate studies support the possibility that physical activity in older people is associated with mood enhancement and improved mental health and a few, diverse studies are now reviewed. However, as Berger (1984a) and Folkins and Sime (1981) have noted, there are methodological problems in this newly developed area of research. Restricting the number of studies to those employing older subjects further limits the quality of developmental research. Locating a large number of participants, randomly assigning participants to treatments, and periodical testing of the same subjects would greatly enhance psychological studies of exercise and elderly populations. Shephard and Sidney (1979) have described a few experimental concerns that tend to result in "false positive" psychological results of exercise:

1) favorable attitudes to exercise prior to initiation of the study,
2) attitudes reflected by program advertising, and exercise leaders,
3) medical and personal attention received during training and testing, and
4) desire to please investigators.

## Fitness and Personality: The Research

Comparing regular and non-regular exercisers during a four year period, Young and Ismail (1977) concluded that the relationship between fitness and self-confidence is stable over a long period of time. Participants ($N$ = 48) with a mean age of 43 years were separated into three groups:

- those who were regularly active before and after 1971 (Group 1, $n$ = 16),
- those who were inactive before 1971, participated in a semester-long exercise program, and remained active for the subsequent 3½ years (Group 2, $n$ = 16), and
- those who were inactive before 1971, participated in the fitness program for a semester, and became inactive again (Group 3, $n$ = 16).

As expected, the first two active groups improved in physical fitness during a four year period (Young & Ismail, 1977). The group that was most active of the three was significantly more confident and emotionally secure as measured by the Cattell 16 Personality Factor Questionnaire, *16 PF* (Cattell, Eber, & Tatsuoka, 1970) administered at the beginning of the study than was Group 3. The group that was physically active prior to the study continued to report more confidence and security than the other two groups even after four years of exercise. From these results, it seems that people who seek exercise may differ in personality from those who do not.

In a second study, Young and Ismail (1978) further investigated the relationship between fitness and mental health. Men between 21 and 61 years of age were divided into high ($n$ = 14) and low ($n$ = 14) fitness groups. All subjects were participants in a four month program of jogging, calisthenics, and recreational activities and volunteered to be in the study. As indicated by their scores on the Cattell 16 PFQ, the high-fitness group was more unconventional, imaginative, adventurous, and trustful than those in the low fit group when measured at the beginning of the study and after four months of participation. Again, highly fit individuals reported more positive personality characteristics than those who were less fit. These initial differences, however, were not affected by a four month exercise program. The 16 PFQ may not be an appropriate inven-

tory to measure change since it measures stable personality characteristics.

Further illustrating an association between exercise and personality,
middle-aged (40 to 59 years) runners and joggers who exercised three
days a week and covered at least two miles a session were significantly
more intelligent, imaginative, self-sufficient, reserved, sober, shy and
forthright than the general population as measured by the Cattell 16
PFQ (Hartung & Farge, 1977). Employing self-selected joggers, however
*prohibited a causal interpretation.* Individuals who are intelligent, self-
sufficient, and imaginative may be more able and motivated to schedule
exercise as part of their daily routine than those who are not.

## Exercise and Life Satisfaction

There is an impressively high correlation between physical activity
and life satisfaction (Heinzelman & Bagley, 1970; Schaie & Geiwitz,
1982). These studies suggest that older people who are physically active
have more positive attitudes toward work, are in better health, report
more stamina, and report greater ability to cope with stress and tension.
More specifically, Heinzelman and Bagley reported that men (N = 381)
between the ages of 45 and 59 significantly improved in a variety of life
qualities after exercising three times a week for 18 months. Major
changes reported by the exercisers were in

1) increased work performance and in attitudes toward work,
2) personal health such as increased stamina, stress reduction, and
   more positive feelings about weight reduction, and
3) habit behavior which reflected increased walking, stair use, and
   decreased use of the automobile.

The relationship between exercise, life satisfaction, and personality
is complex in people of all ages. As reported by Neugarten, Havighurst,
and Tobin (1968), people with well-adjusted, "integrated" personalities
usually are satisfied with life *regardless of their activity levels.* In contrast, people with "unintegrated" personalities often are dissatisfied with their
lives regardless of their exercise levels. Exercise and activity in general
have the greatest influence on life satisfaction in people who are between
these two extremes. For example, people with "armored" personalities
(ambitious and striving individuals who need to control impulses and
emotions) use high activity levels to defend against the idea of growing
old.

Low levels of activity are very disturbing to these people. Similarly,
passive-dependent persons need interactions; they need people to
talk to, people to help them make decisions. Without activity, they
fall into apathy and depression (Schaie & Geiwitz, 1982, p. 263).

**Happiness:** Recently, Rosenberg (1986) has cast doubt on the direct correlation between membership in sport groups and happiness in adults between 55 and 75+ years of age (N = 468). There was a significant, positive relationship between the number of voluntary associations (regardless of type) in which one was a member and avowed happiness. When examining only the number of sport associations to which one belonged, however, there was no relationship to happiness. Older people in three different age groups (55 to 64; 65 to 74; 75+) were no happier if they had a membership in a sports group than if they had memberships in non-sport organizations. This finding is not surprising. Formal membership in sports organizations—especially at 65 years of age—may be quite different from being physically active. A problem with this interesting study was the small cell frequencies for those participating in sports groups which detracted from the power of the statistical analyses.

**Self-Efficacy:** One way that physical activity is associated with life satisfaction is by an increase in self-efficacy. Self-efficacy is the belief that one is capable of executing a particular task. In other words, self-efficacy denotes personal feelings of competency and ability. People who feel competent generally attempt to perform a wider variety of activities than those who feel less competent. Because of ageism in American society, older people often hold misconceptions about their physical abilities (Hogan & Santomier, 1984). Enhanced feelings of physical self-efficacy seem likely to increase the activity levels of the elderly.

In the only psychological study of swimming and older adults (age 60 and older) of which we are aware, beginning swimmers met for five weeks of instruction at a local YMCA (Hogan & Santomier, 1984). In comparison to a non-swimming group of controls (n = 33), swimmers (n = 32) reported significantly larger changes in self-efficacy regarding swimming. In addition, 78% of the swimmers reported increased feelings of competency in general. Examples of the generalizations from swimming to other skills included, "I am able to do things more easily now—swimming and chores" (Hogan & Santomier, 1984, p. 295).

**Self-Concept, Self-Esteem, and Body Image:** Another way in which exercise might increase life satisfaction in the elderly is by enhancing the participant's body image, self-concept, and self-esteem. (See Berger [1984b] for a general discussion of these concepts and their relationship to physical activity.) Researchers have observed a positive and significant correlation between physical activity and self-concept in a wide range of exercisers: male rehabilitation clients (Collingwood, 1972), obese male teenagers (Collingwood & Willett, 1971), and elementary school children of both sexes (Martinek, Cheffers, & Zaichkowsky, 1978).

Attitudes in regard to the physical image and the capabilities of one's body are important determinants of overall self-concept and body image (e.g., Berger, 1984b). In one of the few studies of body image and exercise in an older population, nursing home residents participated in rhythmic breathing, slow stretching, and upright exercises for eight weeks (15 sessions). Their body image scores improved significantly (Olson, 1975). Sidney and Shephard (1976) also reported increases in body image scores for elderly subjects (mean age = 66) following a program consisting of endurance activities for one hour per day, four days a week over a 14 week period. Exercise seems to be associated with increased feelings of pride and self confidence in a variety of populations including the elderly.

**Life Quality:** Life quality refers to "the degree to which an individual or a society is able to satisfy its perceived psychophysiologic needs" (Dalkey, Lewis, & Snyder, 1972). The Pflaum Life Quality Inventory has been employed in several exercise studies, and measures the degree to which the environment is perceived as facilitating one's functioning in four general areas of daily living: biophysical, self-concept, primary social (personal relationships), and secondary social (relationships in institutional settings such as work, personal reputation), (Pflaum, 1973). As noted by Morris et al. (1982), "life quality" refers to a state of excellence.

Improvement in life quality has been reported by college students who participated in an endurance conditioning program (Morris & Husman, 1978). Recently, Morris et al. (1982) reported on the life quality of 10 women athletes who were in Masters competition, were at least 40 years of age, and were of national caliber. The runners were significantly higher in life quality ($p < .01$) than the normative group of nonrunning adults. Although there are no data concerning life quality and exercise in the elderly, it would seem that life quality in this group would be affected by exercise as the participants noticed and enjoyed the psychophysiological changes. A study at Brooklyn College is presently underway to test this possibility (Berger et al., 1988).

## Decreased Stress After Exercise

Research on exercise and mental health emphasizes that systematic exercise helps to reduce physical and psychological stress symptoms (e.g., Berger, 1987; deVries, 1981; Long, 1983; Morgan, 1987). Stress is a pervasive health problem in modern Western societies. It occurs within the individual in response to events that excite, frighten, irritate, confuse, or endanger. Stress results from a person's negative appraisal of a situation. It causes a variety of psychological and physical responses (Berger, 1983/1984).

Certainly not all stress is to be avoided! Some stress adds zest to life and has been called "eustress" to distinguish it from "distress." However, too much stress results in increased illness and mortality rates (Benson, 1975; Lynch, 1975). Coronary heart disease, stroke, ulcers, rheumatoid arthritis, and even cancer are a few diseases which occur more frequently in stressed than in relaxed individuals (e.g., Levy, 1983).

The elderly are just as prone to stress as are younger members of the population. In fact, the elderly encounter numerous stressful events:

- retirement
- inflation and the economic woes of living on fixed incomes
- decreased physical abilities such as decreased visual and auditory acuity
- undesirable changes in appearance (wrinkles, loss of muscle tone, increased body fat, age spots, and skin blemishes)
- arthritic joints
- chronic illnesses
- the death of spouse and friends

**Exercise: Ideal for Stress Reduction:** Because of its psychological and physiological benefits, exercise is an ideal stress reduction technique for older adults. It is accompanied by reductions in anxiety, depression, and anger—three common psychological stress symptoms. Exercise also improves several other psychological stress symptoms by enhancing the participants' vigor and clear-mindedness (decisiveness). In addition, regular exercise reduces several physical stress symptoms: elevated heart rate, blood pressure, obesity, and general muscular tension (deVries, 1981; Sharkey, 1984).

Exercise has specific advantages when it is compared to other stress reduction techniques. In contrast to biofeedback, it requires no complicated equipment. The side effects of drugs are avoided, and a variety of physical benefits accrue: weight reduction, improved appearance, and increased energy and cardiovascular endurance (Berger, 1986).

**Decreases in Anxiety and Muscular Tension:** People from "normal" populations, i.e., those who are not clinically anxious, report short-term or "acute" decreases in state anxiety, but no long-term reductions in anxiety after exercising (e.g., Berger, 1984a; Berger, Friedmann, & Eaton, in press). Thus, people from nonclinical populations need to exercise regularly to maintain the acute benefits. In contrast, people who are clinically anxious report both "chronic" (long-term) and acute decreases in anxiety after exercising (Berger, 1984a, 1987; Morgan 1979; Sachs & Buffone, 1984).

Although much of the research has focused on college students and other young adult populations, there is little reason to assume that the psychological benefits of exercise are age related. If the benefits are physiologically based (increased strength and endurance, decreased systolic blood pressure, improved appearance, increased body temperature, practiced stress response), the benefits should exist for the old as well as the young. If the benefits of exercise are primarily psychological ("time out" from worries, feelings of accomplishment, social interaction, and the psychological concomitants of delaying the aging process) they should occur in the elderly as well as in younger populations. However, rather than extrapolate the results of studies on younger people, further research is needed to directly investigate the psychological benefits of exercise in the elderly. Results of a few studies of the stress reducing benefits of exercise for older people suggest that properly conducted exercise programs for older populations are stress reducing and are accompanied by a host of psychological benefits such as the reduction of anxiety and depression (e.g., Blumenthal et al., 1982; Long, 1983).

In an unusually well-designed study, Long (1983) compared the stress reduction benefits of a walk-jog program with those of stress innoculation (changing self-statements in anxiety producing situations) and a waiting list control group. As illustrated in Figure 6-7, participants in both the walk-jog and stress innoculation programs reported significantly less tension, state anxiety, and trait anxiety after 10 weeks of practice. The men and women ($N$ = 73) in the two stress reduction activities met for an hour and a half once a week in supervised sessions during the 10 weeks. In addition, the exercisers were required to practice independently at least twice a week. Results of this study are particularly interesting because it is one of the few to focus on exercise and stress reduction in older individuals. Participants were volunteers who ranged in age between 24 and 65 years, with a mean age of 39.9. The subjects felt that they were unusually stressed and needed help to reduce their stress levels. Results indicated that exercisers who were in the top half of fitness improvement at the end of the program reported no greater stress reduction benefits than those whose fitness levels improved less. Because of this, Long concluded that the psychological aspects rather than the actual amount of change in aerobic fitness were responsible for the reductions in stress.

In one of the few studies of muscular tension and exercise in older adults, deVries and Adams (1972) investigated the tranquilizing effects of exercise. Volunteers (6 men; 4 women) in the study ranged in age from 52 to 70 years. They were recruited by advertisements for individuals who felt that they had sleep difficulties. They were generally nervous, tense, irritable, restless, panicky, worried, and under stress. These subjects scored in the 87th percentile for anxiety on the Taylor Manifest Anxiety Scale (Taylor, 1953) and served as their own controls in a double blind study. The participants were tested before and after each of the following five treatment conditions. Subjects were assigned randomly to treatment and were tested three times for the same treatment for a total of 15 trials. The treatments were as follows:

1) 400 meg meprobamate,
2) placebo,
3) 15 minutes of walking at a heart rate of 100 beats per minute,

*AGING AND MOTOR BEHAVIOR*

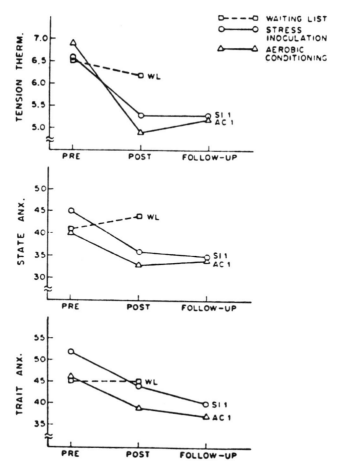

**FIGURE 6.7.** *Mean ratings of change on measures of stress before and after treatment, and at a three-month follow-up. (From Long, 1983, p. 180). Reprinted by permission.*

4) 15 minutes of walking at a heart rate of 120 beats per minute or,
5) a control situation in which the subjects read (deVries & Adams, 1972).

Electromyographic recordings from the biceps indicated the subjects' muscle action potential, a physiological measure of stress. The participants' muscle action potential was tested at rest and following "mental stress" induced by asking the subjects to perform a mental arithmetic task. Electrical muscle activity decreased significantly after walking for fifteen minutes at a heart rate of 100 beats per minute, but not after walking at a rate of 120 beats per minute. Neither the placebo or control groups also reported any changes. Meprobamate, a common tranquilizer,

*PSYCHOLOGICAL WELL-BEING*                                                      **143**

did not produce a relaxation effect. It should be noted, however, that the 400 mg dosage was very low. Low intensity exercise of only 15 minutes produced a desirable tranquilizing effect as indicated by EMG recordings.

**Decreases in Depression:** In a classic study of depression and exercise, Morgan et al., (1970) administered the Zung Self-Rating Depression Scale (Zung, 1965) to men ($N$ = 67) between 26 and 55 years of age (mean = 40 years). No relationship was observed between depression and age, or the physiological parameters of weight, percent body fat, grip strength or physical work capacity. These subjects and an additional 34 participants (total $N$ = 101) then were presented with the option of participating in either a jogging, swimming, treadmill-running, or bicycle ergometry training program three times a week for six weeks, or to serve as sedentary controls. Results indicated that exercise was not associated with changes in the depression scores of these subjects. However, the eleven participants who scored high in depression (50 or more on the Zung Depression Scale) at the beginning of the study reported significant decreases in depression. Thus, training was beneficial to those who initially were quite depressed.

In a study of older adults between the ages of 60 and 80 years, Uson and Larrosa (1982) reported that 70% of those who exercised for an hour twice a week for nine months reported reductions in depression as measured by Zung's Depression Inventory Scale. In contrast, 40% of age-matched individuals who belonged to clubs for retired persons increased in depression. The authors provided no explanation of the increase in depression other than it was "a fact which gives an idea of the rapid deterioration of these persons" (Uson & Larrosa, 1982). The supervised exercise program included warm-ups, flexibility and abdominal strength exercises, and a slowly paced 10-minute run. Exercisers also improved on measures of neuroticism and reported decreases in the number of psychosomatic complaints and doctor visits.

Valliant and Asu (1985) also investigated the influence of exercise on depression and locus of control in men and women who were between the ages of 50 and 80 ($N$ = 114). Participants in a 12-week supervised exercise program met twice a week for sixty minutes ($n$ = 30). Three other groups were employed for the purpose of comparing pre-activity scores of participants in differing types of activity: one group exercised independently on their own; one group was socially active in weekly parties, cards and bingo; and the final group was composed of individuals who never engaged in physical activity. The $n$'s were not provided for any of these last three groups.

Results of the pre-, post-exercise program indicated that participants in the supervised exercise group decreased in body fat, body weight and depression as measured by the Minnesota Multiphasic Personality Inventory (Dahlstrom, Welsh, & Dahlstrom, 1979). Since only one set of scores were collected for the other three groups (non-exercisers, the socially active group, and the independent exercisers), no change data were available. Examining pre-activity scores of the four groups, it was concluded that when age was employed as a covariate on the initial scores, the two groups of exercisers (supervised and independent) were significantly more depressed and thinner than the non-exercisers and more socially active. This observation of initially high depression scores in exercisers indicated that the elderly who were "less satisfied with life" were more motivated to exercise than were the comparison groups.

In another study of exercise and depression, Bennett, Carmack, & Gardner (1982) evaluated the effects of exercise in 38 elderly nursing home residents and senior community center participants. The participants included three males and 35 females between the ages of 50 and 98 years. The eight-week exercise program included two 45 minutes sessions a week. The relatively mild program included only balance and flexibility exercises. Exercisers who showed signs of clinical depression on the Zung Self-Rating Depression Scale reported significantly less depression at the end of the eight weeks of exercise.

Results of a final study of exercise and depression supported a decrease in depression for an older psychiatric population (Martinsen, Medhus, & Sandvik, 1985). Depressed male and female psychiatric patients ranging in age from 17 to 60 years (mean age = 40) were randomly assigned to an occupational therapy-control group ($n$ = 19) or to an exercise group ($n$ = 24). Exercisers participated in supervised aerobic exercise at 50 to 70% of their maximum aerobic capacity three times a week. Initially, the two groups did not differ in depression as measured by the Beck Depression Inventory and the Psychopathological Rating Scale (Asberg et al., 1978; Beck et al., 1961). After exercising for nine weeks, the exercisers increased in aerobic capacity and decreased in depression. Thus among exercisers of all ages, a moderate-intensity training program has been associated with significant antidepressive benefits—particularly among the highly depressed.

## Attitudes of the Elderly Toward Exercise: Ageism

Many older individuals do not have accurate information about exercise that would enable them to exercise independently on their own. Ageism—prejudicial and discriminatory views about aging—is rampant in American society, and is especially pronounced in the context of exercise (Ostrow, 1983). Thus, organized exercise programs, individualized for the needs of various subpopulations, are greatly required to combat the exercise stereotypes. Investigation of the attitudes of senior citizens toward activity show that the elderly believe that the need for activity declines with age (Conrad, 1976). As previously noted, older people tend to consider exercise to be dangerous. Since the elderly vary widely in physical ability, there is a great need for supervised, individualized exercise programs. Graded exercise programs should be designed to help the elderly to develop and discover their physical capabilities, to increase their strength and energy levels, and to promote flexibility and cardiovascular efficiency.

The elderly have been stereotyped as being generally in poor health, decrepit, forgetful, withdrawn and isolated, incapable of learning new things, and less likely to participate in physical activities (e.g., McTavish, 1971; Ostrow, 1983). As reported by Ostrow (1983),

> These diminished self-expectancies, coupled with social expectations that one should act his age and that one should be less competitive and expect less from a competitive outcome, lead many individuals to gradually disengage from sport and physical activity as they grow older (p. 159).

Supporting the stereotype of a decreased need for physical activity with increasing age, Ostrow, Jones, & Spiker (1981) reported that a person's age significantly predicted whether nursing students ($N$ = 93) considered exercise to be appropriate for that individual. The Activity Appropriateness Scale was especially designed to investigate the nurses' perception of the appropriateness of twelve different sport activities such as archery and marathoning for various age groups (Ostrow, Jones, & Spiker, 1981). Results indicated that the student nurses viewed physical activity as increasingly "less appropriate" as the participant increased in age from 20 to 40 to 60 to 80 years. In fact, the participant's age was a far more important influence on exercise appropriateness than was the participant's sex. Thus, it seems that age role expectations are learned early in life. These results are particularly important because nurses often determine the activities that are available to the elderly living in nursing homes.

As noted earlier in this chapter, research on age-grading among preschool children (Ostrow, Keener, & Perry, 1986-87) and among older adults themselves (Ostrow & Dzewaltowski, 1986) supported the pervasiveness of ageism in reference to exercise. Age-grading by older adults would seem to be a major barrier to increasing the number of elderly who exercise and to increasing exercise intensity among those who are physically active.

## EXERCISE PROGRAMS TO ENHANCE THE PSYCHOLOGICAL BENEFITS

Although the relationship between exercise and mood is not fully understood, the psychological benefits are impressive. Exercise is associated with decreases in anxiety, depression, anger, confusion, and fatigue, and with increases in self-concept, self-esteem and vigor (e.g., Berger, 1984a, 1984b, 1987; Blumenthal et al., 1982; Morgan, 1987; Morgan & Goldston, 1987; Sachs & Buffone, 1984). However, *not all types of exercise* are stress reducing. In fact, athletic competition and exhausting exercise are stress producing!

Maximal psychological benefits can be gleaned if exercise programs are tailored to the needs of various subgroups in the elderly population. Individualization of exercise programs according to *individual psychological needs* maximize the benefits. The most successful participants in physical activity are those who exercise in programs where attainable performance goals are set (Ostrow, 1984). Unrealistic goal setting and under or overestimation of performance ability cause frustration and lead to failure.

Emphasis on educating the elderly regarding the benefits of exercise should include descriptions of the psychological and physiological benefits and guidelines for obtaining these effects. In addition, competent exercise leaders with the adjunct support of sport psychologists can help the elderly discover and develop new physical capabilities, decrease anxiety and depression, and improve their self-concepts, self-image, self-efficacy, and the quality of life. Feelings of mastery and personal choice as well as exercise adherence are enhanced when exercise programs include novelty and freedom of choice (Wankel & Kreisel, 1985; Whitehouse, 1977). Involvement of friends or spouses provide mutual support and serve as motivators for regular exercise participation (Franklin, 1978).

**Enjoyment is a Critical Feature:** A general requirement of programs for enhancing psychological well-being is that the exercise sessions are enjoyable (Berger & Owen, 1987; Wankel & Kreisel, 1985). Although exercise has been shown to be mood enhancing, it does not occur in *all* situations or for all individuals! Unpleasant environmental influences such as extreme heat or cold, and exercising so intensely that it becomes unpleasant can negate the stress reduction benefits (Berger & Owen, 1986, 1987, 1988). For example, in a study conducted during an intense, five week summer school session, Berger and Owen (1986) were surprised to find no evidence of the expected relationship between mood and swimming. It seemed that the accidentally hot air and water temperatures (over 90° on the day of testing) negated the previously observed stress reducing benefits associated with swimming (Berger & Owen, 1983, in press).

Results of another study investigating the mood benefits of swimming, body conditioning, Hatha yoga, and fencing in college students indicated that exercise that is too intense may not be stress reducing (Berger & Owen, 1988). Body conditioning, a combination of jogging and weight training, was associated with significant increases in fatigue, but with no other mood benefits. The absence of stress reduction benefits was surprising because jogging (½ of the course) is stress reducing, and weight training has been positively related to self concept and positive moods (e.g., Freedson et al., 1983; Morgan & Goldston, 1987; Sachs & Buffone, 1984). Inspection of class procedures indicated that the exercise intensity was high rather than moderate. A goal of the instructor, an exercise physiologist, was to facilitate maximal aerobic and muscular fitness. Thus, the jogging portion was not long, slow distances, but interval training at 90% age-adjusted maximal heart rate. This rigorous approach to exercise was reflected in the significant increase in fatigue scores and the significantly larger number of students (12 of an initial 28) who dropped out of the course. Results of a recent study of swimmers supported the likelihood that fatigue producing exercise may not be mood enhancing (Berger & Owen, 1988). The absence of mood changes in intense exercise further supported the suggestion that exercise be pleasing and of moderate intensity. Additional research is needed to determine the exercise parameters of intensity, duration, and frequency that enhance the psychological benefits of exercise.

If one type of exercise is unpleasant to an older person, she or he would be well-advised to seek alternate forms of activity. For example, a person who is bored with walking could try walking with a partner, Hatha yoga, aerobic dance, or swimming. Some people enjoy the social atmosphere of exercising in a group; others might feel self-conscious and prefer exercising at home alone. In addition to the enjoyment quality, physical activities that promote abdominal breathing, are non-competitive, and predictable are likely to promote exercise and mood alteration and psychological well-being.

**Rhythmical Abdominal Breathing, or the "Aerobic" Requirement:** The need for aerobic exercise is frequently cited in the literature (e.g., Berger, 1986; Berger & Owen, 1983, 1988; Goldwater & Collis, 1985). However, there is little research directly investigating the need for an aerobic quality to enhance the psychological benefits of exercise. The psychological effects of non-aerobic activities have been neglected except for a study comparing the mood benefits of swimming, Hatha yoga, body conditioning, and fencing (Berger & Owen, 1988). Hatha yoga clearly is not aerobic, yet the participants in two different classes reported significant decreases in psychological stress. More specifically, they reported less anxiety, tension, depression, anger, and confusion immediately after yoga sessions than before class on three different occasions. Hatha yoga and many aerobic types of exercise facilitate rhythmical, abdominal breathing.

Perhaps it is the rhythmical breathing, rather than the aerobic quality, that facilitates stress reduction. Since the elderly tend to be cautious about taxing their hearts with aerobic exercise, it is encouraging to note

that aerobic exercise may not be a prerequisite for stress reduction benefits. Additional research is clearly needed to directly investigate the aerobic facet of exercise prescription for influencing mental health. At the
present time, it seems that older individuals can "ease" into exercise with
a moderate program, reap some of the psychological benefits, condition
their bodies, and gain confidence before contemplating aerobic programs
for cardiorespiratory conditioning.

**Absence of Interpersonal Competition:** Physical activities provide
opportunity for competition against one's self, but they vary widely in
the necessity of competing against others. Since interpersonal competition often is stress producing, competition should be avoided *if relaxation is
a major goal.* (An exception to this requirement can be made for individuals
who are noncompetitive in activities such as tennis and ping-pong.)

Glasser (1976) has noted the importance of an absence of competition in his discussion of exercise and positive addictions. [Positive addiction (PA), in direct contrast to negative addiction, leads to confidence,
creativity, happiness, and health]. Glasser emphasized, "Not only *must we
not compete with others,* we must learn *not to compete with ourselves* [italics added]
if we want to reach the PA state" (p. 57).

**Closed, Predictable Activities:** Highly predictable activities such as
swimming, jogging, and calisthenics have been described as "closed,"
"temporally and spatially certain," and "predictable" (e.g., Berger, 1972;
Singer & Gerson, 1981). Self-paced, predictable activities allow participants to "tune out" or to disassociate from the environment. In closed
activities, exercisers can engage in free association while exercising, and
temporarily escape from daily stressors and hassles. This "time-out" opportunity may be especially beneficial to older people who are beseiged
with seemingly insurmountable problems such as illness and dwindling
fixed incomes.

Glasser (1976, p. 93) supported the importance of predictability
when he noted that activities which do not require great mental effort
are likely to become positive addictions. Swimming, jogging, and Hatha
yoga are highly predictable activities. Swimmers often note appreciation
of the creativity of thoughts produced while exercising, of the empty
time for focusing on their own thoughts, and of the solitude; Hatha yoga
participants enjoy the quiet, inward focus of their exercise activity.

**Exercise Frequency:** Participants become progressively more fit and
able to enjoy the physical exertion when they exercise regularly (Berger,
1986; Glasser, 1976; p. 123). In practical terms, this means there is a need
·to exercise in the same activity at least twice, and preferably three times a
week. Habitual exercisers learn to pace themselves, to relax while exercising, and to interpret various physical sensations. These abilities are
especially important for the elderly who may be unaccustomed to exercising. Another reason for the need to exercise regularly is that in members

of a psychologically "normal" population, the psychological benefits are short-term. Thus most participants need to exercise frequently to retain the benefits.

**Moderate Intensity:** It is not clear exactly whether a person needs light, moderate, or high intensity exercise to maximize the psychological benefits. At the present time, moderate exercise seems to be the best choice. Some researchers indicated that *high intensity* exercise (80 to 100% age adjusted maximal heart rate) may be stress reducing. (See Berger, (1984a) and Dishman (1986) for reviews of this literature.) deVries (1981) has recommended *low intensity* exercise for older people as reflected by 30 to 60% of the difference between resting and maximal heart-rate values. As previously noted, elderly men and women who walked for 15 minutes at a relatively low exercise heart rate of 100 beats per minute significantly reduced electrical activity in their muscles (deVries & Adams, 1972). Exercise that is between 50 and 65% of one's age-adjusted maximal heart rate generally is considered to be *light in intensity*.

Research supports the likelihood of stress reduction with *moderate intensity exercise* (60 to 75% of one's age-adjusted maximal heart rate). Dishman (1986) recently concluded, "it appears that an intensity exceeding *70% of $\dot{V}O_2max$ or age-adjusted HR* for *at least 20 minutes* [italics added], is needed to insure an accurate reduction [in anxiety] (p. 311). For the elderly, and possibly for younger populations, exercise intensity probably should be moderate, rather than mild or intense (Berger, 1986; Berger & Owens, 1987). High intensity exercise (75% + of age-adjusted maximal heart rate) probably does not help reduce stress for most participants (e.g., Berger & Owen, 1987; 1988). The relationship between exercise intensity and mood alteration needs further clarification.

**Duration: At Least 20 to 30 Minutes:** Initially 20 to 30 minutes might seem to be a long time for exercising to many older persons. However by beginning gradually, monitoring their target heart rates, and slowly increasing the duration, most healthy people in their 60's, 70's, and even 80's can exercise for this length of time. In the study of exercise and aging presently underway at Brooklyn College, several different groups of exercisers have increased their initial exercise sessions of 20 minutes to nearly 75 minutes (Berger et al., 1988). The 20 to 30 minute session is a minimal amount of time suggested (Berger, 1986). Glasser (1976) has suggested an hour, and habitual exercisers may choose to exercise for this length of time to maximize the psychological benfits.

## CONCLUSIONS AND DIRECTIONS FOR FUTURE RESEARCH

The conceptualization of old age as a time for rest and disengagement is changing. New role models are evolving as the healthy old are exploring unchartered possibilities and are challenging society's rules and norms. With the aid of a physically active lifestyle, a person can be physically capable, energetic, and an exercise participant *long beyond* the ages of 50, 60, and 70! With advancing age, exercise becomes increasingly important as a way to maintain psychological and physical well-being.

It is hoped that this chapter will serve as a catalyst for professionals now working with the elderly to develop exercise programs that encourage the elderly to *explore, develop, and extend their physical capabilities.* Most older individuals need encouragement and supervision in their exercise programs if strenuous physical activity is to become an integral part of their lives.

Throughout this chapter, we have presented our beliefs as well as the research data that suggest exercise can enhance the quality of life in older individuals, and perhaps extend life expectancy. We are the first to recognize, however, that there are many research issues that need resolution before exercise programs can be designed that maximize the exciting psychological benefits. Despite the never ending need for additional research, there are enough data which suggest that certain types of exercise promote psychological and physical well being. It is time to develop exercise programs based on the present state of knowledge.

We have summarized much of the psychological literature related to exercise in the elderly to integrate a diverse body of literature. One purpose of this review and synthesis was to enable researchers focusing on the psychosocial aspects of exercise for the elderly to explore a wide variety of issues and topics. It is hoped that a new generation of researchers will continue to explore the following areas:

1) The role of exercise and diet in preventing, delaying, and possibly reversing *osteoporosis,*
2) The influence of exercise on *cognitive functioning* throughout the lifespan,
3) The influence of *previous exercise and sport experiences* on current exercise beliefs and habits in the elderly,
4) The complex interrelationships between *psychological stress, exercise, and the aging process,*
5) *Therapeutic use of exercise* in treating elderly patients with anxiety and depression,
6) The relationships between exercise and *self-concept, self-esteem, and body-image* in older adults,
7) The influence of exercise on *life satisfaction and quality of life* in the elderly,
8) The influence of *gender* on the type and extent of psychological benefits associated with exercise in senior citizens,
9) Delineation of *exercise modes* (e.g., aerobic versus anaerobic, com-

petitive versus noncompetitive) that are stress reducing in the elderly,

10) *Intensity, duration, and frequency guidelines* for exercise programs that promote mood alteration in older populations,

11) Possible *mechanisms* that mediate the relationship between exercise and mood alteration in senior citizens,

12) The interrelationship between *psychological factors* (e.g., feelings of competency, need for stimulation, and locus of control) *and physical activity* throughout the lifespan,

13) Factors that promote *exercise adherence* in the elderly,

14) The value of appropriate exercise *role models* on the extent and type of exercise participation in the elderly, and

15) Specific social-psychological benefits of exercise for the institutionalized old.

## SUMMARY

The physiological, psychological, and social benefits of exercise are inextricably related to the aging process. This chapter provides experimental evidence that exercise is increasingly important as one ages. For example, biological signposts of aging such as cardiorespiratory fitness, bone density, muscular strength and endurance, body composition, and reaction time are markedly improved with regular and vigorous physical exercise—regardless of a person's chronological age! The training effects of exercise in the elderly are similar to those in younger individuals. A longer life expectancy has been associated with a combination of a stimulating social environment, exercise, a healthful physical environment, genetic factors, nutrition, and sexual activity.

Preliminary research data indicate that the psychosocial effects of exercise for older adults may include such benefits as increased happiness, life satisfaction, and life quality. The number of research studies that have focused on elderly populations, however, is quite small, and are plagued by methodological inelegancies. Considerable effort is needed to examine the 15 areas of needed research outlined in the preceeding section. However, it does seem many psychological benefits are associated with exercise. The elderly report decreases in stress, especially anxiety and depression, after exercising. In a study of older adults who volunteered to participate because of difficulties with anxiety, worry, and sleep, there also was a decrease in muscular tension after exercise. In addition, older members of psychiatric populations report decreases in depression. Such benefits are associated with exercise despite the ageism attached to physical activity.

Organized exercise programs for the elderly, individualized for the needs of various subpopulations, are greatly needed to combat the stereotypes that are rampant in American society. Diminished self-expectancies coupled with social expectancies that one should "act his or her age" greatly reduce the amount of exercise most older individuals pursue. Thus to enhance the psychological benefits of exercise, the supervised program should be enjoyable! In addition it should promote abdominal breathing and be noncompetitive. By exercising three times a week or more, the senior citizen can be comfortable with the moderate level of exercise intensity which seems to promote mood alteration. To maximize the likelihood of the psychological benefits, the older individual should participate for 20 to 30 minutes.

George Sheehan (1978), cardiologist and noted writer who is in his 70's, has described the psychic energy and up-beat emotions people of all ages can gain from exercise.

My fight is not with age. Running has won that battle for me. Running is my fountain of youth, my elixir of life. It will keep me young forever. When I run, I know there is no need to grow old. I know that my running, my play, will conquer time.

And there on the roads, I can pursue my perfection for the rest of my days, and finally, as his wife said of Kazantzakis dead at seventy-four, be mowed down in the first flower of my youth (Sheehan, 1978, pp. 122-123).

## REFERENCES

American College of Sports Medicine (1986). *Guidelines for exercise testing and prescription* (3rd ed.). Philadelphia: Lea and Febiger.

Andres, R., Bierman, E.L., & Hazzard, W.R. (1985). *Principles of geriatric medicine.* New York: McGraw Hill.

Asberg, M., Perris, C., Schalling, D., & Sedvall, G. (1978). The CRPS-development and applications of a psychiatric rating scale. *Acta Physiologica Scandinavia,* 227(Suppl.), 1-27.

Bahrke, M.S., & Morgan, W.P. (1978). Anxiety reduction following exercise and meditation. *Cognitive Therapy and Research, 2,* 323-334.

Beck, A.T., Ward, C.H., Mendelson, M., Mock, J., & Erbauch, H. (1961). An inventory for measuring depression. *Archives of General Psychiatry,* 561-571.

Bennett, J., Carmack, M.A., & Gardner, V.J. (1982). The effect of a program of physical exercise on depression in older adults. *Physical Educator, 39,* 21-24.

Benson, H. (1975). *The relaxation response.* New York: Avon.

Berger, B.G. (1972). Relationships between environmental factors of temporal space uncertainty, probability of physical harm, and nature of competitions and selected personality characteristics of athletes. *Dissertation abstracts international, 33,* 1014A. (University Microfilms No. 72-23689, 373).

Berger, B.G. (1983/1984). Stress reduction through exercise: The mind-body connection. *Motor Skills: Theory into Practice, 7,* 31-46.

Berger, B.G. (1984a). Running away from anxiety and depression: A female as well as male race. In M.L. Sachs & G.W. Buffone ( Eds.), *Running as therapy: An integrated approach* (pp. 138-171). Lincoln: University of Nebraska Press.

Berger, B.G. (1984b). Running toward psychological well-being: Special considerations for the female client. In M.L. Sachs & G. Buffone (Eds.), *Running as therapy: An integrated approach* (pp. 172-197). Lincoln: University of Nebraska Press.

Berger, B.G. (1986). Use of jogging and swimming as stress reduction techniques. In J.H. Humphrey (Ed.), *Current selected research in human stress.* (Vol 1) (pp. 169-190). New York: AMS Press.

Berger, B.G. (1987). Stress reduction following swimming. In W.P. Morgan & S.E. Goldston (Eds.), *Exercise and mental health* (pp. 139-143). Washington, DC: Hemisphere Publishing.

Berger, B.G., Friedmann, E., & Eaton, M. (in press) Comparison of jogging, the relaxation response, and social support for stress reduction. *Journal of Sport and Exercise Psychology.*

Berger, B.G., Michielli, D., & Cohen, K. (1988). Life quality and exercise in the elderly. Manuscript in preparation.

Berger, B.G., & Owen, D.R. (1983). Mood alteration with swimming — swimmers really do "feel better." *Psychosomatic Medicine, 45,* 425-433.

Berger, B.G., & Owen, D.R. (1986). Mood alteration with swimming: A re-evaluation. In L. Vander Velden, & J.H. Humphrey, (Eds.), *Current selected research in the psychology and sociology of sport* (Vol. 1) (pp. 97-114). New York; AMS Press.

Berger, B.G., & Owen, D.R. (1987). The stress reducing benefits of swimming: Exploration of a causal relationship. *Association for the Advancement of Applied Sport Psychology Abstracts, 1987.*

Berger, B.G., & Owen, D.R. (in press). Anxiety reduction with swimming: Relationship between exercise and state, trait, and somatic anxiety. *International Journal of Sport Psychology.*

Berger, B.G., & Owen, D.R. (1988). Stress reduction and mood enhancement in four exercise modes: Swimming, body conditioning, Hatha yoga, and fencing. *Research Quarterly for Exercise and Sport, 59,* 56-67.

Blumenthal, J.A., Williams, R.S., Needels, T.L., & Wallace, A.G. (1982). Psychological changes accompany aerobic exercise in healthy middle-aged adults. *Psychosomatic Medicine, 44,* 529-536.

Bortz, W.M. (1982). Disuse and aging. *Journal of the American Medical Association, 248,* 1203-1208.

Brown, J.R., & Shephard, R.J. (1967). Some measures of fitness in older female employees of a Toronto department store. *Canadian Medical Association Journal, 97,* 1208-1213.

Canada Fitness Survey (1982). *Fitness and aging.* Ottawa: Fitness Canada.

Cattell, R.B., Eber, H.W., & Tatsuoka, M. (1970). Handbook for the sixteen personality factor questionnaire (16PF). In *Clinical educational, industrial and research psychology.* Champaign, IL: Institute for Personality and Ability Testing.

Collingwood, T.R. (1972). The effects of physical training upon behavior and self attitudes. *Journal of Clinical Psychology, 28,* 583-585.

Collinwood, T.R., & Willett, L. (1971). The effects of physical training upon self-concept and body attitude. *Journal of Clincial Psychology, 27,* 411-412.

Collins, G.L. (1987, April 2). As nation grays, a mighty advocate flexes its muscles. *The New York Times,* pp. C1, C8.

Comfort, A. (1979) *The biology of senescence.* (3rd Ed.), New York: Elsevier Press.

Conrad, C.C. (1976). When you're young at heart . *Aging, 258,* 11-13.

Costill, D. (1986). *Inside running: Basics of sports physiology.* Indianapolis: Benchmark.

Dahlstrom, W., Welsh, G., & Dahlstrom, L. (1979). *An MMPI handbook. Vol. 1: Clinical Interpretation.* Minneapolis: University of Minnesota Press.

Dalkey, N.C., Lewis, R., & Snyder, D. (1972). *Studies in life quality.* Boston: D.C. Heath.

deVries, H.A. (1981). Tranquilizer effects of exercise: A critical review. *The Physician and Sportsmedicine, 9*(11), 46-55.

deVries, H.A., & Adams, G.M. (1972). Electromyographic comparison of single doses of exercise and meprobamate as to effects on muscular relaxation. *American Journal of Physical Medicine, 51*(3), 130-141.

Dishman, R.K. (1986). Mental health. In V. Seefeldt (Ed.), *Physical activity and well-being* (pp. 304-341). Reston, Va: American Alliance for Health, Physical Education, Recreation, and Dance.

Era, P. & Heikkinen, E. (1984, July). Postural sway during standing and unexpected disturbance of balance in men at different ages. Paper presented at the 1984 Olympic Scientific Congress, Eugene, OR.

Folkins, C.H., & Sime, W.E. (1981). Physical fitness training and mental health. *American Psychologist, 36,* 373-389.

Franklin, B.A. (1978). Motivating and educating adults to exercise. *Journal of Physical Education and Recreation, 49,* 13-17.

Freedson, P.S., Mihevic, P.M., Loucks, A.B., & Girandola, R.N. (1983). Physique, body composition, and psychological characteristics of competitive female body builders. *The Physician and Sportsmedicine, 11*(5), 85-90.

Fries, J.F. (1980). Aging, natural death, and the compression of morbidity. *The New England Journal of Medicine, 303*(3), 130-135.

Fries, J.F., & Crapo, L.M. (1981). *Vitality and aging.* San Francisco: W.H. Freeman.

Gallagher, D., Thompson, L.W., & Levy, S.M. (1980). Clinical psychological assessment of older adults. In L.W. Poon (Ed.), *Aging in the 1980s* (pp. 19-40). Washington, DC: American Psychological Association.

Gatz, M., Smyer, M.A., & Lawton, M.P. (1980). The mental health system and the older adult. In L.W. Poon (Ed.), *Aging in the 1980s* (pp. 5-18). Washington, DC: American Psychological Association.

Glasser, W. (1976). *Positive addiction.* New York: Harper & Row.

Goldwater, B.C., & Collis, M.L. (1985). Psychologic effects of cardiovascular conditioning: A controlled experiment. *Psychosomatic Medicine, 47,* 174-181.

Goodrick C. (1980). Effects of long-term voluntary wheel exercise on male and female Wistar rats I: Longevity, body weight, and metabolic rate. *Gerontology, 26,* 22-33.

Greist, J.H., Klein, M.H., Eischens, R.R., Faris, J., Gurman, A.S., & Morgan, W.P. (1979). Running as treatment for depression. *Comprehensive Psychiatry, 20*, 41-54.

Haber, P., Honiger, B., Klicpera, M. & Neiderberger, M. (1984). Effects in elderly people 67-76 years of age of 3-month endurance training on a bicycle ergometer. *European Heart Journal, 5*(Suppl. E.), 37-39.

Hartung, G.H., & Farge, E.J. (1977) Personality and physiological traits in middle-aged runners and joggers. *Journal of Gerontology, 32*(5), 541-548.

Heinzelman, F., & Bagley, R.W. (1970). Response to physical activity programs and their effects on health behavior. *Public Health Report, 85*, 905-911.

Helson, R., & Moane, G. (1987). Personality change in women from college to midlife. *Journal of Personality and Social Psychology, 53*, 176-186.

Hogan, P.I., & Santomier, J.P. (1984). Effect of mastering swimming skills on older adults' self-efficacy. *Research Quarterly for Exercise and Sport, 55*(3), 294-296.

Holloszy, J.O., Smith, E.K., Vining, M., & Adams, S. (1985). Effect of voluntary exercise on longevity of rats. *Journal of Applied Physiology, 59*(3), 826-831.

Jette, A.M., & Branch, L.G. (1981). The Framingham disability study: II. Physical disability among the aging. *American Journal of Public Health, 71*, 1211-1216.

Johannessen, S., Holly, R.G., Lui, H., & Amsterdam, E.A. (1986). High-frequency, moderate-intensity training in sedentary middle-aged women. *The Physician and Sportsmedicine, 14*(5), 99-102.

Kavanagh, T., & Shephard, R.J. (1977). The effect of continued training on the aging process. In R. Milvy (Ed.), *Annals of the New York Academy of Sciences, 301* (pp. 656-670). New York: New York Academy of Sciences.

Kavanagh, T., Shephard, R.J., Tuck, J.A., & Qureshi, S. (1977). Depression following myocardial infarction: The effects of distance running. In R. Milvy (Ed.), *Annals of the New York Academy of Sciences, 301* (pp. 1029-1038). New York: New York Academy of Sciences.

Krumpe, P.E., Knudson, R.J., Parsons, G., & Reiser, K. (1985). The aging respiratory system. *Clinics in Geriatric Medicine, 1*, 143-175.

Lakatta, E.G. & Yin, F.C.P. (1982). Myocardial aging: Functional alterations and related cellular mechanisms. *American Journal of Physiology, 242*, H297.

Larsson, B., Renstrom, P., Svardsudd, K., Welin, L., Grimby, G., Eriksson, H., Ohlson, L.O., Wilhelmson, L. & Bjorntorp, P. (1984). Health and aging characteristics of highly physically active 65 year old men. *European Heart Journal, 5* (Suppl. E.), 31-35.

Levinson, D., Darrow, C.M., Klein, E.B., Levinson, M.H., & McKee, B. (1978). *The seasons of a man's life*. New York: Knopf Books.

Levy, S.M. (1983). Host differences in neoplastic risk: Behavioral and social contributions to disease. *Health Psychology, 2*, 21-44.

Lin, N., Ensel, W.M., Dean, A. (1986). The age structure and the stress process. In N. Lin, A. Dean, & W.M. Ensel (Eds.), *Social support, life events, and depression* (pp. 213-231). New York: Academic Press.

Lobstein, D.D., Mosbacher, B.J. & Ismail, A.H. (1983). Depression as a powerful discriminator between physically active and sedentary middle-aged men. *Journal of Psychosomatic Research, 27*, 69-76.

Long, B.C. (1983). Aerobic conditioning and stress reduction: Participation or conditioning? *Human Movement Science, 2*, 171-186.

Lynch, J.J. (1975). *The broken heart: The medical consequences of loneliness*. New York: Basic Books.

Martinek, T.J., Cheffers, J.T., & Zaichkowsky, L.D. (1978). Physical activity, motor development and self-concept; Race and age differences. *Perceptual and Motor Skills, 46*, 147-154.

Martinsen, E.W., Medhus, A., & Sandvik, L. (1985). Effects of aerobic exercise on depression: A controlled study. *British Medical Journal, 291*, 109.

Mazess, R.B. (1982). On aging bone loss. *Clinical Orthopaedics, 165*, 239-252.

McPherson, B.D. (1986). Sport, health, well-being, and aging: Some conceptual and methodological issues and questions for sport scientists. In B.D. McPherson (Ed.), *Sport and aging* (pp. 3-23). Champaign, IL: Human Kinetics.

McTavish, D.G. (1971). Perceptions of old people: A review of research methodologies and findings. *The Gerontologist, 11*, 90-108.

Morgan, W.P. (1979). Anxiety reduction following acute physical activity. *Psychiatric Annals, 9*, 141-147.

Morgan, W.P. (1980, July ). Test of champions; The iceberg profile. *Psychology Today*, pp. 92-99; 101; 108.

Morgan, W.P. (1987). Reduction of state anxiety following acute physical activity. In W.P. Morgan & S.E. Goldston (Eds.), *Exercise and mental health* (pp. 105-109). Washington, DC: Hemisphere.

Morgan, W.P., & Goldston, S.E. (1987). *Exercise and mental health*, Washington, DC: Hemisphere.

Morgan, W.P., Roberts, J.A., Brand, F.R., & Feinerman, A.D. (1970). Psychological effect of chronic physical activity. *Medicine and Science in Sports, 2*, 213-217.

Morris, A.F., & Husman, B.F. (1978). Life quality changes following an endurance conditioning program. *American Corrective Therapy Journal, 32*, 3-6.

Morris, A.F., Lussier, L., Vaccaro, P., & Clarke, D.H. (1982). Life quality characteristics of national class women masters long distance runners. *Annals of Sports Medicine, 1*, 23-26.

Naughton, J. (1985). Cardiac Rehabilitation: Current status and future possibilities. In N.K. Wenger (Ed.), *Exercise and the heart. Cardiovascular clinics* [Vol. 15 (2), pp. 185-192]. Philadelphia: F.A. Davis.

Neugarten, B.L., Havighurst, R.J., & Tobin, S.S. (1968). Personality and patterns of aging. In B.L. Newgarten (Ed.), *Middle age and aging* (pp. 173-177). Chicago: University of Chicago Press.

Nordin, B. (1979). Treatment of postmenopausal osteoporosis. *Drugs, 18,* 484-492.

Olson, M.I. (1975). The effects of physical activity on the body image of nursing home residents. Unpublished master's thesis, Springfield College, MA.

Ostrow, A.C. (1983). Age-role stereotyping: Implications for physical activity participation. In G. Rowles & R. Ohta (Eds.). *Aging and milieu: Environmental perspectives on growing old* (pp. 153-170). New York: Academic Press.

Ostrow, A.C. (1984). *Physical activity and the older adult: Psychological perspectives.* Princeton, NJ: Princeton Book Company.

Ostrow, A.C., & Dzewaltowski, D.A. (1986). Older adults' perceptions of physical activity participation based on age-role and sex-role appropriateness. *Research Quarterly for Exercise and Sports, 57,* 167-169.

Ostrow, A.D., Jones, D.C., & Spiker, D.D. (1981). Age role expectations and sex role expectations for selected sport activities. *Research Quarterly for Exercise and Sport, 52,* 216-227.

Ostrow, A.C., Keener, R.E., & Perry, S.A. (1986-87). The age grading of physical activity among children. *International Journal of Aging and Human Development, 24,* 101-111.

Paffenbarger, R.S., Hyde, R., Wing, A., & Hsieh, C. (1986). Physical activity, all-cause mortality, and longevity of college alumni. *New England Journal of Medicine, 314,* 605-613.

Paffenbarger, R.S., Wing, A., & Hyde, R. (1978). Physical activity as an index of heart attack risk in college alumni. *Journal of Epidemiology, 108,* 161-175.

Pelletier, K.R. (1981). *Longevity: Fulfilling our biological potential.* New York: Dell.

Pflaum, J.H. (1973). Development of a life quality inventory. Unpublished doctoral dissertation, University of Maryland.

Porcari, J., McCarron, R., Klein, G., Freedson, P.S., Ward, A., Ross, J.A., & Rippe, J.M. (1987). Is fast walking an adequate aerobic training stimulus for 30-to 69-year-old men and women?, *The Physician and Sportsmedicine, 15,* 119-129.

Rockstein, M., Chesky, J., & Lopez, T. (1981). Effects of exercise on the biochemical aging of mammalian myocardium I: Actomyosin ATPase. *Journal of Gerontology, 36,* 294-297.

Rodeheffer, R.J., Gerstenblith, G., Becker, L.C., Fleg, J.L., Weisfeldt, M.L., & Lakatta, E.G. (1984). Exercise cardiac output is maintained with advancing age in healthy human subjects: Cardiac dilation and increased stroke volume compensate for a diminished heart rate. *Circulation, 69,* 203.

Rosenberg, E. (1986). Sport voluntary association involvement and happiness among middle-aged and elderly Americans. In B. McPherson (Ed.), *Sport and aging* (pp. 45-52). Champaign, IL: Human Kinetics.

Rosenfeld, A.H. (1978). *New views on older lives: A sampler of NIMH-sponsored research and service programs.* (DHEW Publication NO. ADM 78-687). Washington, DC: U.S. Government Printing Office.

Sachs, M.L. & Buffone, G.W. (Eds.). (1984). *Running as therapy: An integrated approach.* Lincoln: University of Nebraska Press.

Saltin, B., Blomquist, G., Mitchell, J., Johnson, R., Wilderthal, K., & Chapman, C.B. (1968). Response to exercise after bedrest and after training. A longitudinal study of adaptive changes in oxygen transport and composition. *Circulation, 33*(Suppl. 7), 1-78.

Sapolsky, R.M., Krey, L.C., & McEwen, B.S. (1985). Prolonged glucocorticoid exposure reduces hippocampal neuron number: Implications for aging. *Journal of Neuroscience, 5,* 1222-1227.

Schaie, K.W., & Geiwitz, J. (1982). *Adult development and aging.* Boston: Little, Brown & Company.

Seals, D.R., Hagberg, J.M., Ehsani, A.D., & Holloszy, J.O. (1984). Effects of training on glucose tolerance and plasma lipid levels in older men and women. *Journal of the American Medical Association, 252,* 445-449.

Sharkey, B.J. (1984). *Physiology of fitness* (2nd ed.), Champaign, IL: Human Kinetics.

Sheehan, G.A. (1978). *Running and being: The total experience.* New York: Simon and Schuster.

Sheehey, G. (1976). *Passages.* New York: Bantam Books.

Shephard, R.J. (1978). *Physical activity and aging.* Chicago: Yearbook Medical Publishers.

Shephard, R.J. (1986a). Physical activity and aging in a post-industrial society. In B.D. McPherson (Ed.), *Sport and aging* pp. 37-43). Champaign, IL: Human Kinetics.

Shephard, R.J. (1986b). Physiological aspects of sport and physical activity in the middle and later years of life. In B.D. McPherson (Ed.), *Sport and aging* (pp. 221-232). Champaign, IL: Human Kinetics.

Shephard, R.J. & Sidney, K.H. (1979). Exercise and aging. In R. Hutton (Ed.), *Exercise and sport science reviews* (pp. 1-57). Philadelphia: Franklin Press.

Sidney, K.H., & Shephard, R.J. (1976). Attitudes toward health and physical activity in the elderly: Effects of a physical training program. *Medicine and Science in Sport, 8,* 246-252.

Sidney, K.H., & Shephard, R.J. (1978). Frequency and intensity of exercise training for elderly subjects. *Medicine and Science in Sport, 10,* 125-131.

Singer, R.N., & Gerson, R.F. (1981). Task classification and strategy utilization in motor skills. *Research Quarterly for Exercise and Sport, 52,* 100-112.

Smith, E.L. (1981). Age: The interaction of nature and nurture. In E.L. Smith & R.C. Serfass (Eds.) *Exercise and aging: The scientific basis* (pp. 11-17). Hillside, NJ: Enslow Publishers.

Smith, E.L. & Gilligan, C. (1986). Exercise, sport, and physical activity for the elderly: Principles and problems of programming. In B.D. McPherson (Ed.), *Sport and aging* (pp. 91-105). Champaign, IL: Human Kinetics.

Smith, E.L., Sempos, C.T., & Purvis, R.W. (1981). Bone mass and strength decline with age. In E.L. Smith and R.C. Serfass (Eds.), *Exercise and aging: The scientific basis* (pp. 59-87). Hillside, NJ: Enslow Publishers.

Spirduso, W.W. (1980). Physical fitness, aging, and psychomotor speed: A review. *Journal of Gerontology, 35*(6), 850-865.

Spirduso, W.W. (1982). Effects of physiological fitness on the aging motor system. In J.A. Mortimer, F.J. Pirozzolo, & G.J. Maletta (Eds.), *The aging motor system*. New York: Praeger Scientific.

Spirduso, W.W. (1985). Age as a limiting factor in human neuromuscular performance. In D.H. Clarke & H.M. Eckert (Eds.), *Proceedings of the fifty-sixth annual meeting of the American academy of physical education* (pp. 57-69). Champaign, IL: Human Kinetics.

Spirduso, W.W. (1986). Physical activity and the prevention of premature aging. In V. Seefeldt (Ed.), *Physical activity and well-being* (pp. 142-160). Reston, VA: American Alliance for Health, Physical Education, Recreation, and Dance.

Spirduso, W.W., & Clifford, P. (1978). Replication of age and physical activity effects on reaction and movement time. *Journal of Gerontology, 33*, 26-30.

Spurgeon, H.A., Steinbach, M.A., & Lakatta, E.G. (1983). Chronic exercise prevents characteristic age-related changes in rat cardiac contraction. *American Journal of Physiology, 244*, H513-H518.

Starnes, J.W., Beyer, R.E., & Edington, D.W. (1983). Myocardial adaptations to endurance exercise in aged rats. *American Journal of Physiology, 245*, H560-H565.

Stillman, R.J., Lohman, T.G., Slaughter, M.H., & Massey, B.H. (1986). Physical activity and bone mineral content in women aged 30 to 85 years. *Medicine and Science in Sports and Exercise, 18*, 576-580.

Taylor, J.A. (1953). A personality scale of manifest anxiety. *Journal of Abnormal and Social Psychology, 48*, 285-290.

Uson, P.P., & Larrosa, V.R. (1982). Physical activities in retirement age. In J. Partington, T. Orlick, & J. Samela (Eds.), *Sport in perspective* (pp. 149-151), Canada: Coaching Association of Canada.

Valliant, P.M., & Asu, M.E. (1985). Exercise and its effects on cognition and physiology in older adults. *Perceptual Motor Skills, 61*, 1031-1038.

Wankel, L., & Kreisel, P.S. (1985). Factors underlying enjoyment of youth sports: Sport and age group comparisons. *Journal of Sport Psychology, 7*, 51-64.

Weisfeldt, M. (1985). The aging heart. *Hospital Practice*. 115-130.

Wells, C. (1985). *Women, sport, and performance: A physiological perspective*. Champaign, IL: Human Kinetics.

Wells, C. (1986). Menstruation, pregnancy, and menopause. In V. Seefeldt (Ed.), *Physical activity and well-being* (pp. 212-234). Reston, VA: American Alliance for Health, Physical Education, Recreation, and Dance.

Whitehouse, F. (1977). Motivation for fitness. In R. Harris & L.J. Frankel (Eds.), *Guide to fitness after 50*. New York: Plenum Press.

Young, J.R., and Ismail, A.H. (1977). Comparison of selected physiological and personality variables in regular and nonregular adult male exercisers. *Research Quarterly, 48*(3), 617-622.

Young, J.R., and Ismail, A.H. (1978). Ability of biochemical and personality variables in discriminating between high and low physical fitness levels. *Journal of Psychosomatic Research, 22*, 193-199.

Zung, W. (1965) Self-rating depression scale. *Archives of General Psychiatry, 12*, 63-70.

*PSYCHOLOGICAL WELL-BEING*

# 7

## The Effects Of Age On Physiological And Psychological Responses To A Training And Detraining Program In Females

PEGGY A. RICHARDSON

BETH S. ROSENBERG

## ABSTRACT

Participation in aerobic training leads to positive cardiovascular changes in females (Drinkwater, 1984) which often leads to favorable psychological feelings (Buffone, 1980). Equally important, however, are responses to detraining, an area which has received limited attention (Wilmore, 1982). Therefore, the purposes of the present investigation were to: (1) determine the effects of training and detraining on aerobic performance, perceived exertion, and state anxiety; and (2) determine if these effects are related to age in sedentary females.

Thirty female subjects classified into under 40 and over 40 age-groups participated in a 14-week walk-jog training and detraining program. Aerobic indicators included heart rate, blood pressure, treadmill time and oxygen uptake. Psychological parameters included ratings of perceived exertion and state anxiety. Data were analyzed by 2x3 ANOVA's with the following results: 1) older women had higher blood pressures prior to training but after conditioning and deconditioning their pressures decreased to a level similar to younger women, 2) older subjects demonstrated healthier psychological profiles throughout the study and had lower ratings of perceived exertion, and 3) maximal heart rate in older women decreased with training and increased after detraining, while heart rate in younger women was unchanged with training but decreased with detraining; however, the interaction with age was not statistically significant.

## INTRODUCTION

There is a clear distinction between chronological and physiological age. Physiological age is described as a person's ability to adapt to the environment in normal life situations or life crises. There is, however, a reduction in adaptability in general physiological function over chronological time. According to Smith and Serfass (1981), an individual reaches peak maturity at about age 30, and thereafter there is a functional capacity decline at a rate of 0.75% per year. Thus, work capacity is reduced by approximately 30% between the ages of 30 and 70 years in both men and women.

While genetic components of age control the life span, research suggests that the quality of life is controlled by how a person interacts with his/her environment and that up to 50% of the work capacity decline exhibited in physiological aging may be attributed to inactivity or sedentary lifestyles (Goldman & Rockstein, 1975; Morse & Smith, 1981; Shephard, 1978). Thus, participation in physical activity or training programs can result in positive physiological adaptations in flexibility, strength and power, speed and agility, and endurance and relaxation (Pollock, 1973).

These physiological health-related changes often lead to favorable psychological feelings (Morgan, 1976). In recent years, investigators have indicated that a direct relationship exists between psychological benefits and fitness training. For example, Buffone (1980) reported that an increase in cardiovascular functioning following training was associated with self-reports of increases in sense of well-being; Solomon and Bumpus (1978) argued that physical fitness improvements gave individuals a feeling of mastery and control over bodily functions; and Morgan (1979) explained that exercise provides distractions from anxiety-provoking cognitions. El-Naggar and Ismail (1986) reported that in middle aged men (ages 40-65 years) regular exercise positively influenced cognitive functioning and emotional health.

A bridge between physiological and psychological sensations experienced during physical exertion is the Rating of Perceived Exertion (RPE). Robertson (1982) suggested that RPE's expressed during exercise are mediated by the duration and the intensity of activity. Borg (1982) pointed out that a close relationship exists between RPE and heart rate (HR); however, he cautioned that HR might be influenced by factors other than physical strain or exertion, such as age, exercise mode, environment, and anxiety. While physiological cues play a major role in perception of exertion, psychological variables appear to interact with the physiological responses, and both have effects on self-reports of exertion (Rejeski, 1981).

Extensive information is available on types of training programs, frequency of participation, duration of training sessions and programs, performance intensities, and fitness levels of participants (Clausen, 1977; Fox, 1979; Fox & Mathews, 1974). Yet an area that is equally important but has received only limited attention is that of detraining. What happens to the conditioned performer when activity ceases? Do the physical and psychological detraining rates reflect a reversed training curve? Do certain physiological and/or psychological parameters decline more rapidly than others? Similarly, there is a paucity of research concerning physical training and subsequent detraining in females, specifically on the effects of age on physiological and/or psychological responses to detraining.

Much of the existing literature has extrapolated information about females in general from studies which used male subjects (deVries, 1974; Wilmore, 1982); or from studies that examined highly trained, competitive females (Drinkwater & Horvath, 1972). Several studies have examined detraining responses in relatively young (17 to 28 years) subjects (Fringer & Stull, 1974; Pederson & Jorgensen, 1978; Smith & Stransky, 1976). All found that the physiological improvements that occurred with training (resting heart rate, maximum heart rate, and maximal oxygen uptake) reversed themselves, returning to nearly pretraining levels after a period of detraining. The consensus in the literature appears to be that after a period of detraining equal in length to the training period, most physiological parameters will return to pretraining levels. Only one study was reviewed that dealt with detraining in older than college-aged women. Sadamoto, Fuchi, Taniguchi and Miyashita (1986) examined the responses of middle-aged women ($M=40.90$ years) to equal length training and detraining periods. They reported that heart rate during sleep declined significantly during a detraining period while resting heart rate while awake underwent no significant change.

According to Smith and Stransky (1976), training status prior to cessation of activity might also influence the rate of detraining. If this is true, then one might hypothesize that younger individuals might detrain more rapidly than older individuals (at least initially) due to their higher functional capacity, even if sedentary. Yet, subjective observations from many older individuals indicate that perhaps age and rate of detraining are positively correlated.

The present study was designed to examine these problems. Therefore, the purposes of the investigation were: (1) to determine the effects of training and detraining on aerobic performance, perceived exertion, and state anxiety in females; and (2) to determine if the effects are associated with age in sedentary females.

## METHODS

The subjects for this investigation were 30 sedentary females ranging in age from 20 to 63 years ($M=42.27$ years, $SD=8.28$ years). These women were healthy but were not active in a program of regular aerobic exercise prior to the study. The total group was divided into two subgroups: under 40 ($<40$) which included 12 women ($M=29.42$ years, $SD=5.98$ years), and 40 plus (40+) which included 18 women ($M=49.11$ years, $SD=5.36$ years). Age at the beginning of the investigation was used to classify subjects into one of the two groups. The breakpoint of 40 years was selected since this is within the period of physiological decline that typically starts at 30 years of age (Smith & Gilligan, 1983). All subjects were cleared for participation in this study by their personal physicians and each gave informed consent prior to inclusion in this investigation.

Each subject was pretested (T1), then underwent a seven-week walk/jog program, was tested again (T2), then was asked to discontinue all regular aerobic activity for seven weeks, after which a final test (T3) was performed.

## Measurement of Dependent Variables

Subjects reported to the lab for each testing session dressed in comfortable, loose fitting clothes and walking/jogging shoes. They were asked to refrain from eating, smoking, and drinking caffeinated beverages for three hours prior to each session. At the beginning of each testing session (T1, T2, T3), subjects were asked to sit quietly for a minimum of 10 minutes. At the conclusion of the 10-minute rest period, resting pulse and blood pressure were measured and recorded. The subjects then completed the Competitive State Anxiety Inventory (CSAI-2) (Martens, et al., 1981). This inventory was selected because the 27 items make reference to physical performance and measure three separate components of state anxiety. Subsequently, subjects were weighed.

During T1, T2 and T3 each subject performed a symptom-limited maximum modified Balke treadmill test. This test was performed on a motor driven treadmill at a constant speed of 3.5 m.p.h. (94m/min.) with elevation increasing by 2.5% every 2 minutes. Heart rate (HR), blood pressure, and rating of perceived exertion (RPE) were measured and recorded during the last 30 seconds of each minute while maximum oxygen uptake ($\dot{V}O_2$max) was monitored throughout the test via a Beckman Metabolic Measurement Cart which was calibrated prior to each test.

## Training Program

The training program was a seven-week walk/jog program with individually determined intensity levels (based on T1-pretest performance). All sessions were supervised by research assistants. The initial intensity was 60% of the individual's maximal capacity. This relatively low intensity was selected because the subjects were sedentary. Subjects started with a one mile walk, three days per week during the first week and progressed to a combination of walking and jogging for two miles at 75% of maximal capacity three days per week during the seventh week. Subjects were instructed by the trained assistants to obtain their pulse rates prior to, midway through, and at the conclusion of each exercise session to help keep their activity level within their training range. These measures were recorded. At the end of the seventh week of training, subjects were retested (T2). Following T2, subjects were asked to refrain from taking part in any regular aerobic activities (walking, jogging, cycling, or dancing) for seven weeks. Additionally, subjects were told to outline, in diary form, the type and amount of daily physical activity during the detraining period. This information was assessed prior to the final test (T3).

The data were analyzed by 2x3 (Age Group x Testing Time) analysis of variance with repeated measures on the last factor. All F ratios were tested at the .05 level of significance. Significant differences between tests were further examined by simple paired t tests. Additionally, simple F tests were performed on several of the dependent variables (maximum heart rate, maximum treadmill time, maximum oxygen uptake) to test the significance of the quadratic trends for these variables.

## RESULTS

The physiological and psychological responses of 12 women in a <40 group were compared to the responses of 18 women in a 40+ group. The groups were not significantly different with respect to height or weight but were different with respect to age ($p<.01$) as might be expected. Table 7-1 summarizes pretest descriptive information for the group as a whole, with comparative subgroup data.

Resting heart rate (RHR), systolic blood pressure (RSBP), and anxiety state reported as three subscales (A-state somatic—AS; A-state self-confidence—ASC; A-state cognitive—AC), as well as maximal physiological and psychological exercise responses (maximum heart rate—MAXHR; maximum treadmill time—TMAX; maximum systolic blood pressure—MAXSBP; maximum oxygen uptake in $ml.kg^{-1}.min^{-1}$—$\dot{V}O_2$max; maximum rating of perceived exertion—MAXRPE) were measured on three occasions. Table 7-2 depicts the physiological and psychological responses to training and detraining for the group as a whole, as well as for the two subgroups. Significant group differences are noted where appropriate.

No significant group, test effects, or interactions were demonstrated for RHR, AC or MAXSBP. Although no significant interactions occurred

**TABLE 7.1.** *Pretest (T1) Sample Characteristics.*

| Group | n | Age (Yrs.) | Preweight (KG.) | Height (CM.) |
|---|---|---|---|---|
| <40 | 12 | 29.42±5.98 | 63.02±13.30 | 163.92±8.03 |
| 40+ | 18 | 49.11±5.36 | 65.48±8.97 | 162.11±4.85 |
| TOTAL | 30 | 42.27±8.28 | 64.50±10.88 | 162.83±6.29 |
| | | ($p<.01$) | (NS) | (NS) |

**TABLE 7.2.** *Data Summary.*

*Ages:* <40: 22-38, M = 29.42±5.98
40+: 40-60, M = 49.11±5.36

| Variable | Group | T1 | T2 | T3 |
|---|---|---|---|---|
| RHR | <40 | 86.67± 14.47 | 73.50± 11.67 | 77.50± 11.63 |
| | 40+ | 78.89± 10.09 | 77.67± 10.50 | 79.67± 9.06 |
| | TOTAL | 80.00± 11.87 | 76.00± 10.98 | 78.80± 10.03 |
| | | (NS) | (NS) | (NS) |
| RSBP | <40 | 114.25± 8.93 | 115.25± .605 | 114.33± 4.96 |
| | 40+ | 126.94± 12.10 | 121.67± 10.27 | 117.39± 6.73 |
| | TOTAL | 121.87± 12.49 | 119.10± 9.27 | 116.17± 6.18 |
| | | ($p<.01$) | (NS) | (NS) |
| AS | <40 | 16.17± 3.07 | 14.33± 4.36 | 13.92± 4.91 |
| | 40+ | 12.83± 4.08 | 11.78± 3.02 | 11.61± 3.33 |
| | TOTAL | 14.17± 4.01 | 12.80± 3.76 | 12.53± 4.12 |
| | | ($p<.03$) | (NS) | (NS) |
| ASC | <40 | 25.58± 2.91 | 27.25± 4.79 | 26.50± 6.25 |
| | 40+ | 28.83± 4.44 | 30.67± 4.61 | 31.06± 5.27 |
| | TOTAL | 26.73± 5.30 | 29.30± 4.91 | 29.23± 6.02 |
| | | ($p<.01$) | (NS) | ($p<.05$) |
| AC | <40 | 13.50± 3.37 | 12.00± 5.22 | 12.58± 5.70 |
| | 40+ | 12.22± 5.59 | 11.39± 3.03 | 10.50± 2.90 |
| | TOTAL | 12.73± 4.80 | 11.63± 3.98 | 11.33± 4.28 |
| | | (NS) | (NS) | (NS) |
| MAXHR (BPM) | <40 | 186.50± 10.74 | 185.92± 8.81 | 181.58± 14.22 |
| | 40+ | 170.89± 17.09 | 162.67± 20.16 | 165.22± 18.67 |
| | TOTAL | 177.13± 16.60 | 171.97± 20.05 | 171.77± 18.64 |
| | | ($p<.01$) | ($p<.01$) | ($p<.02$) |
| TMAX (MIN) | <40 | 10.23± 3.92 | 11.68±39 | 11.13± 3.02 |
| | 40+ | 7.23± 2.18 | 8.02± 2.05 | 7.71± 2.44 |
| | TOTAL | 8.42± 2.98 | 9.48± 3.19 | 9.07± 3.14 |
| | | ($p<.02$) | ($p<.01$) | ($p<.01$) |
| MAXSBP (mmHg) | <40 | 170.50± 15.11 | 174.17±12.81 | 163.50± 19.17 |
| | 40+ | 168.22± 16.46 | 173.22± 20.56 | 169.11± 16.65 |
| | TOTAL | 169.13± 15.71 | 173.60± 17.61 | 166.87± 17.60 |
| | | (NS) | (NS) | (NS) |
| MAXRPE | <40 | 19.08± 0.79 | 19.67±0.49 | 19.42± 0.79 |
| | 40+ | 18.11± 2.22 | 18.22± 2.16 | 18.06± 1.01 |
| | TOTAL | 18.50± 1.83 | 18.80± 1.83 | 18.60± 1.75 |
| | | (NS) | ($p<.04$) | ($p<.04$) |
| $\dot{V}O_2MAX$ (ml/min) | <40 | 1669.10± 406.21 | 1877.55±349.00 | 1638.90± 272.68 |
| | 40+ | 1710.64± 479.32 | 1871.31± 502.13 | 1635.47± 273.67 |
| | TOTAL | 1697.42± 448.03 | 1873.30± 450.44 | 1636.59± 266.79 |
| | | (NS) | (NS) | (NS) |

*AGING AND MOTOR BEHAVIOR*

**TABLE 7.2.** *Data Summary. (continued)*

| $\dot{V}O_2MAX$ | | | | | | | | |
|---|---|---|---|---|---|---|---|---|
| $(ml.kg^{-1}.min^{-1})$ | <40 | 29.16± | 5.75 | 31.88±3.58 | | 27.50± | 3.47 | |
| | 40+ | 25.69± | 6.30 | 27.89± | 5.95 | 24.98± | 5.03 | |
| | TOTAL | 26.89± | 6.30 | 29.49± | 5.42 | 25.79± | 4.67 | |
| | | (NS) | | (NS) | | (NS) | | |

KEY:

RHR (Resting heart rate)
RSBP (Resting systolic blood pressure)
AS (State anxiety somatic scale)
ASC (State anxiety self confidence scale)
AC (State anxiety cognitive scale)
MAXHR (Maximum heart rate)
TMAX (Maximum treadmill time)
MAXSB (Maximum systolic blood pressure)
MAXRPE (Maximum rate of perceived exertion)
$VO_2MAX$ (Maximal oxygen uptake)

for most variables, significant group and/or test effects were seen in the remaining dependent variables.

Significant group and test effects were found for RSBP, AS, ASC, TMAX and MAXHR. The older women had significantly higher RSBP's ($p<.01$) than younger women prior to conditioning, but decreased toward the younger women's levels with aerobic conditioning and remained there even after seven weeks of detraining. A significant interaction was observed for RSBP ($p<.01$) which is presented in Figure 7-1.

Somatic anxiety was significantly lower in the older women prior to conditioning and, while it remained slightly lower in this group after conditioning (T2) and after deconditioning (T3), the difference failed to reach significance. However, the decrease in AS was significant for both old and young age groups ($p<.02$) and, as is depicted in Figure 7-2, was similar for both groups.

Figure 7-3 depicts the results for ASC. The older group demonstrated greater self-confidence than the younger women at the beginning of the study (T1) and at the end of the study (T3). However, after conditioning (T2) neither the difference between the two age groups nor the interaction effect was significant ($p=.91$). The improvement in ASC was significant over time ($p<.01$), but as is shown in Figure 7-3, continued during detraining only in the 40+ group. The ASC of the <40 group experienced a decline during detraining.

The TMAX results (Figure 7-4) demonstrated significant group differences (<40 exceeding 40+) throughout the study: T1–$p<.02$; T2–$p<.01$; T3–$p<.01$. It should also be noted that an overall test effect was demonstrated ($p<.01$) indicating that the TMAX during the pretest (T1) was significantly lower than on the subsequent post-conditioning (T2) or post-deconditioning tests (T3). This indicates a significant training effect

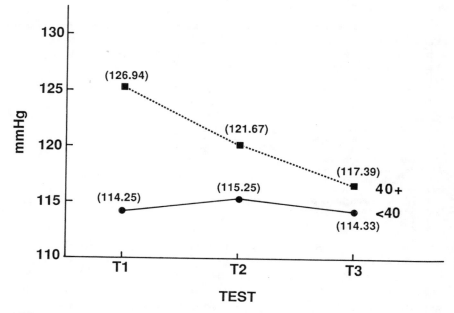

**FIGURE 7.1.** *Resting Systolic Blood Pressure.*

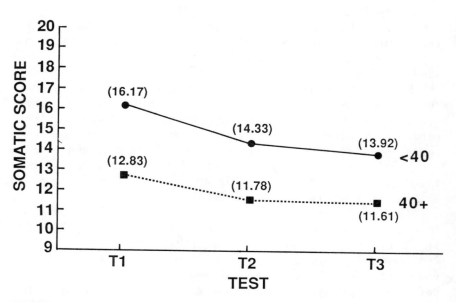

**FIGURE 7.2.** *State Anxiety—Somatic Scale.*

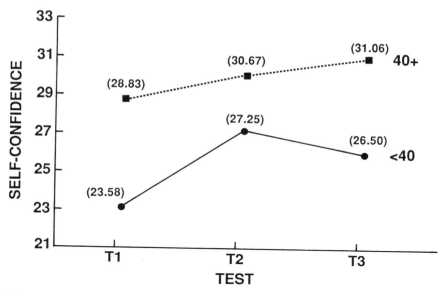

**FIGURE 7.3.** *State Anxiety—Self Confidence Scale.*

but a lack of significant loss with detraining. The interaction effect, however, was not significant ($p = .47$).

Similarly, MAXHR, which is included in Figure 7-5, demonstrated significant group differences with the <40 group having higher maximum heart rates than the 40+ group throughout the study ($p < .02$). Significant test differences ($p < .01$) were demonstrated as reduction in MAXHR occurred with training and increase in MAXHR occurred with detraining. Simple $t$ test results indicated that for the group as a whole, MAXHR was significantly lower at T2 ($p < .01$) and T3 ($p < .01$) than at T1. However, it is of interest to note in Figure 7-5 that while the older group followed the above mentioned pattern, the <40 group had a somewhat dissimilar pattern. Although the patterns were dissimilar, the interaction was not significant ($p = .12$).

Significant group effects were demonstrated only by MAXRPE (Figure 7-5). The difference between the two groups (<40 exceeding 40+) was significant at the post conditioning (T2 – $p < .04$) and post deconditioning (T3 – $p < .04$) test intervals. However, no significant interaction was indicated ($p = .44$).

Maximal oxygen uptake ($\dot{V}O_2$max) surprisingly demonstrated no significant group differences; however, significant test differences were demonstrated. Between T1 and T2, $\dot{V}O_2$max increased ($p < .05$) and between T2 and T3, $\dot{V}O_2$max declined ($p < .01$). Figure 7-6 depicts the

*PHYSIOLOGICAL AND PSYCHOLOGICAL RESPONSES*        **167**

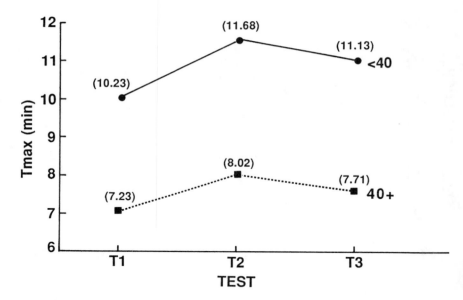

**FIGURE 7.4.** *Maximum Treadmill Time.*

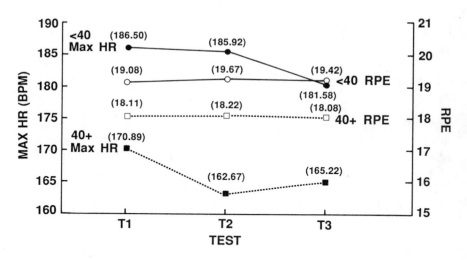

**FIGURE 7.5.** *Maximum Heart Rate and Maximal Rating of Perceived Exertion.*

$\dot{V}O_2$max results for oxygen uptake equalized for body weight. The gross $\dot{V}O_2$max (ml/min.) are included in Table 7-2. It should be noted that gross $\dot{V}O_2$max demonstrated a pattern nearly identical to $\dot{V}O_2$max equalized for body weight, as is indicated by a significant test effect ($p = <.03$) when

*AGING AND MOTOR BEHAVIOR*

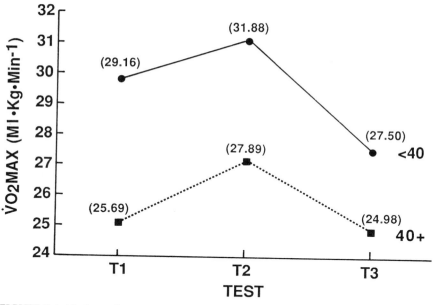

**FIGURE 7.6.** *Maximum Oxygen Uptake.*

analyzed by the ANOVA; this indicates that changes in oxygen uptake were, in fact, due to changes in cardiovascular efficiency and not merely changes in body weight.

The post hoc trend analyses performed on MAXHR, TMAX and $\dot{V}O_2$max (ml.kg.min$^{-1}$) revealed: (1) that MAXHR did not demonstrate a significant quadratic trend; and (2) that significant quadratic trends were present for TMAX and $\dot{V}O_2$max but that these trends were statistically equal across the age groups.

## DISCUSSION

The effects of training and detraining appear to be equivocal for both physiological and psychological measures. Several of the variables demonstrated no age group or test differences (RHR, AC, MAXSBP). Others that were reflective of improved resting or psychological states (RSBP, AS, ASC, MAXRPE) or maximal functional capacity (MAXHR, TMAX, $\dot{V}O_2$max) confirmed the findings of earlier investigators (Fringer & Stull, 1974; Morgan, 1979; Pederson & Jorgensen, 1978; Smith & Stransky, 1976).

The decrease in RSBP demonstrated by the older group of women lends support to the contention that aerobic exercise of moderate intensity may be efficacious in lowering blood pressure (Pollock, Wilmore & Fox, 1984, p. 54). The interaction which resulted from the 40+ group declining while the <40 group remained constant confirms the selective benefit of regular aerobic exercise in individuals exhibiting above average blood pressures, versus the lack of effect on individuals with average or sub-average blood pressure (Pollock, Wilmore, & Fox, 1984, p. 20).

The significant quadratic trends demonstrated by TMAX and $\dot{V}O_2$max lend support to the belief that seven weeks of aerobic conditioning followed by seven weeks of inactivity (deconditioning) will result in significant changes in functional capacity regardless of age. An interesting finding was the lack of significant age group differences for $\dot{V}O_2$max. All subjects were previously sedentary, so it was anticipated that there would be age group differences at least at the outset. The lack of significant age group differences in $\dot{V}O_2$max is substantiated by Wessel and Van Huss (1969) who found that in studying women between the ages of 20 and 69 years, physical activity level had a greater effect on oxygen uptake while age was a more critical factor for other performance variables such as ventilation volume. The two groups examined in this study were significantly different with respect to age; however, they were similar with respect to activity level (sedentary).

The MAXHR and MAXRPE responses in this study are among the most interesting findings. As anticipated, MAXHR was significantly higher in the <40 group than in the 40+ group. However, with training, the group as a whole demonstrated significant improvements (lower MAXHR). It appears (see Figure 7-5) that the 40+ group contributed more to this decrease (demonstrating an 8 bpm decrease) than the <40 group (which demonstrated a negligible decrement of 0.57 bpm). Following detraining a reversal of these trends occurred insofar as the 40+ group increased slightly (2.55 bpm) while the <40 group decreased slightly (4.34 bpm). Although the interaction was not significant, the unique trend demonstrated in this study warrants further investigation, perhaps with larger samples. These findings concur with those of Drinkwater and Horvath (1972) who reported a lack of significant change in maximum heart rate with detraining in younger, highly trained, competitive female subjects.

The change in MAXRPE over time was not significant, but there were differences between the two groups at T2 and T3. One very interesting aspect of MAXRPE in this study is that while the anticipated parallelism with heart rate may be observed in the younger group (see Figure 7-5), this relationship appears to be absent in the 40+ group. This supports the warnings of Borg (1982), that while a close relationship tends to exist between RPE and heart rate, heart rate may be influenced by many other factors, including age.

The improvements in the somatic and self-confidence anxiety state subscales after seven weeks of physical conditioning provide evidence for the link between aerobic conditioning and improved psychological status.

In the present study, subjects reported that they felt better physically. Further, they expressed a sense of satisfaction gained by their commitment to an exercise regime. It appears that reciprocal physical and psychological benefits were obtained by young and old subjects. For example, subjects felt better when exercising and believed they were improving their physical fitness. These feelings in turn probably led to increases in confidence and a reduction in somatic anxiety. This link is strengthened by the tendency for the group as a whole to decrease in the self-confidence subscale during the detraining period, with the younger group accounting for the reduction in self-confidence. It was interesting to note that where group differences existed, the 40+ group had more favorable psychological scores or RPE's while the <40 had more favorable physiological responses.

## SUMMARY

In summary, the effects of training and detraining on aerobic performance, perceived exertion, and state anxiety of young and middle-aged women are: (1) older subjects had higher resting systolic blood pressures than younger subjects prior to conditioning, but after seven weeks of training followed by seven weeks of detraining, their pressure decreased to a level not significantly different from younger subjects; (2) older subjects demonstrated healthier psychological profiles (with respect to anxiety states) although the somatic anxiety states of the younger subjects improved after seven weeks of aerobic conditioning; (3) maximal rating of perceived exertion was lower in the older group after seven weeks of training and remained lower after seven weeks of detraining; and (4) the trends for maximal rating of perceived exertion and maximal treadmill time were similar in the two groups examined, but maximal heart rate trends were not. Training resulted in sizeable decreases in maximal heart rate in older subjects, with a reversal in this trend seen after detraining; while in younger subjects, maximal heart rates remained virtually unchanged with training but decreased subsequent to detraining. Although interactions were not significant for this variable, it might be anticipated that studying larger samples and/or employing lengthier training/detraining periods might result in significance.

Based on the results of this study, it appears that the psychological correlates changed concomitantly with conditioning and deconditioning and that the changes were, for the most part, similar in older (40+ years) and younger (<40 years) women who were previously sedentary. Future research in this area should attempt to examine a wider spectrum of ages (particularly older age groups) and a wider spectrum of physical activity levels (sedentary, minimally trained, moderately trained, and intensely trained).

# REFERENCES

Borg, G.A.V. (1982). Psychophysical bases of perceived exertion. *Medicine and Science in Sport and Exercise, 14*, (5), 377-381.

Buffone, G.W. (1980). Exercise as therapy: A closer look. *Joural of Counseling and Psychotherapy, 3*, 101-115.

Clausen. J.P. (1977). Effect of training on cardiovascular adjustments to exercise in man. *Physiological Review, 57*, 779-815.

deVries, H.A. (1974). *Physiology of exercise for physical education and athletics*, (2nd ed.). Dubuque, IA: Wm. C. Brown.

Drinkwater, B.L. (1984). Women and exercise: Physiological aspects. In R.L. Terjung (Ed.), *Exercise and sport science reviews* (pp. 21-51), Lexington, MA: D.C. Heath & Co.

Drinkwater, B.L., & Horvath, S.M. (1972). Detraining effects on young women. *Medicine and Science in Sports, 4*, (2), 91-95.

El-Naggar, A., & Ismail, A.H. (1986). Cognitive processing, emotional health, and regular exercise in middle-aged men. In B.D. McPherson (Ed.), *Sport and aging.* (pp. 205-209), Champaign, IL: Human Kinetics Publishers, Inc.

Fox, E.L. (1979). *Sports physiology,* Philadelphia: W.B. Saunders.

Fox, E.L., & Mathews, D.K. (1974). *Interval training: Conditioning for sports and general fitness.* Philadelphia: W.B. Saunders.

Fringer, M.N., & Stull, G.A. (1974). Changes in cardio-respiratory parameters during periods of training and detraining in young adult females. *Medicine and Science in Sports, 6* (1), 20-25.

Goldman, R., & Rockstein, M. (Eds.) (1975). *The physiology and pathology of human aging.* New York: Academic Press.

Martens, R., Burton, D., Veeley, R., Smith, D., & Bump, L. (1981). The development of the competitive state anxiety inventory - 2 (CSAI). Paper presented at the annual meeting of North American Society for the Psychology of Sport and Physical Activity, Monterrey, CA.

Morgan, W.P. (1976). Psychological consequences of vigorous physical activity and sport. Paper presented at the Annual Meeting of The American Academy of Physical Education, Milwaukee, WI.

Morgan, W.P. (1979). Anxiety reduction following acute physical activity. *Psychiatric Annals, 9,* 141-147.

Morse, C.E., & Smith, E.L. (1981). Physical activity programming for the aged. In E.L. Smith & R.C. Serfass (Eds.) *Exercise and aging.* (pp. 109-120). Hillsdale, N.J.: Enslow Publishers.

Pederson, P.K., & Jorgensen, K. (1978). Maximal oxygen uptake in young women with training, inactivity and retraining. *Medicine and Science in Sports, 10* (4), 233-237.

Pollock, M.L. (1973). Quantification of endurance training programs. In J.H. Wilmore (Ed.), *Exercise and sport science reviews, vol. I.* (pp. 155-188). New York: Academic Press.

Pollock, M.L., Wilmore, J.H. & Fox, S.M. (1984). *Exercise in health and disease-evaluation and prescription for prevention and rehabilitation.* Philadelphia: W.B. Saunders Company.

Rejeski, W.J. (1981) The perception of exertion: A social psychophysiological integration. *Journal of Sport Psychology, 4,* 305-320.

Robertson, R.J. (1982). Central signals of perceived exertion during dynamic exercise. *Medicine and Science in Sports and Exercise, 14,* 390-396.

Sadamoto, J., Fuchi, T. Taniguchi, Y., & Miyashita, M. (1986). Effect of 8 weeks submaximal conditioning and deconditioning on heart rate during sleep in middle-aged women. In B.D. McPherson (Ed.), *Sport and aging.* (pp. 233-240). Champaign, IL: Human Kinetics.

Shephard, R.J. (1978). *Physical activity and aging.* Chicago: Year Books Medical Publishers.

Smith, D.P., & Stransky, F.W. (1976). The effect of training and detraining on the body composition and cardiovascular response of young women to exercise. *Journal of Sports Medicine, 16,* 112-120.

Smith, E.L., & Gilligan, C. (1983). Physical activity prescription for the older adult. *The Physician and Sports Medicine, 11* (8), 91-101.

Smith, E.L., & Serfass, R.C. (Eds.) (1981). *Exercise and aging: The scientific basic.* Hillside, N.J.: Enslow Publishers.

Solomon, E.G., & Bumpus, A.K. (1978). The running meditation response: An adjunct to psychotherapy. *American Journal of Psychotherapy, 32,* 583-592.

Spielberger, C.D., Gorsuch, R.L., & Lushene, R.E. (1970). *S.T.A.I Manual.* Palo Alto, CA: Consulting Psychologists Press, Inc.

Wessel, J.A., & Van Huss, W.D. (1969). The influence of physical activity and age on exercise adaptation of women, 20-69 years. *Journal of Sports Medicine, 9,* 173-180.

Wilmore, J.H. (1982). *Training for sport and activity.* Boston: Alyn & Bacon.

# 8

# The Psychological Effects of Chronic Exercise in the Elderly

JEFFREY S. HIRD

JEAN M. WILLIAMS

## ABSTRACT

This review critically evaluates research examining the relationship of exercise and psychological benefits in older adults. Most studies of older adults have explored the influence of exercise on either general well-being, psychological mood states, locus of control, body image, self-efficacy, or cognitions. Although many studies of older adults do not report significant changes as a result of exercise, most of the findings are in a positive direction and this, in itself, is encouraging. Numerous methodological imperfections and conceptual shortcomings are discussed in an effort to help interpret the equivocal results of existing research and to improve future research. Variations amongst studies in the dimensions of exercise (mode, frequency, intensity, duration) also are identified. These differences create difficulties in comparing and analyzing research results, and produce the need to contrast these variables in future research. For example, what are the preferred types, frequency, intensity, and duration of exercise programs needed to both assure psychological benefits and insure adherence in the elderly? Finally, underlying mechanisms that may account for psychological benefits are identified and discussed. Suggestions for future research directions are addressed throughout the chapter.

## INTRODUCTION

Many researchers have labored to identify the relationship between exercise and psychological improvement in nonelderly populations, while only a few have focused on the role of habitual exercise in fostering psychological benefits in older persons. Conclusions from the general field of research are obscured by many methodological imperfections, conceptual shortcomings, and contradicting theorizations. These problems, which will be discussed later, become even more acute in research with the elderly because there are fewer studies involving this age group and there are additional limitations associated with studying older adults.

The shortage of research on the elderly is unfortunate. Older adults, who are often a sedentary group, may in fact exhibit more psychological and physiological benefits from regular aerobic activity because they may be in poorer physical and emotional health compared to their nonelderly counterparts. The elderly, therefore, may be more likely to undergo significant changes with exercise (Folkins, Lynch, & Gardner, 1972).

This chapter will critically review existing literature in an attempt to identify the status and quality of research evaluating the relationship of exercise and psychological improvement in older adults. The effects of exercise on well-being, personality and cognition in the elderly will be evaluated. Also, this chapter will identify and discuss methodological and conceptual concerns that need to be considered when interpreting the results of current research. Finally, the underlying mechanisms that may account for psychological benefits will be presented. Suggestions for future research directions are addressed throughout the chapter.

## SUMMARY OF RESEARCH

This section will review research seeking to identify the relationship between habitual exercise and psychological improvement in older adult populations. The effects of exercise on well-being, personality, and cognition will be examined. Although a limited number of studies with older adults exist, many with considerable methodological and conceptual differences, research results have established a primary data base upon which future research on the elderly can build. See Table 8-1 for a summary of the studies in this area.

### Well-Being

Many terminologies exist in the literature for well-being as each tool that measures well-being has its own operational definition for the term (Kozma and Stones, 1978). Generally, these definitions deal with some type of positive change in attitude, whether in the form of a feeling, behavioral tendency, or thought. Specifically, operationalization of this concept typically has encompassed the constructs of life satisfaction, happiness, and/or morale.

Several of the studies of older adults have looked, with mixed results, for changes in well-being following exercise intervention. Hogan and Santomier (1984) and Perri and Templer (1985) informally asked subjects if they had noticed changes in their attitude as a result of an exercise program. Both groups of researchers reported that subjects commented positively. Typical responses were: "I am more confident," "I sleep better," "I feel more certain of my ability," and "I eat better". Blumenthal et al. (1982) noted similar results following an 11-week ergometer-riding program. Normal elderly adults between the ages of 65 and 85 ($M$ = 69.3 years) filled out a retrospective general health survey which assessed physical functions and ten psychological characteristics. The researchers, however, did not statistically analyze these data, electing in-

**TABLE 8.1.** Experimental Studies On The Psychological Effects Of Exercise In The Elderly

| Research Study | Subjects: Sex and Age | Fitness Program | Psychological Effect Studied | Instrument | Outcome |
|---|---|---|---|---|---|
| Barry et al. (1966) | Males and Females 55-78 yrs. $M = 69.5$ | Ergometer 3×/wk., 3 mos. | Personality | Myers-Briggs Type Indicator | No change |
| | | | Memory | Short Term Retention | No change |
| | | | Mental functioning | Ravens Progressive Matrices: Simple Addition | No change |
| Blumenthal et al. (1982) | Males and Females 65-85 yrs. $M = 69.3$ Old-old $= \geqslant 70$ Young-old $= \leqslant 70$ | Ergometer 3×/wk., 16 wks. | Type-A behavior | Jenkin's Activity Survey | No change |
| | | | active, vigorous, impulsive, dominant, sociable, reflectable | Thurstone Temperament Schedule | No change |
| | | | | General Health Survey | ↑ Mood, satisfaction, self-concept, achievement |
| | | | | POMS | ↓ Anger |
| Coleman et al. (1985) | Females 55-81 yrs. | Swimming, walking, aerobics, flexibility 3×/wk. | Locus of control | Rotter's Locus of Control Scale | No difference from control |
| Elsayed et al. (1980) | Males 24-68 yrs. Young: $M = 35$ Old: $M = 53$ | Progressive running, self-selected recreation, 3×/wk., 16 wks. | Fluid intelligence | Culture Fair Intelligence Test Scale 3, Form A | ↑ in 3 of 5 measures |
| | | | Crystallized intelligence | Cattell 16-PF Factor B | No chan... |

**TABLE 8.1** (continued)

| Research Study | Subjects: Sex and Age | Fitness Program | Psychological Effect Studied | Instrument | Outcome |
|---|---|---|---|---|---|
| Hogan & Santomier (1984) | Males and Females M = 67.0 years | Swimming 5×/wk., 12 wks. | Self-efficacy | Swim Skills Efficacy Scale | ↑ Self-efficacy |
| Perri & Templer (1985) | Males and Females 60-79 yrs. M = 65.6 | Walking, jogging 3×/wk., 14 wks. | Depression | Zung's SDS | No change |
| | | | Anxiety | Zuckerman's MAACL (anxiety) | No change |
| | | | Self-concept | Fitt's Tennessee Self-Concept Scale | ↑ Self-concept |
| | | | Locus of control | Rotter's Locus of Control Scale | ↑ Internal locus of control |
| | | | Memory | Key Auditory Verbal Training Test | No change |
| Powell (1974) | Male & Female Mental Patients 59-89 yrs. M = 69.3 | Brisk walking/ calisthenics 5×/wk., 12 wks. | Mental functioning | Raven's Progressive Matrices | ↑ Mental functioning |
| | | | Memory | Memory for Designs Test Wechsler Memory Scale | No change ↑ Memory |
| | | | Behavior | Nurses observation Geriatric Assessment Scale | No change |
| Riddick & Freitag (1984) | Females 50-70 yrs. | Exercise & dance routines 2×/wk., 8 wks. | Body image | My Body Index | ↑ Body image |
| Rottella & Bunker (1978) | Males | Tennis | Locus of control | Rotter's Locus of Control Scale | No difference from control |

**TABLE 8.1** *(continued)*

| Research Study | Subjects: Sex and Age | Fitness Program | Psychological Effect Studied | Instrument | Outcome |
|---|---|---|---|---|---|
| Sidney & Shephard (1976) | Males & Females Males $M$ = 66.2 yrs. Females $M$ = 65.7 yrs. | Walking/jogging 0-4 wk., 14 wks. | Trait anxiety | Taylor's Manifest Anxiety Scale | ↓ Anxiety |
| | | | Body image | Kenyon's Body Image Scale | ↑ Body image (hi frequency low intensity group) |
| | | | | McPherson's Real Me Test | ↑ Body image (all groups except low freq./low intensity) |
| | | | Self-concept, mood, goal achievement | Life Satisfaction Index | No change (only low freq./ low intensity) |
| Stamford et al. (1974) | Male & Female Mental patients $M$ = 71.5 yrs. Continuous hospitalization $M$ = 21 yrs. | Walking 5×/wk., 12 wks. | Intelligence | Wechsler Adult Intelligence Scale Digit Span Test General Information Test | No change No change ↑ Intelligence |
| | | | Sensitivity, self-concept, judgement, impulse, regulation | Draw-A-Person Test | No change |
| Valliant & Asu (1985) | Males & Females 50+ yrs. | Calisthenics, flexibility 2×/wk., 12 wks. | Depression | MMPI Depression Scale | ↓ Depression |
| | | | Locus of control | Rotter's Scale | No change |
| | | | Self-esteem | Coopersmith Self-Esteem Inventory | No change |
| | | | Fear | Motivational Analysis | No change |
| | | | Assertiveness | Motivational Analysis | No change |

stead to merely present percentages. A third of the patients indicated that their physical health had improved, while about half claimed it to be about the same. Between 40% and 50% reported improved mood, satisfaction, achievement and self-confidence. In contrast, 10% to 15% actually indicated a decrease in psychological and physiological well-being

Sidney and Shephard (1976) measured mood, behavior and feeling patterns in 42 normal older adults before and after an aerobic fast walking/running program. Five components of psychological well-being and morale were appraised using Neugarten's Life Satisfaction Index. Scores showed little or no change after training. Nevertheless, Sidney and Shephard claimed that 83% of the subjects reported improved well-being, which was not validated by their measuring instruments. Stamford, Hambacher, and Fallica (1974) and Powell (1974) also found nonsignificant changes in well being in geriatric mental patients.

Individual claims of well-being often have not been verified by psychological testing instruments. For the most part, well-being improvements only have been found in methods that are nonrepresentative of systematic data collection, such as informal interviewing (Blumenthal et al., 1982; Perri and Templer, 1985). Often these methods tend to be suggestive, thus potentially confounding the responses of the subjects interviewed. Are psychometric instruments insensitive to the subtle changes in well-being that are subjectively reported, or are subjects simply led to expect changes to occur and respond accordingly? Future research needs to address this issue.

## Psychological Mood States

Psychological mood states refer to an individual's feelings and emotions at a particular time, and as such they are transitory constructs. Aerobic activity has been found to modify these mood states, particularly the states of depression (Blue, 1979; Brown, Ramirez, & Taub, 1978; Gardner, Bennett, & Carmack, 1982; Greist et al., 1978; Kavanagh, Shephard, & Tuck, 1975; Perri & Templer, 1985; Valliant & Asu, 1985) and anxiety (Blumenthal et al., 1982; Folkins, 1976; Morgan, 1973; Perri & Templer, 1985; Sidney & Shephard, 1976).

The effect of exercise on depression in older adults was assessed in only a few of the preceeding named studies. Perri and Templer (1985) found nonsignificant depression changes in elderly subjects between the ages of 60 and 79 ($M$ = 65.5 years) who participated in a flexibility and walking/jogging program for a 14-week period. Valliant and Asu (1985) obtained a significant decrease in depression from participants in a 12-week structured exercise program who were involved in calisthenic and flexibility exercises.

Blumenthal et al. (1982) used the Profile of Mood States (POMS) to assess depression in elderly subjects, as well as the states of tension, anger, vigor, fatigue, and confusion. At the conclusion of the 11-week ergometer-riding program, scores on the anger subscale decreased significantly. Univariate analyses on depression and the four other POMS subscales failed to reach significant levels. In addition, subjects displayed a nonsignificant decrease in Type A behavior patterns, as measured by the Jenkins Activity Survey.

Is exercise an effective treatment for relieving anxiety in the elderly? The effect of exercise on anxiety was studied by Sidney and Shephard (1976). Since these researchers employed Taylor's Manifest Anxiety Scale, a tool that measures the established personality consistencies of trait anxiety, fewer (if any) recordable changes in anxiety would be expected than if a state anxiety instrument was used. Exercise participation in volunteer geriatric subjects was categorized retrospectively by frequency (attendance) and intensity (pulse rate and observed activity patterns of exercise participation). Levels of frequency and intensity were self-selected by the subjects. There was a significant decrease in manifest anxiety with training, due largely to the frequent, low-intensity exercise group. Anxiety also decreased in the same group as measured by the Cornell Medical Index-Health Questionnaire. In another anxiety study, researchers claimed that exercise produced a nonsignificant decline in anxiety (Perri & Templer, 1985).

In summary, exercise-suppressed depression and anxiety have not been significantly substantiated in the elderly. Research with nonelderly populations has been much more successful in finding significant anxiety and depression reductions (Mihevic, 1982). The mood changes with the nonelderly were most likely to occur in studies in which depressed and anxious populations were studied, or in studies in which aerobic activity was done at high intensities and across a long time interval. Perhaps the potential for positive effects of exercise in the elderly have been masked by the study of primarily "normal" elderly, and the failure of these exercise programs to last long enough or to be sufficiently intense. The very nature of most sedentary elderly populations, however, necessitates a longer initial period of low intensity workouts compared to nonelderly populations. By lengthening exercise programs, sufficient time is allowed to safely increase exercise intensity to more vigorous levels.

It also has been suggested that exercise decreases somatic anxiety more than cognitive anxiety (Schwartz, Davidson, and Goldman, 1978). If this is true, perhaps older subjects with high somatic anxiety would derive more benefit from exercise than older subjects with high cognitive anxiety. Previous studies with the elderly have not employed measurement tools that distinguished between somatic and cognitive anxiety. This, and other individual variables that may influence the effects of aerobic activity on elderly populations, needs to be investigated in future research.

## Locus of Control

A number of researchers have examined whether or not exercise affects the personality construct locus of control. Individuals with a more internal, as opposed to external, locus of control perceive causality within themselves and assume more responsibility for their environments. Phares (1971) (cited in Rotella and Bunker, 1978) has argued that older adults may display a more external locus of control than the norm for younger individuals because, as a group, the elderly often return to the helplessness of childhood. One also might conjecture that elderly individuals who choose to participate in an exercise program have a more internal causality than their nonexercising peers, and participation in an exercise program also may lead to an increase in internal locus of control.

Rotella and Bunker (1978) failed to support any of these hypotheses. Both their "super senior" male tennis players and their social control group, which was involved in a senior's volunteer program, displayed internal causality, with the tennis players having slightly higher internal locus of control. Similarly, an internal causality was found by Coleman, Washington and Price (1985) for both exercising and control groups of adult women between the ages of 55 and 81. The exercising women showed no significant changes in locus of control when compared to the control group. Valliant and Asu (1985) also reported nonsignificant pretest to posttest changes from external to internal locus of control for their structured exercise group, but Perri and Templer (1985) found significant pretest to posttest shifts in internal causality for elderly exercise subjects, while no changes occurred in the nonexercising control group.

In summary, most elderly subjects in these studies, whether they were exercisers or nonexercisers, were more likely to have an internal than external locus of control. Whether or not exercise participation leads to a more internal locus of control remains to be demonstrated, but these mixed findings merit further investigation.

## Body Image

The influence of aerobic activity on body image (and its counterpart self-concept) also has been examined more closely in younger adult age groups (Collingwood, 1972; Collingwood & Willett, 1971; Folkins, 1976; Hilyer & Mitchell, 1979; Johnson, Fretz, & Johnson, 1968; McGowan, Jarman, & Pederson, 1974) than in older adult populations (Olson, 1975; Perri & Templer, 1985; Riddick & Freitag, 1984; Sidney & Shephard, 1976; Stamford, Hambacher, & Fallica, 1974; Valliant & Asu, 1985). One study of the elderly, Sidney and Shephard (1976), used two instruments to measure body image of their older subjects. On Kenyon's Body Image Scale, which measures the difference between desired and perceived body images, subjects who trained more frequently with a high level of intensity had a significant increase in perceived body image, bringing it closer to their ideal. Individuals who either trained more frequently at a lower intensity or less frequently at a higher intensity level had no significant increases in actual body image. Subjects who exercised at a low frequency and low intensity actually had a widening between actual and ideal images, but these negative changes were nonsignificant. The second measure of body image, McPherson's Real Me Test, yielded similar results. Subjects with little or no gain in aerobic power had lower "Real Me" scores at the end of the fitness program. Those with large to moderate improvements in maximum oxygen intake increased their "Real Me" scores significantly. These findings suggest that positive changes in body image may occur only when exercise programs are sufficiently rigorous to cause significant improvements in aerobic function. Frequency and intensity differences between individuals when exercising may influence other psychological changes as well.

Riddick and Freitag (1984) compared perceived body images of a control group to normal women 50 years and older participating in an eight-week aerobics program. Aerobic class members tested significantly higher on body image following the program than the body image scores on the pretested controls. Strangely enough, no pretest measures were obtained for the experimental group, and no posttest measures were performed on the controls who were on a waiting list to get into the program. Since the two groups could not be tested for preexperimental or postexperimental differences, body image changes within and between the groups could not be adequately determined, thus making interpretation of their results somewhat difficult.

Olson (1975) found elderly nursing home patients increased their perceived body image as a result of fitness training. In addition, participants in research conducted by Perri and Templer (1985) improved significantly in self-concept. Valliant and Asu (1985) found conflicting results in subjects 50 years and older participating in a 12-week structured exercise program. Stamford, Hambacher, and Fallica (1974) reported nonsignificant results in geriatric mental subjects. However, the tool that the preceding researchers used was not a specific self-concept measure, but rather a general psychological measure. In summary, for the most part, correlations between body image and exercise in the elderly have been encouraging.

## Self-Efficacy

Self-efficacy is the strength of an individual's conviction that he/she can successfully perform a specific task. Self-efficacy greatly influences the decision to produce a behavior, as well as the effort spent and persistence maintaining it during adversities and setbacks (Bandura, 1977). Hogan and Santomier (1984) have been the only researchers to investigate changes in self-efficacy in older adults following an exercise program. These researchers believed achievement in activity settings may improve efficacy, resulting in positive changes in behavioral intentions that generalize to numerous other behavioral settings. Activities previously thought to be beyond physical or cognitive abilities may now be considered achievable.

Hogan and Santomier (1984) found self-efficacy improved for older adults (M age =67.01 years) after a five-week beginning swim class. A Swim Skills Efficacy Scale (SSES) that measured self-efficacy for specific swimming skills was developed by the investigators. The experimental group showed significant improvement in self-efficacy, while no significant changes were found in a control group. In addition, 14 of 18 experimental subjects indicated a positive change in attitude concerning their ability to perform or achieve as a result of the swimming experience.

Until there is verification through future research, these results should not be generalized to running or to other nonswimming exercise programs. There may be something unique in a swimming program, such as the sense of mastery that might accompany the acquisition of swimming skills, which contributes to the development of self-efficacy compared to what occurs in programs such as running and general exercising.

## Cognition

A number of researchers have looked at changes in mental functioning and cognition in the elderly as a consequence of participation in physical activity (Barry et al., 1966; Elsayed, Ismail, & Young, 1980; Perri & Templer, 1985; Powell, 1974; Stamford, Hambacher, & Fallica, 1974). Cognitive changes as a result of exercise have been studied in other age groups as well (Fretz, Johnson, & Johnson, 1969; Weingarten, 1973; Young, 1979).

Stamford, Hambacher, & Fallica, (1974) found intellectual improvement on two of three cognitive tests following aerobic conditioning in elderly mental patients (M age=71.5 years). On both the Wechsler Adults Intelligence Scale (WAIS) (general information) and another similar questionnaire developed by the researchers, statistically significant intellectual improvement was obtained for the experimental group. The experimental group underwent a 12-week exercise program consisting of daily walking. Daily walking sessions were lengthened from six minutes to 20 minutes through the duration of the study. A social control group who gathered in a room instead of exercising showed no significant cognitive changes.

The Stamford, Hambacher, & Fallica (1974) results may have been influenced by the fact that the subjects were institutionalized elderly mental patients. Browman (1981) suggested elderly adults admitted to mental rehabilitation centers are exceedingly lower in physical fitness compared to similarly aged individuals who are emotionally stable. Thus, the institutionalized elderly may be more apt to show physiological and psychological changes as a result of exercise. Along with the caution in generalizing these results to a noninstitutionalized elderly population, the Stamford, Hambacher, & Fallica investigation was limited to only nine subjects under the treatment condition. In addition, mean scores and the difference in psychological pre-test and post-test scores were not reported in the results. Thus, discretion should be taken in generalizing these results to other elderly mental patients.

Elsayed, Ismail, & Young (1980) claimed older male subjects showed more improvements on three of four fluid intelligence factors as a result of a 16-week exercise program than younger male subjects in both high fit and low fit groups. The program involved Purdue University male faculty and staff as well as local businessmen between the ages of 24 and 68, and consisted of three 90-minute sessions per week of jogging, calisthenics, progressive running, and self-selected recreational activities. *Fluid intelligence* reflects the capacity for abstract reasoning. Fluid intelligence is not influenced by experience and decreases after adolescence. *Crystallized intelligence* is the ability to understand relationships, make judgements, and solve problems based on learned cultural information and skills. As such, crystallized intelligence may increase steadily after adolescence. Older subjects in the Elsayed, Ismail, & Young study had much lower fluid intelligence scores than younger subjects based on pre-testing, so the difference in the amount of change may merely represent statistical regression. That is, individuals with more outlying scores are more likely to regress toward the mean than individuals who initially score closer to the mean.

Barry et al. (1966) measured the effect of exercise on cognition as measured by a three-test battery. Cognitive ability was examined by means of performance on an abstract problem solving test, a short term retention task, and simple addition exercises. Eight normal adults between the ages of 55 and 78 ($M$=69.5 years) trained on an ergometer for three months. These subjects performed a series of two or three minute work periods with varying loads for a total of 10 to 15 minutes, followed by 6 to 10 minutes of loads representing near-maximum effort. No significant changes were found in the experimental and control groups. Perri and Templer (1985) also found no significant changes in short-term memory from a 14-week aerobic exercise program. They had 23 senior citizens participating in calisthenics and walking/jogging while a control group maintained their normal lifestyles.

Powell (1974) looked at mental functioning in geriatric mental patients between the ages of 59 and 89 ($M$ age=69.3 years). Eleven subjects participated in a 12-week program which included brisk walking, calisthenics, and rhythmic movements. Results showed improved mental functioning in the exercise group, and only negligible changes in a control group and social interaction control group. Exercise seemed to improve cognition as measured by the Wechsler Memory Scale and Raven's Progressive Matrices Test, a broad measure sensitive to intellectual impairment.

In summary, the preceding research sought to establish correlations between exercise involvement and changes in mental functioning such as abstract reasoning, problem-solving and retention. Several of the researchers found positive changes in cognition while other researchers found no changes. Future research is needed to clarify what type of cognitive functioning is influenced by exercise, what type of exercise is needed for changes to occur, and what individual characteristics may influence these changes. It also should be emphasized that nearly one-half of the research in this area has been performed with elderly subjects who were institutionalized for psychological impairments. Generalizing of these findings to normal older adults is highly suspect, at best.

## METHODOLOGICAL AND CONCEPTUAL ISSUES

A number of methodological and conceptual problems have occurred in the elderly research reported in the preceding section. Some of these problems are resolvable and, by focusing upon them here, hopefully future researchers will be less likely to make the same mistakes. Other problems may not be resolvable, but there is still merit in identifying the problems so at least appropriate precautions can be taken in interpreting the results of current and future research.

### Age Differences

The elderly do not represent a homogenous group (Blumental et al., 1982). A few years difference in age between "younger" senior citizens and "older" senior citizens could be rather significant, both physically and psychologically. Thus, the selection of subjects may have a major impact on findings (Neugarten, 1975).

Shephard (1978) proposed that old age exists between 65 to 75 years. This is the period immediately following retirement when functional impairment is still relatively minimal. Very old age occurs at 75 to 85 years when functional impairment becomes more significant, but individuals can still live somewhat independently. Ages 85 and older constitute extreme old age, when greater functional impairment and institutional care takes place.

In addition to Shephard's age categorizing, Ostrow (1984) cited research by Birren and Renner (1977) who distinguished three types of aging. *Biological age* is the functional capacity of the life-limiting individual, and *psychological age* is the functional capability in every day environmental

*AGING AND MOTOR BEHAVIOR*

situations. *Social age* refers to the roles and habits a person performs compared to others in the culture. It should be pointed out that the use of age categories does not consider interindividual and intraindividual differences between biological, psychological, and social aging (Ostrow, 1984).

Young-old, those less than 70 years, and old-old, those 70 or older, were age categories delineated in testing by Blumenthal et al. (1982). These were the only researchers to make an effective age distinction with an elderly population. It should be noted, however, that individuals working in the field of gerontology would be more likely to operationalize 80+ years as old-old. Riddick and Freitag (1984) also compared age groups but their groupings were 50 to 54 and 55 and older, making their age comparisons not very meaningful due to the potential differences that can be found within the 55 and older category.

Blumenthal et al. (1982) found significant main effects for age. Individuals 70 years or older showed higher vigor scores than the younger subjects as measured by the Thurston Temperament Schedule, but scored lower on the active scale. Other subscales measuring impulsiveness, dominance, stability, sociability and reflectiveness yielded nonsignificant results. Those 70 years or older also had significantly lower scores on the Type-A behavior pattern measure. Age differences on the POMS, which measures six psychological mood states, were not significant.

Problems caused due to differences in age can be remedied in the future if individual researchers would study a sufficiently large numbers of elderly subjects across a wide enough age range that meaningful age comparisons can be made. Such studies would determine if there are differential effects and considerations for say young-old, middle-old and old-old. For example, one might be able to build the case that external locus of control would be more prominent in the old-old than in the young-old or middle-old. If this type of subject selection is not possible, researchers should at least attempt to draw all their subjects from a homogenous age grouping. When this cannot be done, some attempt should be made to statistically control for differences in age.

## Gender Differences

Consideration for gender differences are not made frequently enough in research. For example, older women have a less secure perception of their body image when compared to older men (Riddick & Freitag, 1984; Sidney & Shephard, 1976), and possibly vary in other personality dimensions as well (Sidney & Shephard, 1976). Body weight, waist girth, hip width, and body fatness increase as an individual ages, and women appear to be more self-conscious about these changes than men.

Lower self-concept and a tendency toward external causality also have been suggested to appear more often in women than men (Valliant

& Asu, 1985). This may influence research results, and should be kept in mind when reviewing studies. For example, Blumenthal et al. (1982) had 18 female subjects and only six male volunteers. Hogan and Santomier (1984) had 11 elderly males compared to 27 females. Perri and Templer (1985) had twice as many women as they did men in their control and treatment groups. Sidney & Shephard (1976) had similar numbers in their study.

Whether this mixture in gender influenced the results in any of the preceding studies is unknown because the experimenters did not analyze for potential sex differences. Without such analyses, we cannot assume the men and women responded the same to exercise. For example, perhaps self-efficacy improvements from participation in a swimming program occurred for only the females in the Hogan and Santomier study. If women have a lower body image and self-concept, as some researchers have found, then they also may be more receptive than men to self-efficacy changes following exercise. Because women comprised over 70 percent of the subjects, their changes alone could have carried the whole group. Until we control and analyze for gender, we cannot answer such questions.

## Volunteerism

The subjects in the studies of older adults were all volunteers who joined primarily for health improvement reasons. Although many of the volunteers may have been in poor health to begin with, perhaps those who did not volunteer had an even lower level of fitness, health consciousness, motivation, or simply different personality characteristics altogether. In a study by deVries (1970), individuals who were previously least active made the greatest gains physiologically. Psychological changes may occur similarly. If there is a difference in fitness levels between volunteers and nonvolunteers, this might cloud the applicability of results obtained with volunteers to those who do not volunteer. On the other hand, exercise volunteers may be interested in the activity or concerned about their physiological or psychological well-being, and therefore may have a certain degree of expectation regarding exercise. Positive expectations may have a significant impact on testing results.

There is no easy solution to the volunteerism problem. Consequently, most future studies also will probably employ volunteers. Some researchers, however, may have access to a retirement community, nursing home, insurance unit, or some other group whereby they could randomly select and assign participants to control and exercise groups. Of course, some type of incentive to participate in the study, such as free medical exams or being eligible at the end of the study for a drawing of some prize, may be necessary to maximize participation rates.

## Physical Screening

Older adults must pass a thorough physical examination before being accepted as potential subjects in exercise research. This ensures their capability to withstand the demands of an aerobic-exercise program. Such screening may reject poorly fit individuals who have certain physical health limitations. Again, this population group may be the most receptive to psychological benefits from aerobic exercise.

The screening issue is more serious than many realize. For example, Sidney and Shephard (1976) rejected 23% of their subjects prior to research and Blumenthal et al., (1982) excluded 35% of their older subjects on the basis of an unsatisfactory physical history and examination. Stamford, Hambacher, & Fallica (1974) eliminated 44% of their patients because of discomfort, EKG abnormalities during exercise, or poor past medical history. Elsayed, Ismail, & Young (1980) eliminated nearly half of their volunteers because of the physical exam results, while Powell (1974), Barry et al. (1966), and Hogan and Santomier (1984) also rejected subjects. Differences in the preceding studies in standards for rejecting subjects may have influenced the findings from these various studies.

There is no way to avoid thorough medical screening when selecting elderly subjects for an exercise study because not all elderly can safely participate in exercise programs. The reader, therefore, is merely advised to be aware of this restriction, and the different criteria used in selecting subjects, when interpreting the results of studies with the elderly. Better standardization could occur in future studies if the sports medicine community would establish guidelines identifying physical limitations serious enough to exclude the elderly from exercise.

## Attrition

Not only is the selection process from physical screening a potential problem, but also is the dropout rate of subjects approved for participation. Although Perri and Templer (1985) failed to cite physical exam rejections in their study, they indicated a 43% dropout rate from their exercise program. Of the 124 elderly volunteers that Sidney and Shephard (1976) began with, 82 were eliminated because of physical exam rejection, dropout, poor health, or late recruitment. Valliant and Asu (1985) noted that only 58% of the subjects in their structured exercise program attended on a regular basis. Many of the other studies failed to mention participation or dropout rates.

Perhaps the positive effects of some of these exercise programs have been exaggerated, in that maybe the dropouts were not experiencing the same positive physical and psychological benefits as those individuals who opted to adhere to the exercise program. Future researchers might be able to lessen the dropout contaminant if they implemented exercise programs that incorporated some of the suggestions for reducing recidivism, currently being proposed by researchers studying exercise adherence. See Dishman (1984), Shephard (1985), and Buffone, Sachs, and Dowd (1984) for suggestions for lowering exercise attrition rates.

## Socioeconomic Background

Coleman, Washington, & Price (1985) found that social background variables explained differences in well-being, rather than exercise participation itself. Results did not support the hypothesis that older women participating in exercise would have a better sense of well-being than nonparticipants. Instead, there were significant main effects for the social variables of occupation, employment status, and education.

This supports Kozma and Stones' (1978) research which claimed social variables such as socioeconomic position, marital state, education level, and occupational status play an important role in older adults' self-perceived well-being. In addition, Riddick and Freitag (1984) found that the perceived body image of participants in an exercise group fluctuated significantly with sociodemographic variables such as perceived satisfactory health status and number of friends in the program. Future studies should test and control for differences in socioeconomic background.

## Duration, Intensity, and Frequency of Exercise

Exercise programs in research studies on the elderly were substantially varied in terms of duration, intensity, frequency, and/or type. Differences in these exercise dimensions may create variances in interpreting psychological improvements among programs. As an example, the length of many of the exercise programs may not have been sufficient to establish definite conclusions regarding improvements in personality, psychological well-being, or mental functioning. Five weeks of exercise, which was the length of some of the exercise programs, may be too short a time for any meaningful or lasting physiological or psychological effects to occur. Obviously, the longer the exercise intervention the greater the likelihood that psychological effects will take place. Further research is necessary to determine the minimal length of exercise intervention necessary to initiate psychological changes. Future research also needs to establish if greater improvements in psychological variables will occur with longer participation (Browman, 1981), and finally to determine if these psychological changes last over time.

Differences amongst the various exercise programs occur most often with the intensity-level variable. Some researchers created vigorous physical activity intensities (approximately 70% to 85% of maximum heart rate) within their exercise programs (Blumenthal et al., 1982; Riddick & Freitag, 1984; Sidney & Shephard, 1976; Stamford, Hambacher, & Fallica, 1974), and other researchers had their subjects exercise at only

40% to 50% of maximum heart rate (Perri & Templer, 1985) or simply take part in flexibility exercises (Valliant & Asu, 1985). A few researchers failed to report intensity levels in their studies (e.g., Powell 1974; Rotella & Bunker, 1978). For aerobic benefits to occur, Sachs (1984) proposed that physical activity should maintain an intensity of 70% to 80% of maximum heart rate, and last at least 15 to 20 minutes. If these minimal exercise standards must be achieved for significant physiological benefits to take place, then perhaps the same exercise standards must be met for significant psychological changes to occur.

For the most part, researchers who studied the elderly established minimal acceptable standards for exercise frequency levels. Each program had exercise sessions scheduled at least three times per week, except for the regimens developed by Riddick and Freitag (1984) and Valliant and Asu (1985) where subjects exercised biweekly. Variations in frequency, intensity, and duration amongst exercise programs may have contributed to differences in results, as suggested by the results of the Sidney and Shephard (1976) study in which intensity and frequency level were intentionally manipulated.

Varying types of aerobic exercise amongst studies may also impact on research results, both physiological and psychological. Sachs (1984) emphasized that aerobic activities such as running, walking, cycling, and swimming provide rhythmic, continuous movement, and thus may more readily permit physiological and psychological benefits compared to activities such as basketball, tennis, and racquetball. Physical activity has many potential operationalizations, and future research should distinguish between the psychological changes they induce (Ostrow, 1984).

Variations in duration, intensity, and frequency among exercise programs have been noted in the elderly literature, with greatest variations occurring within the intensity (Barry et al., 1966; Blumenthal et al., 1982; Elsayed, Ismail, & Young, 1980; Hogan & Santomier, 1984) and duration dimensions (Stamford, Hambacher, & Fallica, 1974; Valliant & Asu, 1985). Comparisons between different levels within each variable and across each variable have been relatively ignored in research examining psychological variables. This needs to be addressed in the future.

## Research Design

Because most of the studies of older adults incorporated different methodologies in their experimentation, it is difficult to compare results across studies. A lack of clarity and specificity in describing the treatment conditions, aerobic levels, subject characteristics, and other aspects of research also make interpretation of results within given studies a most formidable task. A case in point is the study by Valliant and Asu (1985). These researchers did not report subject characteristics and posttested only one of four groups of the study's participants. These limitations make it difficult to show clear comparisons between their groups and to know for whom these findings may be most likely to occur.

Additional problems in interpreting the data from past studies on exercise with the elderly have occurred because of inadequate research designs. It is essential that future research designs be appropriate for examining the stated purpose(s) of the study. This usually means researchers should pretest and posttest all groups so both between and within group comparisons can be made at the end of the study. Examples of studies that failed to do this are Coleman, Washington, & Price, 1985; Riddick & Freitag, 1984; Rotella & Bunker, 1978; and Valliant & Asu, 1985. Although there may be times when pretesting cannot be done, such testing should occur whenever possible.

A design imperative for studies proposing to assess whether the psychological benefits of exercise are a consequence of the physical benefits of exercise is the measurement of all subjects both psychologically and physiologically. This has occurred (Barry et al., 1966; Blumenthal et al, 1982; Elsayed, Ismail, & Young, 1980; Sidney & Shephard, 1976; Stamford, Hambacher, & Fallica, 1974) in less than half of the research with the elderly. Without such documentation it is impossible to know if the exercise condition, and only the exercise condition, elicited a physiological training effect. Also, when no psychological improvements are obtained, we will know it is not the fault of an inadequate exercise program if physiological measurements confirm a training effect.

Variations in the parameters of exercise (frequency, intensity, and duration) provide one of the strongest arguments for measurement of a physical training effect. By evaluating the physiological influence of these exercise variables, researchers can determine the appropriate levels of each necessary to achieve minimal and maximal amounts of psychological improvement (Morgan & Goldston, 1987). Identifying the minimal amount of each dimension necessary to cause psychological benefits may be of particular significance to the elderly. First, only the lower levels of exercise may be within the physical capabilities of some older adults. Second, it may be easier for some elderly individuals to adhere to a more moderate exercise program (Morgan & Goldston, 1987).

Another research design imperative for studies intending to determine if improvements in physical fitness account for psychological benefits is the inclusion of both a control group and a placebo control group. Individuals in the control group would merely continue with their everyday lifestyles, thus serving as a baseline to be compared with both the placebo control group and exercise group(s). When studying population extremes such as the depressed or anxious, the inclusion of a control group is particularly critical in order to rule out effects from the mere passage of time and potential regression to the mean.

A placebo control group is necessary in order to rule out the Hawthorne effect, that is, changes occurring merely as a consequence of the attention given when one receives some type of treatment within an experiment. Designing a placebo control group that incorporates a social condition would be particularly desirable because inclusion of such a group, assuming no psychological benefits occur for it, would help eliminate the criticism that the benefits of group exercise result from increases in social contacts and social reinforcement rather than the physiological benefits of exercising.

Some researchers (Barry et al., 1966; Coleman, Washington, & Price, 1985; Hogan & Santomier, 1984; Perri & Templer, 1985; Riddick & Freitag, 1984) have compared an exercise group to a non-social placebo control group, but this did not eliminate the effects of social interaction. Other studies (Rotella & Bunker, 1978; Stamford, Hambacher, & Fallica, 1974) developed a social control group, but no simple control to establish a baseline for measurement. Unfortunately, Blumenthal et al. (1982) had neither a social interaction nor a non-social placebo control group.

A number of the studies with older adults used a nonequivalent control group design (Coleman, Washington, & Price, 1985; Hogan & Santomier, 1984; Riddick & Freitag, 1984; Rotella & Bunker, 1978; Valliant & Asu, 1985). That is, no randomization of subjects occurred; rather, the control and exercise groups were naturally assembled collectives (Campbell & Stanley, 1966). When this occurs, preexperimental differences such as history and selection biases cannot be ruled out. Pretesting is particularly critical when there is no random assignment. When initial differences are identified, appropriate statistical tools, such as covariance analyses, need to be employed.

The Powell (1974) study would be an excellent research model to emulate, except for its limitation of failing to physiologically pretest and posttest subjects. Powell used a randomized block design that equalized differences in age, gender and ward residence among his three groups: a treatment group that participated in 12 weeks of walking, calisthenics, and rhythmic movements; a placebo control social therapy group that was involved in games, crafts, music, and social interaction with no physical activity; and a normal control group that served as a baseline. Finally, Powell pretested and posttested all subjects on the psychological variables.

## Inappropriate Psychological Measurement

Ismail (1987) reported that the frequent occurrence of nonsignificant psychological results in exercise research may be partially due to the insensitivity of many psychometric tests. Folkins and Sime (1981) noted that a number of researchers measured aspects of personality that are unlikely to change following short-term exercise intervention. An additional measurement problem when doing research with the elderly is that many of the psychological instruments have not been designed or validated with older adult populations, and thus may fail to account for conditions that frequently appear in the elderly while stressing others that tend not to occur with older adults (Brink et al., 1982). In support of this measurement concern, Brink et al. indicated depression measures, including the Zung scale, have given incorrect psychological evaluations for older adults.

Wolber (1980) recommended 11 instruments that may be appropriate for older adults. Yet, test scores from the elderly on these instruments may still be influenced by slowed motor ability, fatigue, and visual and auditory problems that can cause anxiety and poor communication skills. Therefore, the suitability of even these measures will vary based on the individual needs and abilities of the subjects. Related to these measurement problems is the lack of normative data on the elderly.

Barry et al. (1966) used a barrage of nine tools to measure personality, motivation, perception, and cognition. A "shotgun-type" approach is not highly advocated because some tested components may by chance alone show signs of improvement in posttesting, and many subjects will experience problems such as fatigue, concentration lapses, and other factors often associated with taking too many tests at one time.

In addition to the methodological differences that exist between studies, it is difficult to compare psychological variables across research because of the potpourri of measurement instruments. If standardization in measurement was to occur, the Profile of Mood States (POMS) may be one tool worth considering because it has the advantage of measuring six transitory states (tension, depression, anger, vigor, fatigue, and confusion) by rating 65 adjectives, on a five-point semantic differential scale. While this tool has proven quite effective in identifying the psychological benefits of exercise in younger adults, to date only Blumenthal et al. (1982) used the POMS in research with the elderly. When there is interest in measuring changes in somatization as well as psychological variables, the Hopkins Symptom Check List (HSCL) (Derogatis et al., 1971) may be an appropriate tool. This instrument has good validity and reliability, and has been used extensively in the general health literature.

In summary, factors such as subject selection, nonadherence, history, maturation, test-taking effects, and statistical regression can be extremely difficult to control, and clearly hinder both long-term and short-term research with the elderly. Nevertheless, the potential benefits from controlling these factors more than outweigh the difficulties that need to be overcome to create a sound methodology. If greater consideration is given to the methodological improvements suggested here, future research may come closer to effectively evaluating the relationship between exercise and positive psychological change.

## ADDITIONAL RESEARCH NEEDS

Researchers in this area must give greater consideration to the methodological, conceptual, and design issues previously presented if future research is to better clarify the psychological benefits of exercise. This section will address additional research needs which should be considered.

### Elderly Response to Exercise

We reported earlier that Folkins, Lynch, & Gardner (1972) suggested older adults may exhibit more psychological and physiological benefits from exercise because they may initially be in poorer physical and mental health. This suggestion may be true for some elderly, but it certainly is not valid for the elderly who are physically active. A different perspective is that beginning elderly exercise participants may have extensive psychosocial and behavioral histories which make them resistant to immediate psychological changes from exercising. Although there is no direct empirical evidence to support this claim, other than the failure of many studies to find positive changes, it represents a necessary consideration for future researchers. As noted earlier, we also may need to allow longer time intervals for initial psychological improvements to occur in the elderly (Blumenthal et al., 1982).

The preceding propositions are feasible competing explanations for both the timing of and the degree of psychological improvements that may appear in older adults. Future research with the elderly should assess the time interval between the commencement of an exercise program and initial signs of psychological improvements, and any individual differences that may influence these effects. The results of such research would help exercise leaders and participants have a better understanding of when exercise typically can be expected to have an impact on psychological functioning.

### Exercise for Prevention and Rehabilitation

In a recent book, Morgan and Goldston (1987) contended that the only sensible approach to the control of today's major health problems is through prevention, not just treatment. McGinnis (1985) also reported that disease prevention and health promotion are central concerns in recent policy efforts at the federal level. In the final chapter of their edited book, Morgan and Goldston proposed several directions for future research regarding identification of the role of habitual physical activity in the prevention and rehabilitation of emotional and physical disorders.

Because of the relevance of these suggestions to the elderly, who most would agree are at considerably greater risk for at least physical breakdown, three of Morgan and Goldston's specific research questions are included here:

(1) "What is the role of exercise in the management of mental stress in physical disorders such as cancer, diabetes, renal failure and arthritis?" (p. 158); (2) "What is the effect of exercise in comparison to, and in combination with, other approaches to stress reduction such as drug therapy, psychotherapy and other stress management programs?" (p. 157); and (3) "What are the effects of exercise on the following disorders: substance abuse, schizophrenia, personality disorders (esp. antisocial and borderline), sleep disorders, eating disorders, psychosexual disorders, psychosomatic disorders, bipolar disorders, and severe unipolar depression?" (p. 158).

The aforementioned research questions raise many new issues for individuals interested in conducting research with the elderly on the effects of participation in physical activity. To date, very little research has been conducted with younger adults regarding these issues. The relevance of these questions to older adults cannot be denied.

## Mechanisms Underlying Exercise Effects

Several hypotheses have been proposed to identify potential mechanisms underlying the psychological benefits achieved from exercise. The most commonly stated, or implied, hypothesis is that the positive psychological effects are a direct consequence of improvement in cardiovascular functioning. Even if psychological changes are a consequence of improvements in physical fitness, researchers do not know, from a mechanistic standpoint, exactly what physiological changes cause the psychological effects. Discussion of research into some of the proposed physiological mechanisms (beta-endorphins, catecholamines, and increased blood flow to the brain) behind the exercise-emotion-cognition effects is beyond the scope of this chapter. Instead, competing psychological hypotheses such as emotional release, social reinforcement, and self-efficacy/mastery will be addressed.

Although there has been minimal research with the elderly regarding the competing psychological hypotheses for explaining the benefits achieved from exercising, understanding of what might be causing the psychological benefits is as critical with older adults as it is with younger adults. Clarifying which of the hypotheses, and with what types of individuals, offer the best explanation of psychological benefits could have major ramifications for designing optimal exercise environments for given individuals.

Bahrke and Morgan (1978) proposed that fundamental exercise could serve as a channel for the release of stored emotions. Results from Valliant and Asu (1985) suggested that more fearful, depressed, and assertive elderly subjects appeared to seek out physical activity. Many individuals look forward to their retirement years and growing old, but many others experience frustration, anxiety and depression imposed by a decreased ability in performing basic skills and many other factors. This may cause older individuals to turn aggression and anger inward against themselves. Such building internalization, without the emotional release that exercise provides, may lead to psychosomatic illnesses (Kreitler & Kreitler, 1970).

Hughes (1984) proposed still a different hypothesis for explaining the psychological benefits of exercise. This researcher believes individuals experience anxiety-related symptoms (sweating, heart palpitation, and hyperventilation) during exercise, but not the subjective state of anxiety. When these symptoms continue to be present without feelings of anxiety, subjects will start to feel less anxious. Hughes suggested this may be due to several psychological processes: reattribution of symptoms, cognitive dissonance, counter-conditioning, or extinction.

Riddick and Freitag (1984) proposed that social reinforcement and interaction may be the underlying mechanism to best explain the relationship between exercise and mood. In non-elderly populations, this has been one of the most frequently suggested explanations as an alternative to the physiological benefits hypothesis. This explanation may be even more viable for older adults, because of the decreasing social support resources found with the elderly due to the greater likelihood of death of a spouse or friends, retirement from a job, retired friends moving to a warmer climate, and so forth. An individual participating in a group exercise program often receives liberal encouragement and other types of social support from others, which makes the activity all the more enjoyable; morale increases dramatically. There may be individual differences in how important the social environment is to achieving the psychological benefits of exercise in an elderly population. Brown, Ramirez, & Taub (1978), in studying younger adults, reported that some runners claimed they felt better after jogging by themselves, rather than with a group.

Through chronic aerobic exercise, psychological benefits may occur because young and old alike could develop better perception and more conscious control over their own bodily reactions. The mind initiates contact with the body and the two begin working as a single system. A sense of internal mastery arises because the individual builds control over functions such as heart rate, breathing, and so forth. These increased feedback cues (Sidney & Shephard, 1976) become more reassuring as the individual becomes more fit. Self-confidence and an internal locus of control may be enhanced; anxiety and depression may decrease. Perri and Templer (1985) offered some support for this concept. They suggested that confidence and reassurance developed in their older subjects when they became involved in physical activities normally reserved for younger individuals. The internal mastery that develops with prolonged exercise may eventually generalize to several external behavioral situations. In short, aerobic activity may be a form of positive biofeedback that contributes to a sense of mastery and confidence (Hollandsworth, 1979).

Mastery may not only arise from internal control of physiological processes, but also from improved self-efficacy on a particular task. For example, Hogan and Santomier (1984) found that self-efficacy increased for older adults in a swim class, and this self-efficacy improvement was displayed across other tasks and behavioral situations, such as routine housework and extended outdoor activities like walking. Therefore, increases in self-efficacy also may be a mechanism to explain psychological change due to exercise. If so, perhaps the task mastery and resulting self-efficacy effects need not occur in just aerobic activities such as swimming. Learning skills such as bowling or fly fishing may be equally effective in promoting the psychological benefits of exercise.

Kreitler and Kreitler (1970) speculated on another mechanism for the psychological changes brought on through exercise. These researchers believed that physically inactive people see their bodies as being broader and heavier than they actually are. Feelings of awkwardness, anxiety, depression, and insecurity can then develop within these individuals, causing bodily activities to seem increasingly strenuous. The desire to exercise and perceived body image fall even lower in the elderly when they begin to identify with social-stereotyped misconceptions of old-aged behavior (Hogan & Santomier, 1984), creating a circular effect of decreasing activity and declining body image. Exercise may serve to break this continuous self-defeating pattern. As Sidney & Shephard (1976) suggested based on results from their research, improvements in body image as a result of exercise motivate an individual to continue in a fitness program. Through aerobic conditioning older adults begin slowly rebuilding confidence in their physical and cognitive capabilities, achieving a fulfillment in these activity situations that was nonexistent before.

The mechanisms proposed for mediating the beneficial effects of exercise warrant further investigation, for each supposition has merit. Studies designed to compare and contrast different theoretical explanations are particularly needed. While no answer currently exists for explaining whether exercise itself or other factors associated with the exercise experience cause the benefits derived from exercising, additional research may shed light on explanations which appear to be the most viable and with what types of populations.

## CONCLUSIONS AND SUMMARY

Most elderly and exercise research has focused on either general well-being; personality constructs such as mood states, locus of control, body image, and self-efficacy; or cognitive functioning. An increased sense of well-being has not been verified with standardized testing instruments, but does appear frequently when well-being is measured informally such as through interviews. Changes in psychological mood states have been reported, but with more equivocal results than what has been found in nonelderly populations. There is some evidence with the elderly for decreases in anger and anxiety with exercise, but also no evidence for decreased depression in elderly subjects. This may be because most of the research has been conducted with "normal" populations rather than with mildly or moderately depressed populations. Locus of control appears to become more internal through participation in aerobic activity and, while positive changes occur in body image, these changes were as often nonsignificant as they were significant. Cognitive changes also were observed after an exercise program, but this particularly contingent on the measurement tools being used and the nature of the subject population.

Contradictory results have been reached in nonelderly age groups partly because of the existence of many methodological imperfections, conceptual and research design shortcomings, and contradictory theorizations. Unfortunately, these problems also have occurred with research on the elderly. Issues such as volunteerism; differences amongst studies in physical entrance standards and attrition rates; individual differences in age, gender, occupation, employment, marital status, and other sociocultural background variables; and initial psychological and physical variables may significantly influence the psychological changes that occur through exercise. These issues need to be addressed in interpreting the results of existing research and in planning future research if we are to better clarify exactly who might benefit the most from exercise and what benefits are most likely to occur.

Where feasible, suggestions have been offered for eliminating or minimizing some of the preceding problems. Future research directions, based upon these problems and issues, also can be identified. For example: "Do the benefits derived from exercising vary for person's differing in age, gender, socioeconomic background, and so forth"?, "How do the psychological benefits of exercise for elderly in the normal population compare with those persons exhibiting psychopathology or certain physical disorders"?, "What is the role of exercise in the prevention of mental and physical disorders in the elderly"?

Future research also should focus attention on identifying changes between and within the parameters of exercise (type, frequency, intensity, and duration) that are necessary to realize psychological changes. Perhaps some of the exercise programs with the elderly failed to elicit positive psychological changes because the exercise program did not last long enough or the exercise intensity level was too low. The influence of different modes of exercise also needs to be studied more closely. For example, do psychological benefits occur with only rhythmic, aerobic activities? If the answer is no, are any criteria of participation and skill development needed for nonaerobic activities? In short, what are the preferred types, frequency, intensity, and duration of exercise programs needed to both assure psychological benefits and insure adherence in the elderly?

Exactly what might be causing the positive effects of exercise in both elderly and nonelderly populations remains to be determined. Psychological benefits may be a consequence of the physiological changes that occur from improvement in cardiovascular functioning with exercise, or they may be mediated by other factors associated with the exercise experience such as 1) serving as a release for stored emotions; 2) pairing anxiety-related symptoms without the subjective state of anxiety; 3) increasing social contacts and reinforcement, and/or 4) improving self-efficacy/mastery. Studies designed to compare and contrast these different theoretical explanations are particularly needed. Clarifying what mediates the beneficial effects of exercise, and with what types of individuals, has major ramifications for designing optimal exercise programs and environments for given individuals.

Although many elderly do not exhibit significant changes as a result of exercise, most of the results are in a positive direction and this, in itself, is encouraging. If more appropriately designed experiments are conducted in the future, we should be much more able to determine who amongst the elderly are most likely to benefit from exercise, exactly what types of psychological benefits are most likely to occur, and what types of exercise programs are most likely to lead to these benefits.

### REFERENCES

Bahrke, M.S., & Morgan, W.P. (1978). Anxiety reduction following exercise and meditation. *Cognitive Therapy Research, 2,* 323-334.

Bandura, A. (1977). Self-efficacy: Toward a unifying theory of behavioral change. *Psychological Review, 84,* 191-215.

Barry, A.J., Steinmetz, J.R., Page, H.F., & Rodahl, K. (1966). The effects of physical conditioning on older individuals. II. Motor performance and cognitive function. *Journal of Gerontology, 21,* 191-198.

Blue, F.R. (1979). Aerobic running as a treatment for moderate depression. *Perceptual and Motor Skills, 48,* 228.

Blumenthal, J.A., Schocken, D.D., Needels, T.L. & Hindle, P. (1982). Psychological and physiological effects of physical conditioning on the elderly. *Journal of Psychosomatic Research, 26,* 505-510.

Brink, T.L., Yesavage, J.A., Lum, O., Heersema, P.H., Adey, M., & Rose, T.L. (1982). Screening tests for geriatric depression. *Clinical Gerontologist, 1,* 37-43.

Browman, C.P. (1981). Physical activity as a therapy for psychopathology: A reappraisal. *Journal of Sports Medicine and Physical Fitness, 21,* 192-197.

Brown, R.W., Ramirez, D.E. & Taub, J.M. (1978). The prescription of exercise for depression. *The Physician and Sportsmedicine, 6,* 33-45.

Buffone, G.W., Sachs, M.L., & Dowd, E.T. (1984). Cognitive-behavioral strategies for promoting adherence to exercise. In M.L. Sachs & G.W. Buffone (Eds.) *Running as therapy* (pp. 198-214). Lincoln, NE: University of Nebraska Press.

Campbell, D.T., & Stanley, J.C. (1966). *Experimental and quasiexperimental designs for research.* Chicago: Rand McNally.

Coleman, M., Washington, M.A., & Price, S. (1985). Physical exercise, social background and the well-being of older adult women. *Perceptual and Motor Skills, 60,* 737-738.

Collingwood, T.R. (1972). The effects of physical training upon behavior and self-attitude. *Journal of Clinical Psychology, 28,* 583-585.

Collingwood, T.S., & Willett, L. (1971). The effects of physical training upon self-concept and body attitude. *Journal of Clinical Psychology, 27,* 411-412.

Derogatis, L.R., Lipman, R.S., Covi, L., & Rickels, K. (1971). Neurotic symptom dimensions as perceived by psychiatrists and patients of various social classes. *Archives of General Psychiatry, 24,* 454-464.

deVries, H.A. (1970). Physical effects of an exercise training regimen upon men aged 52 to 88. *Journal of Gerontology, 25,* 325-336.

Dishman, R.K. (1984). Motivation and exercise adherence. In J.M. Silva & R.S. Weinberg (Eds.), *Psychological foundations of sport* (pp. 420-434). Champaign, IL: Human Kinetics Publishers.

Elsayed, M., Ismail, A.H., & Young, R.J. (1980). Intellectual differences of adult men related to age and physical fitness before and after an exercise program. *Journal of Gerontology, 35,* 383-387.

Folkins, C.H. (1976). Effects of physical training on mood. *Journal of Clinical Psychology, 32,* 383-388.

Folkins, C.H., Lynch, S., & Gardner, M.M. (1972). Psychological fitness as a function of physical fitness. *Archives of Physical Medicine and Rehabilitation, 53,* 503-508.

Folkins, C.H., & Sime, W.E. (1981). Physical fitness training and mental health. *American Psychologist, 36,* 373-389.

Fretz, B.R., Johnson, W.R., & Johnson, J.A. (1969). Intellectual and perceptual motor development as a function of therapeutic play. *Research Quarterly, 40,* 687-691.

Gardner, V.J., Bennett, J., & Carmack, M.A. (1982). The effect of a program of physical exercise on depression in older adults. *Physical Educator, 39,* 21-24.

Greist, J.H., Klein, M.H., Eischens, R.R., & Faris, J.W. (1978). Running out of depression. *The Physician and Sportsmedicine, 6,* 49-56.

Hilyer, J., & Mitchell, W. (1979). Effect of systematic physical fitness training combined with counseling on the self-concept of college students. *Journal of Counseling Psychology, 26,* 427-436.

Hogan, P.I., & Santomier, J.P. (1984). Effect of mastery swim skills on older adults' self-efficacy. *Research Quarterly for Exercise and Sport, 55,* 294-296.

Hollandsworth, J.G., Jr. (1979). Some thoughts on distance running as training in biofeedback. *Journal of Sport Behavior, 2,* 71-82.

Horley, J. (1984). Life satisfaction, happiness and morals: Two problems with the use of subjective well-being indicators. *The Gerontologist, 24,* 124-127.

Hughes, J.R. (1984). Psychological effects of habitual aerobic exercise: A critical review. *Preventive Medicine, 13,* 66-78.

Ismail, A.H. (1987). Psychological effects of exercise in the middle years. In W.P. Morgan & S.E. Goldston (Eds.), *Exercise and mental health* (pp. 111-115). Washington, D.C.: Hemisphere.

Jasnoski, M.L., & Holmes, D.S. (1981). Influence of initial aerobic fitness, aerobic training and changes in aerobic fitness on personality functioning. *Journal of Psychosomatic Research, 25,* 553-556.

Johnson, W.R., Fretz, B.R., & Johnson, J.A. (1968). Changes in self-concepts during a physical development program. *Research Quarterly, 39,* 560-565.

Kavanagh, T., Shephard, R.J., & Tuck, J.A. (1975). Depression after myocardial infarction. *Canadian Medical Association Journal, 113,* 23-27.

Kozma, A., & Stones, M.J. (1978). Some research issues and findings in the study of psychological well-being in the aged. *Canadian Psychological Review, 19,* 241-248.

Kreitler, H., & Kreitler, S.H. (1970). Movement and aging: A psychological approach. In D. Brunner & E. Jokl (Eds.), *Physical activity and aging* (pp. 302-306). Baltimore: University Park.

McGinnis, J.M. (1985). Recent history of federal initiatives in prevention policy. *American Psychologist, 37,* 1-14.

McGowan, R.W., Jarman, B.O., & Pederson, D.M. (1974). Psychological effects of a competitive endurance training program on self-confidence and peer approval. *Journal of Psychology, 86,* 57-60.

Mihevic, P.M. (1982). Anxiety, depression, and exercise. *Quest, 33,* 140-153.

Morgan, W.P. (1973). Influence of acute physical activity on state anxiety. Paper presented at the meeting of the National College Physical Education Association for Men, Pittsburgh, PA.

Morgan, W.P., & Goldston, S.E. (1987). Summary. In W.P. Morgan & S.E. Goldston (Eds.), *Exercise and mental health* (pp. 155-159). Washington, DC: Hemisphere.

Neugarten, B.L. (1975). The future and the young-old. *The Gerontologist, 15,* 4-9.

Olson, M.I. (1975). The effects of physical activity on the body image of nursing home residents. Unpublished master's thesis. Springfield College.

Ostrow, A.C. (1984). *Physical activity and the older adult.* Princeton, NJ: Princeton Books Company.

Perri, S., & Templer, D.E. (1985). The effects of an aerobic exercise program on psychological variables in older adults. *International Journal of Aging and Human Development, 20,* 167-172.

Powell, R.R. (1974). Psychological effects of exercise therapy upon institutionalized geriatric mental patients. *Journal of Gerontology, 29,* 157-161.

Riddick, C.C., & Freitag, R.S. (1984). The impact of an aerobic fitness program on the body image of older women. *Activities, Adaption and Aging, 6,* 59-70.

Rotella, R.J., & Bunker, L.K. (1978). Locus of control and achievement motivation in the active aged (65 years and older). *Perceptual and Motor Skills, 46,* 1043-1046.

Sachs, M.L. (1984). Psychological well-being and vigorous physical activity. In J.M. Silva & R.S. Weinberg (Eds.), *Psychological foundations of sport* (pp. 435-446). Champaign, IL: Human Kinetics Publishers.

Schwartz, G.E., Davidson, R.J., & Goldman, D.J. (1978). Patterning of cognitive and somatic processes in the self-regulation of anxiety: Effects of meditation versus exercise. *Psychosomatic Medicine, 40,* 321-328.

Shephard, R.J. (1978). *Physical activity and aging.* London: Croom Helm Limited.

Shephard, R.J. (1985). Motivation: The key to fitness compliance. *The Physician and Sportsmedicine, 13(7),* 88-101.

Sidney, K.H., & Shephard, R.J. (1976). Attitudes toward health and physical activity in the elderly: Effects of a physical training program. *Medicine and Science in Sports and Exercise, 8,* 246-252.

Stamford, B.A., Hambacher, W., & Fallica, A. (1974). Effects of daily physical exercise on the psychiatric state of institutionalized geriatric mental patients. *Research Quarterly, 45,* 34-41.

Valliant, P.M., & Asu, M.E. (1985). Exercise and its effects on cognition and physiology in older adults. *Perceptual and Motor Skills, 51,* 499-505.

Weingarten, G. (1973). Mental performance during physical exertion: The benefit of being physically fit. *International Journal of Sport Psychology, 4,* 16-26.

Wolber, G. (1980). A practical approach to the psychological evaluation of elderly patients. *Perceptual and Motor Skills, 51,* 499-505.

Young, R.J. (1979). The effect of regular exercise on cognitive functioning and personality. *British Journal of Sports Medicine, 13,* 110-117.

*AGING AND MOTOR BEHAVIOR*

# 9

## An Exercise Program for Nursing Home Residents

WENDY BLANKFORT-DOYLE

HOWARD WAXMAN

KATHLEEN COUGHEY

FRANK NASO

ERWIN A. CARNER

ELAINE FOX

## ABSTRACT

An exercise program was implemented using ergometer training for impaired nursing home residents. Eight exercise participants and 15 control participants were evaluated primarily for psychological and functional benefits. After 15 months of the program, we have demonstrated the feasibility of exercising this special population of impaired elderly. However, we did not find significant physical, psychological or functional improvements with the designed exercise protocol. Discussion concerns the practical implementation of an exercise program for nursing home residents, the limitations of evaluative research with this unique population, and suggestions for future work in this area.

## INTRODUCTION

Exercise programs have been experimentally used with older adults in a variety of settings. The general premise of such exercise programs is that regular exercise may prevent, retard, or possibly even reverse the physical, psychological, and functional decline that is often seen with aging. Most of these studies and programs have looked at the effects of exercise on relatively healthy, community dwelling elderly. The results of such programs have been mixed, with some showing positive changes

This project was supported by a grant from the William Penn Foundation to Thomas Jefferson University and the Philadelphia Health Management Corporation. Acknowledgement goes to Risa Weinrit, Gerald McCreary, Helene Cohen and Chris Corrigan for their help with this manuscript. Special appreciation goes to the residents and staff of Mercy Douglass Nursing Home for their enthusiasm and cooperation.

attributed to exercise and others showing little or no benefits (Blumenthal et al., 1982; Barry et al., 1966; Gutman et al., 1977; Agate, 1965; Buccola & Stone, 1975). Few programs, however, have examined the influence of exercise on impaired older populations.

One study by Powell (1974) did find significant changes in cognitive status using The Ravens Progressive Matrices Test after 12 weeks of five times per week exercise training on geriatric institutionalized mental patients. The mild exercises included brisk walking at the beginning and end of each session, and calisthenics and rhythmical movements utilizing large muscle movements of the arms, legs, and trunk.

Another study by Stamford, Hambacher, & Falicka (1974), looked at the effects of exercise on nine male geriatric psychiatric patients (average age = 71.5 years). These participants experienced decreased heart rate and systolic blood pressure responses after completing a 12-week program utilizing treadmill and bicycle ergometer exercises. In addition, significant positive changes were shown on the Information Subtest of the Wechsler Adult Intelligence Scale, and on a questionnaire designed to test orientation to hospital and ward routine.

Clark et al. (1975) compared 23 institutionalized geriatric psychiatric patients (average age = 69 years) under three conditions. One group of seven was given a no-treatment condition, a second group of six participated in social and recreational activities, and a third group of 10 exercised daily. These exercises involved light rhythmical activities, stretching, modified weight and circuit training, dancing, and walking performed one hour per day, five days a week, for 12 weeks. Although the exercise group did show a tendency towards increased daily activity levels compared to the social and control groups, these results were not statistically significant.

A study by Karl (1982) tested the effects of a four-week exercise program on self-care activities for institutionalized elderly. Ten elderly residents participated in a range-of-motion exercise program (eight exercise classes), while the control group was not assigned to any exercise regime. Both groups were tested before and after with The Performance Test of Activities, a test that measures 16 different acts of daily living. The group that exercised showed no significant signs of improvement at the post-test; however, two residents individually showed improvement, rising from a somewhat dependent status to an independent one.

A number of different design problems may contribute to these varied results. These include: (1) a sample size that was too small; (2) improper experimental and control group comparisons; (3) exercises that were inappropriate or not of sufficient intensity; (4) duration of the exercises that was inadequate to obtain psychological or functional benefits; (5) specific psychological and functional tests that were not sensitive or appropriate for the elderly population; (6) duration of the program that was too short; and (7) the problem of compliance by the participant.

Approximately four to five percent of Americans over 65 years of age currently reside in a nursing home. Of those over 75 years of age, the proportion increases to about 10 percent. For every five people that live past 65 years of age, it is estimated that one will spend at least part of his or her life in a nursing home (Vladeck, 1980). If the current trend continues, the aged population of nursing home residents should increase by at least 70 percent by the year 2000 (Rubin, 1981). The majority (about 70 percent) of nursing home residents are women; the average age of a nursing home admission is 78 years of age; and the majority (96 percent) are white (Butler, 1975). The average nursing home resident has approximately three to four chronic conditions, with one being psychological (Vladeck, 1980). About half of this population has been diagnosed as having some form of dementia. Between 30 and 40 percent have some type of arthritis and/or rheumatism; approximately 15 percent suffer from diabetes; and more than one in 10 people in nursing homes are at least partially paralyzed (Vladek, 1980). A large proportion also suffer from heart disease, while 16 percent of nursing home residents have some type of serious visual or hearing defect (Butler, 1975).

From this description, it would seem that nursing home residents are often so physically, psychologically and functionally impaired that it is difficult to see potential for improvement, for human experience, or for optimism concerning their existence or future. This common perception may account for the very limited number of physical activity programs in most American nursing homes. Although forms of physical therapy can be found in many nursing homes, few have organized exercise programs for their residents.

Nursing homes are of course plagued by a variety of other problems that may prevent a more opportune climate needed to create change. These include staff morale, staff "burnout," and over-prescribing of medication which may adversely affect instituting an exercise program. Aides suffer from extreme burnout, some of which may be due to the constant and continuing demands put on them with very little acknowledgement or appreciation from the patients and/or their supervisors. In many cases this lack of appreciation from the residents may be due to their physical and emotional constraints. Many staff members also feel that they are up against unreachable goals. This may cause the nurses aides and/or the nurses to do only the minimum that is required for their job. In fact, sometimes a nursing home resident's activity is seen as disruptive by the staff. It is simply easier to care for someone who is rather sedentary than someone who is active (Waxman, Klein & Carner, 1985). In spite of these problems this chapter reports on the design, development, and evaluation of an exercise program for severely impaired nursing home residents, paying close attention to the potential problems of implementing such a program.

## METHOD

### Subjects

Subjects of the following study were residents of a Philadelphia Nursing Home. The majority of residents in the home were in frail health, thus requiring extensive screening. The program's medical director and a rehabilitation specialist, with the assistance of the program nurse, screened all medical charts for potential participants. Next, qualifying residents received a physical examination by a general practitioner and a musculoskeletal examination by the program's medical director. Electrocardiograms were also conducted.

Major exclusionary criteria included: a major organic brain syndrome which would negate a resident's understanding of the program; significant cardiac disease manifested by protracted heart failure or severe angina pectoris; a fragile insulin-dependent diabetic condition; non-ambulatory status because of stroke or bilateral amputations of lower extremities; anemia; and poor kidney function. Of the 180 residents in the home, 23 were medically cleared for the program. Informed consent was obtained from these participants, their doctors, and family members or guardians.

Initially, the participants were randomly assigned to three groups: an Exercise group (n=8), a Nutrition group (n=8) that was to receive a special nutrition program, and a Comparison group (n=7) that received no intervention. However, delays in the implementation of the nutrition program allowed us to combine the Nutrition group with the Comparison group to expand the latter to 15 subjects.

### Apparatus

Equipment purchased for the program included: three ergometer bicycles, a treadmill, and a two-person telemetric system. Two of the bicycles were placed on the floor for lower extremity exercise, and a third was placed on a table, modified as an arm ergometer. Patients could sit in their wheel chairs and exercise their arms by turning the pedals of the bicycle with their hands.

Several other adaptions were made in the equipment to accommodate the physical problems of the residents. Pedal extension tubes were purchased and fastened to the pedals of the bikes extending the pedals away from the cycle, allowing residents with special hip problems to ride. Fastening straps were used to secure the resident's feet in the pedals, particularly for one person who rode the cycle with only one leg. A small stool was needed for some of the patients to get on the bicycles, and cloth bags were designed to hold the telemetric transmitters; these were fastened around the participant's necks.

## Exercise Sessions

Exercise sessions were conducted three times each week for 15 months under the direction of a rehabilitation specialist with the assistance of an exercise physiologist and a nurse. Prior to exercise, the residents' resting heart rates and blood pressures were always recorded; during exercise, heart rates were continually recorded on the telemetry. Residents exercised according to prescribed protocol based on initial stress tests, and according to their physical capacities (i.e. use of upper and lower extremeties). Three of the Exercise group participants could walk independently; the remaining members walked only with the assistance of a device or another person, but for the most part they were sedentary and rarely used their lower limbs. Amputees or individuals with impaired function of the lower limbs exercised with the arm ergometer only. One individual with a fused left knee used the arm ergometer for upper extremity exercise, and rode the exercise bicycle with only the right leg for lower extremity exercise. For the latter, the left pedal of the bicycle was removed allowing for rotation of the right pedal.

As mentioned, for some individuals the use of their lower extremeties had deteriorated to the point where they could not rotate the pedals of the bicycles. Characteristically, these patients would rock the pedals back and forth but were not able to make a complete rotation. In these cases, a pattern was incorporated whereby two staff members knelt by the bicycle and used their hands to assist the residents in completing each cycle. This system was met with early success and these individuals went on to independently ride the bicycles for a duration of five to 10 minutes. On the other hand, the motor skills of the residents' upper extremeties were sufficiently maintained so that no pattern assistance was necessary to teach them to use the arm ergometer, and no fasteners were required to keep their hands on the pedals.

## Physiological Assessment

Prior to the beginning of the program, and at six and 12 month intervals, individuals in both the Exercise and Control groups underwent submaximal stress tests for both upper and lower extremities (where appropriate), and tests for agility. These measures were used as base line data to compare with subsequent measures, and for the development of individual exercise protocols. The program physician, an exercise psychologist, and a nurse were all present during stress testing. Either the treadmill or the bicycle ergometers, whichever was appropriate for the individual, were used for lower extremity tests; upper extremity tests were done on the arm ergometer.

Treadmill stress testing was based on a modified Naughton-Balke Protocol (Wenger & Hellerstein, 1984). This was chosen because it has a very low initial workload and more gradual increments as compared to other protocols. After both resting heart rates and blood pressures were recorded, the residents walked on the treadmill at a constant speed (2mph) beginning at a zero percent grade. Small elevations in the grade (3.5 percent) were made every two minutes. This two minute interval was a modification of the Naughton-Balke Protocol in which each stage was three minutes. At each two minute interval, blood pressures and heart rates were recorded. Heart rates were also monitored throughout the test on the telemetry. Exercise was terminated when the resident experienced fatigue. In the event of a medical problem, exercise would have been terminated immediately; however, no medical problems occurred during any of the stress testing for the program. Resting heart rates were recorded at one, two, four, six, and eight minute intervals after exercise ceased.

Stress tests on the exercise cycles were based on a modified standard bicycle protocol (Pollack, Wilmore & Fox, 1984). Once resting measures were recorded, participants rode the cycles at 40 watts (this is a modification of the standard protocol of 50 watts) with zero resistance. At three minute intervals, resistance was increased by 25 watts and blood pressure and heart rates were recorded. Again, exercise was discontinued when residents experienced fatigue which was usually indicated by the fact they could not maintain 40 watts. At the completion of the test, resting heart rates and blood pressures were again recorded at one, two, four, six and eight minute intervals.

Upper extremity stress tests, based on a modified standard arm ergometer protocol (Hellerstein & Franklin, 1984) also began at zero watts. The subjects were asked to exercise for a three minute warm up period at 40 watts (the standard is 50 watts), rest for two minutes, and then continued to work for four minute intervals, with two minute breaks in between. The reason for the rest periods were twofold: (1) they allowed the test administrator to get an accurate heart rate and blood pressure; and (2) it minimized the local fatigue factor. Because the arms have a much smaller muscle mass than the legs, the local fatigue factor during arm stress tests was greater than during lower extremity tests. Individuals discontinued exercise when they experienced fatigue; recovery heart rates and blood pressure were recorded at that time.

Upper and lower extremity stress tests were always conducted on different days so as not to fatigue the participants, and in addition, to get an accurate measure of their endurance and capability. In a few cases, the residents could not complete the initial stress test. Two of the participants did not have the functional ability to rotate the pedals of the bicycles. A few others simply did not have the endurance to obtain the minimum watts necessary for the stress test or were not able to complete the first stage of the stress test. For these people, beginning measures were unavailable; however, they were all able to complete at least the first stage of the test after six months of regular exercise.

## Psychologial Assessment

Psychological tests were administered by the research assistants before the program and every three months for the duration of the program to all participants. The tests chosen were those either previously used in exercise research with the elderly, or those that had received extensive use in other research with older adults and had been tested for their reliability and validity. Tests were chosen to measure depression, mental status, memory, and functional ability.

The *Geriatric Depression Scale* (Yesavage et al., 1983) is a self-report scale designed to detect depression in older adults. Certain items are scored in reverse in order to eliminate a negative response bias. Cut-off scores had been established in order to divide the population into normal, moderate, and severely depressed groups. Concurrent and discriminant validities of the *Geriatric Depression Scale* have been shown with older psychiatric patients (Hyer & Blount, 1984). The *Cornell Medical Health Index Questionnaire* (Monroe et al., 1965) is a frequently used assessment of general health, and was used here to evaluate somatic complaints which are also an indicator of depression in the elderly (Waxman, Klein, & Carner, 1985). This instrument has been tested for its reliability and validity as a diagnostic instrument (Brodman et al., 1951).

The *Mental Status Questionnaire* (Kahn et al., 1960 A; Kahn et al., 1960B) also has been used extensively in geriatric research. It is correlated with clinical diagnosis of organic brain syndrome and reports an alpha reliability at .84 and a test-retest reliability of .8 (Kahn et al., 1960b). The *Wechsler Memory Scale* (Wechsler, 1945) was developed to create a test that would yield measures that correlated well with intelligence tests, but would not duplicate them in any way. This scale has been tested for reliability and validity on the elderly population, and norms have been obtained for people in their 80's and 90's (Klonoff & Kennedy, 1965). Although The *Wechsler Memory Scale* has been utilized with the elderly, there are still some questions of validity concerning whether the test also measures cooperation, willingness, and/or motivation (Erickson & Scott, 1977).

The *Ravens Colored Matrices* assesses various intellectual processes of mentally deficient people: young children, and very old individuals (Foulds and Raven, 1948). This test is useful in that it is relatively independent of repetitive verbal instruction. *The Colored Matrices Subset* is able to generally assess the ability to complete figures as wholes that are spatially related.

*The Nurses' Observation Scale (NOSIE)* is based on a nurse's observation of a patient over the last three days prior to the administration of the questions (Honigfeld & Klett, 1965). The presently existing measure has been scaled down from its original 100 items in order to eliminate those questions which are not reliable. The scale was originally designed and perfected for use with older schizophrenic patients. The *NOSIE* is divided into seven subsets which measure (1) social competence, (2) social interest (3) personal neatness, (4) cooperation, (5) irritability, (6) manifest psychosis, and (7) psychotic depression. Dye (in press) gives a report on the inter-rater reliabilities for separate factors as very high (above .8). *The Kenny Self-Care Evaluation Scale* (Schoening et al., 1965) measures a patient's ability to function independently in the activities of daily living using objective measures. In addition, it can measure improvement (the progress is depicted numerically) and compare treatment results by looking at whether physical dependency changes, as the number of transfers and the time taken for transfers either increases or decreases. Schoening and Iversen (1968) reported face and content validity; they also found that by using the scale, it is possible to plot a learning curve that can predict rehabilitation time and offer suggestion regarding discharge planning.

## RESULTS

The entire program was conducted for a duration of 15 months. At the end of this time, six of the original eight Exercise participants were still exercising in the program. Two of the participants were hospitalized at about nine months and never re-entered the program. Twelve of the original 15 participants in the Comparison group remained with the program; one left the program after six months and two left after nine months. One was hospitalized for hypertension, another for a respiratory problem, and the third for a condition that was not known to the research staff. One participant in the Comparison group refused psychological and physiological testing at an early portion of the program; however, functional evaluation data by the nurses were available. Thus, there is no indication at all that participants in the Exercise group suffered adverse effects as a result of exercise compared to participants in the Comparison group. Obviously with any nursing home population, it is natural to expect health problems within a 15 month period of time.

Compliance with the exercise protocol was quite high throughout the duration of the program. For example, attendance during month 1 was 96.1%, month 2 was 98.3%, month 7 was 86.5% and month 14 was 98.4%. Our protocol would, of course, be expected to result in higher compliance than a program based entirely on self-initiated exercise (Perkins et al., 1986). The residents' enthusiasm was also quite evident throughout the program, and most of those in the Exercise group really seemed to appreciate the attention and activity.

Table 9-1 shows examples of levels of ergometer performance (measured as watts and time duration) at four points during the program. Both arm and leg activity are shown for four participants, and arm activity only for the other two participants who could not exercise with their legs. The initial low levels of performance seen in the first week of the program may reflect unfamiliarity with the routine and equipment, rather than low capacity. Participants soon reached a higher level of performance once they were more comfortable with the protocol. As can be seen in the table, performance increased uniformly for most participants as the program progressed. Although these results were not evaluated statistically, they are reflected in the increased wattage and/or time duration of exercise. However, the meaning of this increase is not entirely clear. Although it could represent increased physical capacity, it could also reflect increased participant familiarity with the protocol and/or increased staff confidence in allowing the participants to exercise more.

The effects of exercise on stress test performance were determined by evaluating heart rate levels at a standard point, which was two min-

**TABLE 9.1.** *Exercise Performance Level for Six Participants At Four Points in the Program.*

| | First Week | | Month 5 | | Month 9 | | Month 13 | |
|---|---|---|---|---|---|---|---|---|
| | Watts | Time | Watts | Time | Watts | Time | Watts | Time |
| Participant 1 | | | | | | | | |
| Arm Bike | 0 | 7 min. | 25 | 9 min. | 30 | 10 min. | 40 | 10 min. |
| Bicycle | 0 | 0 min. | 0 | 5 min. | 30 | 10 min. | 35 | 10 min. |
| Participant 2 | | | | | | | | |
| Arm Bike | 25 | 5 min. | 45 | 11 min. | 55 | 15 min. | 45 | 15 min. |
| Bicycle | 25 | 10 min. | 45 | 15 min. | 55 | 15 min. | 65 | 15 min. |
| Participant 3 | | | | | | | | |
| Arm Bike | 0 | 3:05 min. | 15 | 10 min. | 40 | 10 min. | 45 | 10 min. |
| Bicycle | 0 | 1:51 min. | 5 | 7 min. | 40 | 10 min. | 45 | 10 min. |
| Participant 4 | | | | | | | | |
| Arm Bike | 0 | 2:23 min. | 0 | 3:45 min. | 35 | 14 min. | 35 | 10 min. |
| Bicycle | 0 | 0 min. | 0 | 3 min. | 35 | 10 min. | 35 | 10 min. |
| Participant 5 | | | | | | | | |
| Arm Bike | 0 | 10 min. 0:30 min. | 50 | 16 min. | 65 | 20 min. | 75 | 20 min. |
| Participant 6 | | | | | | | | |
| Arm Bike | 50 | 20 min. | 35 | 15 min. | 55 | 15 min. | 40 | 10 min. |

utes into the stress test with the arm ergometer (on which all subjects could be tested). T-test comparison of changes of scores in heart rate between the initial and the 12 month stress tests for Exercise and Control groups, however, failed to reveal a significant difference between groups ($t$ = .9 nonsignificant).

Table 9-2 shows the results of the psychological evaluations taken at the beginning of the program (zero months), and at three month intervals throughout the program, as well as corresponding data from the nurses' evaluation of functional activity. Also shown at the bottom of the table are the results of repeated measures two-way ANOVAS comparing Exercise and Comparison participant's scores. As can be seen from the table, there were no obvious effects of exercise over the course of the program as measured by psychological or functional tests.

## DISCUSSION

### Setting Up a Program

After 15 months of the program, much has been learned about conducting an exercise program in a nursing home. This knowledge should be useful to anyone interested in initiating a similar program.

Initially, one would need to not only obtain the approval of the nursing home administrator, but also to have his or her enthusiasm. Mostly this is important for logistical reasons. In addition, the nursing home administrator can help "sell" the idea of an exercise program to the rest of the staff. In our specific program, the administrator was extremely cooperative and enthusiastic, and only voiced a concern about the safety of the residents during exercise. Because a medically trained individual was always present during the exercise sessions, the concern about physical safety diminished.

The most costly part of our program was the purchasing of equipment. This included the bicycles, telemetry, blood pressure cuffs, stethoscope, and filing system. Originally, a treadmill was included in part of the purchased equipment, but was found quite inappropriate for our specific population; the majority of the nursing home residents were not able to walk at even the slowest speed of the treadmill. The cost of one bicycle is approximately $300 and the telemetry can usually be purchased for around $425 (the telemetry is not necessary unless you are monitoring heart rates). Blood pressure cuffs and stethoscopes can usually be found already on site in the nursing home, and materials for filing can be purchased at minimal cost. It is important to maintain a filing system showing the type of exercise performed, increases or decreases in performance, and all medical records.

Our specific program was somewhat staff intensive. The residents involved were frail and often needed one-on-one supervision, therefore

**TABLE 9.2.** *Mean test scores for initial and follow-up psychological and functional assessment for Exercise Group (n = 6) and Comparison Group (n = 11)*

| Test | Group | Month 0 | 3 | 6 | 9 | 12 | 15 | ANOVA Group | Trial | Group × Trial |
|---|---|---|---|---|---|---|---|---|---|---|
| Geriatric Depression Scale | Exercise | 4.3 | 6.0 | 4.5 | 4.6 | 4.6 | 4.3 | 0.01 | 2.36 | 1.82 |
| | Comparison | 4 | 4.7 | 5.3 | 6.1 | 3.8 | 3.0 | | | |
| Somatic Complaints | Exercise | 4.5 | 5.3 | 3.5 | 2.3 | 1.5 | 3. | 2.11 | 5.67** | 1.88 |
| | Comparison | 1.6 | 1.9 | 1.4 | 1.7 | 0.2 | 0.6 | | | |
| Memory Score | Exercise | 1.6 | 1.5 | 2.3 | 1.1 | 0.6 | 0.8 | 0.04 | 0.96 | 1.82 |
| | Comparison | 1.6 | 1.1 | 0.8 | 1.0 | 1.2 | 1.5 | | | |
| Digits Forward | Exercise | 4.0 | 4.8 | 4.6 | 3.0 | 2.8 | 2.1 | 0.90 | 3.49* | 1.09 |
| | Comparison | 3.1 | 3.9 | 2.6 | 1.8 | 2.1 | 3.7 | | | |
| Digits Backwards | Exercise | 2.0 | 1.0 | 1.0 | 1.5 | 1.0 | 1.0 | 1.28 | 1.44 | 0.49 |
| | Comparison | 1.1 | 1.0 | 0.0 | 0.7 | 0.7 | 0.3 | | | |
| Visual Score | Exercise | 1.5 | 1.3 | 1.1 | 0.3 | 0.5 | 0.8 | 0.30 | 1.09 | 1.47 |
| | Comparison | 0.7 | 0.7 | 0.8 | 0.2 | 0.3 | 0.7 | | | |
| Associate Learning | Exercise | 71.6 | 83.8 | 103.5 | 65.3 | 104.0 | 66.3 | 0.24 | 0.89 | 1.12 |
| | Comparison | 67.0 | 70.1 | 71.0 | 93.2 | 82.7 | 90.4 | | | |
| Ravens | Exercise | 0.8 | 0.6 | 0.8 | 0.6 | 1.0 | 0.6 | 0.01 | 2.32 | 0.59 |
| | Comparison | 0.6 | 0.6 | 1.1 | 1.9 | 0.5 | 0.2 | | | |
| MSQ | Exercise | 4.3 | 4.3 | 4.3 | 4.0 | 3.5 | 3.5 | 0.62 | 3.89** | 1.13 |
| | Comparison | 3.2 | 2.8 | 2.8 | 2.2 | 2.3 | 2.5 | | | |
| NOSIE | Exercise | 69.6 | 85.8 | 61.1 | 73.4 | 56.1 | 80.8 | 1.05 | 15.12** | 1.15 |
| | Comparison | 80.6 | 97.7 | 61.5 | 94.0 | 48.0 | 105.6 | | | |
| Kenny Self Care | Exercise | 61.6 | 55.6 | 60.6 | 64.0 | 65.1 | 58.6 | 0.30 | 0.93 | 0.97 |
| | Comparison | 64.5 | 61.2 | 62.7 | 63.5 | 63.5 | 62.5 | | | |

* $p < .05$
** $p < .01$

requiring one or two staff people to work with each resident at any one time. Given these constraints on the staff, it was only possible to exercise two residents at any one time. Considerable time was required to transport the residents from the rooms, get them ready for exercising, conduct the exercises, and transport them back to their rooms. These factors severely limited the number of participants that could be involved in a program of this type. Much time was lost as staff had to wait for the residents to be brought to the program. A lot of waiting around could be avoided through the use of volunteers, such as Physical Therapy and/or Occupational Therapy students who could be involved in all phases of the program. Not only would this be a good learning experience for the students, but it would cut down the cost of hiring additional staffing. Another possibility is to have each aide become responsible for transporting their own patients down to the exercise room. In addition to volunteers, a successful program would need a nurse to monitor heart rates, take blood pressures, and act as a medical supervisor, and an administrator (i.e. - activities director, physical therapist, exercise physiologist, etc.) who could be in charge of the overall running of the program.

Originally, we believed that compliance from the residents would be a major obstacle, but we found this to be only a small problem at the start-up of the program. Exercising quickly became part of the resident's routine and some individuals would arrive in the exercise room on their own. In addition, the continual activity and care of the exercise staff helped to increase the compliance rate. The residents quickly began to look forward to the special attention that they received by being part of the program. The nurses and aides were helpful in maintaining the residents' enthusiasm for the program as it would often become a topic of conversation between staff and residents.

Choosing a time of day for the program can be very important for everyone involved and can directly affect the attendance rate. During most of the program, exercise sessions were conducted in the afternoons as this time was very quiet for the residents in terms of other activities that might interfere. Eventually, the time was changed to early evenings due to staff conflicts, and this time seemed to work well also. The morning is usually not an opportune time as this is when most of the grooming of the residents takes place. Other considerations that might interfere based on an individual basis include visits from relatives, favorite T.V. shows and snack and meal time. If family members chose to visit during the exercise sessions, we would often invite them to watch so they could understand and appreciate our efforts better. It is also important to consider shift changes, although this did not affect us directly as we brought in our own staff.

A few other important points that should be considered became apparent as the program progressed. As the staff got to know the residents

AGING AND MOTOR BEHAVIOR

more on a personal level, they learned more about the "social circles" of each floor. Being aware of which residents were friendly with each other helped in two major ways. One was the task of bringing the patients down off the floors to exercise. If two residents were good friends, it would make the staff's task a lot easier if they approached the two friends together when it was time to exercise. In addition, it was important to know if one friend was sick or had been hospitalized as this change would directly affect the mood and performance of the other friend. Some residents were incontinent, so it was necessary to not only be aware of this condition, but also to make sure that they were brought to the bathroom right before exercising and immediately following the completion of the session. Intermittent illnesses and hospitalizations did occur and it was important to keep abreast of these events. If a resident had just returned from a stay in the hospital, the staff had to be realistic in their expectations of his or her capacity and desire to exercise. As the staff became more familiar with each resident's personality and day-to-day habits, everything seemed to run even more smoothly.

It became apparent that it was important to involve the nurses/aides with the exercise program, even if this simply meant sitting down with the staff and explaining our purpose. By allowing the nursing staff to watch our program, they became much more willing to help with encouraging the residents participation, and in addition were more apt to inform our staff of any particular quirks and/or mood changes of the residents that might affect their performance. Also, most aides and/or nurses are merely involved in the maintenance end of working with the residents and never really get to see any positive changes. Therefore, by involving the nursing staff, it gives them an opportunity to view some positive behavior and beneficial changes in their patients.

Towards the end of the exercise program, we began to work on instituting a walking program for the residents. Although this is still in its initial stages, we are already realizing that a walking program may be easier for some homes to institute as an exercise program. A walking program is less staff intensive, allows more residents to participate, is less costly, and enables the residents to walk outside the home during the nice weather. A walking program is a future possibility that should be explored more fully.

## Physical Effects of Exercise

Five out of six participants who completed 15 months of the program were performing at increasingly higher workloads and for a longer duration as the program progressed. Since exercise limits were determined by monitored heart rate activity, there was some evidence of improved physical performance. This improvement in daily performance, however, was not reflected in significantly improved stress test performance.

Thus, there is no clear-cut evidence of physical benefits to the participants of this program.

## Psychological and Functional Effects of Exercise

As mentioned previously, the Exercise participants showed little if any improvement on the various psychological or functional measures compared to the Control participants. Thus, from this admittedly small study we were unable to find any psychological benefits as a result of exercise among nursing home residents. How should we interpret these results? On the one hand, this was a study with an Experimental and Control group comparison that was conducted for a considerable amount of time. From these considerations, one could justifiably conclude that there are no psychological benefits of exercise for nursing home residents. However, before we come to this conclusion, perhaps prematurely, one should also consider some of the limitations of the study that may have impacted on these findings.

The number of participants in the project was small. Thus, it is possible that a similar program with an increased number of subjects would have showed some statistically significant effect. However, it must be admitted that there is no trend in our data to suggest such an interpretation. Another possible limitation concerns the measuring instruments used in the study. It is possible that the special nature of our participants may have rendered these tests too insensitive or not appropriate enough to measure the psychological effects of exercise. There is a serious shortage of appropriately tested instruments designed specifically for the nursing home population and the development of such tests should be given high priority in aging research. It is also possible that the exercise protocol itself was not one that would yield a maximal impact on the psychological status of our population.

Exercycles were chosen as they had been used in previous research and it seemed easiest to quantify the exercise protocol with this method. However, there is absolutely no reason to expect that riding an exercycle is the best method for yielding psychological benefits for nursing home residents. Of course, psychological effects of exercise have been difficult to demonstrate in all populations.

The functional status of the residents also did not improve as a result of exercise. This admittedly discouraging finding also needs to be interpreted carefully. The finding is discouraging in that one of the major benefits for an exercise program to the nursing home staff would be that exercise would improve the functional status of nursing home residents and thus ease the burden on staff. Many of the same precautions that were given in interpreting the negative psychological effects of exercise should also be included when interpreting the negative functional benefits. Also, there are additional limitations to be applied here.

In this project, program personnel did not have the time to directly observe the functional activities of the residents and rate them. Thus, nursing staff from the nursing home had to conduct the ratings of functional status. This meant that at any one data collection point, different staff had to evaluate different residents; and from one data collection point to another, different staff were also involved in the evaluation of any one resident over time. This less than desirable circumstance arose out of the budget constraints of the project, and the limitations and turnover of the staff in the nursing home itself. Another factor of course could be that the type of exercise itself (e.g. exercycles) did not lend itself to improvements in functional status. It may be that a more targeted program of physical therapy is required to notice improvements in specific functional abilities of residents.

In summary, staff and participants showed great enthusiasm toward the program and compliance was high. Moreover, there were no injuries to participants resulting from program activities during 15 months of exercising. These results suggest that others should be encouraged to pursue exercise research with this population. Although the objective measures in this study did not reveal psychological or functional benefits of exercise, the rather positive subjective observations of the staff, and the participants' enthusiasm for the program indicates that work in this area should continue. Other projects may find new and perhaps more creative methods of exercise and evaluation of the benefits of exercise in nursing home residents.

## REFERENCES

Agate, M. (1965). Case studies of preventive and remedial exercise to improve functional capacity of the well-aging. *Gerontologist, 5,* 30.

Barry, A.J., Daly, J.W., Pruett, E., & Steinmetz, J.R. (1966). The effects of physical conditioning on older individuals. I. Work capacity, circulatory-respiratory function, and work electrocardiogram. *Journal of Gerontology, 21,* 182-191.

Blumenthal, J.A., Page, H.F., Birkhead, N.C., & Rodahl, K. (1982). Psychological and physiological effects of physical conditioning on the elderly. *Journal of Psychosomatic Research, 26,* 505-510.

Brodman, K., Erdmann, A.J., Jr., Lorge, I., & Wolff, H.G. (1951). The Cornell Medical Index - Health Questionnaire II. As a diagnostic instrument. *Journal of the American Medical Association, 145,* 152-157.

Buccola, V.A., & Stone, W.J. (1975). Effects of jogging and cycling programs on physiological and personality variables in aged men. *Research Quarterly, 46,* 134-139.

Butler, R.N. (1975). *Being Old in America* (Chapter 9). New York: Harper and Row Publishers.

Clark, B.A., Wase, M.D., Massey, B.H., & Van Dyke, R., (1975). Response of institutionalized geriatric mental patients to a twelve-week program of regular physical activity. *Journal of Gerontology, 30,* 565-573.

Dye, C.J., D.J. Margen & W.A. Peterson (Eds.)., *Research Instruments in Social Gerontology Vol. I.,* Minneapolis: University of Minnesota (in press).

Erickson, R.C., & Scott, M.L., (1977). Clinical memory testing: A review. *Psychological Bulletin, 84,* 1130-1149.

Foulds, G.A., and Raven, J.C. (1948). Normal changes in mental abilities of adults as age advances. *Journal of Mental Science, 94,* 133-142.

Gutman, M., Brown, S., Herbert, C. (1977). Feldenkrais versus conventional exercise for the elderly. *Journal of Gerontology, 32:* 562-572.

Hellerstein, J.K., and Franklin, B.A. Exercise Testing and Prescription. *Rehabilitation of the Coronary Patient,* Second Edition, Wenger, N.K., and Hellerstein, H.K. eds., John Wiley and Sons, New York, p. 207, 1984.

Honigfeld, A., Klett, C.J. Nurses Observation Scale for Inpatient Evaluation: A New Scale For Measuring Improvement in Chronic Schizophrenics. *Journal of Clinical Psychiatry*, 1965, 21:65-71.

Hyer, L., Blount, J. Concurrent and discriminating validities of the Geriatric Depression Scale with older psychiatric inpatients. Psychological Reports, 1984 (Apr.), Vol. 54 (2), 611-616.

Kahn, R.L., Goldfarb, A.I., Pollack, M., and Gerber, I.E. Relationship of Mental and Physical Status in Institutionalized Aged Persons. *American Journal of Psychiatry*, 1960a, *117*, 120-124.

Kahn, R.L., Goldfarb, A.I., Pollack, M., and Peck, A. Brief Objective Measures for the Determination of Mental Status in the Aged. *American Journal of Psychiatry*, 1960b, *117*, 326-328.

Karl, C.A. The Effects of an Exercise Program on Self-Care Activities for the Institutionalized Elderly. *Journal of Gerontology*, 1982, 8:282-285.

Klonoff, H. and Kennedy, M. Memory and Perceptual Functioning in Octogenarians in the Community. *Journal of Gerontology*, 1965, 20:328-333.

Monroe, R.T., Whiskin, F.E., Bonacich, P. and Jewell, WO III. The Cornell Medical Index Questionnaire as a Measure of Health in Older People. *Journal of Gerontology*, 1965, 20: 18-22.

Perkins, K.A., Rapp, S.R., Carlson, C.R., Wallace, C.E., A behavioral intervention to increase exercise among nursing home residents. *The Gerontologist*, 1986, 26: 479-481.

Pollack, M.L., Wilmore, J.J., & Fox, S.M. III. (1984). *Exercise in health and disease* (p. 173-174). Philadelphia: W.B. Saunders.

Powell, R.R. (1974). Psychological effects of exercise therapy upon institutionalized geriatric mental patients. *Journal of Gerontology*, 29, 157-161.

Rubin, D.L. (1981). Physician care in nursing homes. *Annals of Internal Medicine*, 94, 126-128.

Schoening, H.A., & Angeragg, L., Bergstrom, D., Fonda, M., Steinke N., & Ulrich, P. (1965). Numerical scoring of Self-Care foundation. *Archives of Physical Medicine and Rehabilitation*, 49, 221-229.

Schoening, H.A., & Iversen, I.A. (1968). Numerical scoring of self-care scoring of Self-Care foundation. *Archives of Physical Medicine and Rehabilitation*, 49, 221-229.

Stamford, B.A., Hambacher, W., & Fallica, A. (1974). Effects of daily physical exercise on the psychiatric state of institutionalized geriatric mental patients. *The Research Quarterly*, 45, 34-41.

Vladeck, B.C. (1980). *Unloving Care*. New York: Basic Books Inc.

Waxman, H.M., Klein, M., & Carner, E.A. (1985) Psychotropic medication misuse by nursing homes: An institutional addiction: In E. Gottheil, *Alcohol, drugs and aging*. Springfield, Ill.: Charles C. Thomas Pub.

Wechsler, D.A. (1945). A Standardized memory scale for clinical use. *Journal of Psychiatry*, 19, 87-95.

Wenger, N.K., & Hellerstein, H.K. (Eds.), (1984). *Rehabilitation of the coronary patient*. (p. 416). New York: John Wiley and Sons.

Yesavage, J.A., Brink, T.L., Rose, T.L., Lum, O., Huang, V., Adey, M.B., & Leiver, V.O. (1983). Development and validation of a geriatric depression rating scale: A preliminary report. *Journal of Psychiatric Research*, 17, 27-49.

# Part V
# Aging and Exercise Motivation

## INTRODUCTION

In the preceding sections of this book, research was presented documenting the positive relationship of exercise to the physical and mental health of older adults. Yet, in spite of this mounting evidence, there are also data (e.g., McPherson & Kozlik, 1980; Ostrow, 1980, 1984) that indicate that people disengage from participation in exercise as they grow older, at least within most western, industrialized societies. Furthermore, among middle-aged and older adults who begin participating in a formal program of exercise, compliance and adherence are major impediments to success. It has been estimated that approximately one-half of these individuals will drop out of an exercise program within the first six months of initiation (Dishman, 1984).

A number of demographic, social, and psychological variables have been identified that relate to understanding why people are less active as they grow older. As Shephard and Sidney (1979) noted: "The decline of activity may be due to job promotion, retirement, social and cultural expectations, lack of opportunities for exercise, institutionalization, accidents or illness, rather than to true biological aging" (p. 15). In addition, personal (Dishman, 1984) and situational factors (e.g., Ice, 1985) contribute to the incidence of drop-out from exercise programs. What has been lacking, however, has been a unified attempt to identify theoretically and empirically those factors that are responsible for the decline in exercise motivation with increasing age.

In the chapters that follow, Duda and Tappe focus on the Theory of Personal Investment (Maehr & Braskamp, 1986) as a framework for understanding the motivational orientations of older adults toward exercise participation. Essentially, Duda and Tappe advocate that the subjective evaluation or meaning of the exercise environment dictates the extent to which an individual will invest his or her resources into exercising. Duda and Tappe outline the Theory of Personal Investment. They then present cross-sectional data contrasting young, middle-aged, and older adults, by gender, in terms of their personal incentives toward exercise, sense of physical competence, fitness locus of control, goal directedness, and social identity.

In contrast, Dzewaltowski adopts Bandura's (1986) social cognitive theory as a framework for understanding older adult exercise motivation. Self-efficacy, or the confidence that an individual has that he or she can meet the requirements of an exercise program, is viewed as a central predictor of whether that individual will sustain participation in exercise. Furthermore, the individual's satisfaction or dissatisfaction with the potentially multiple outcomes of an exercise program serves as a motivator for future exercise behavior. Dzewaltowski suggests a number of avenues for future research on older adult exercise motivation based on social cognitive theory.

In many ways, both theoretical orientations are similar. Most significantly, both frameworks emphasize the importance of assessing the older adults' cognitive evaluation of the exercise experience. Levels of confidence and feelings of satisfaction/dissatisfaction are clearly examples of factors that mediate an older persons' evaluation of the exercise experience. What is not clear at this point, however, is the extent to which developmental changes with age, both biological and psychosocial, modify the theoretical approaches we take toward understanding exercise motivation among older adults.

# REFERENCES

Bandura, A. (1986). *Social foundations of thought and action.* Englewood Cliffs, NJ: Prentice-Hall.

Dishman, R.K. (1984). Motivation and exercise adherence. In J.M. Silva and R.S. Weinberg (Eds.), *Psychological foundations of sport* (pp. 420-434). Champaign, IL: Human Kinetics.

Ice, R. (1985). Long-term compliance. *Physical Therapy, 65,* 1832-39.

Maehr, M.L., & Braskamp, L.A. (1986). *The motivation factor: A theory of personal investment:* Lexington, MA: Lexington Press.

McPherson, B.D., & Kozlik, C.A. (1980). Canadian leisure patterns by age. Disengagement, continuity, or ageism:? In V.M. Marshall (Ed.), *Aging in Canada: Social perspectives* (pp. 113-122). Pickering, Ontario: Fitzhenry and Whiteside.

Ostrow, A.C. (1980). Physical activity as it relates to the health of the aged. In N. Datan & N. Lohmann (Eds.), *Transitions of aging* (pp. 41-56). New York: Academic Press.

Ostrow, A.C. (1984). *Physical activity and the older adult: Psychological perspectives.* Princeton, NJ: Princeton Book Company.

Shephard, R.J., & Sidney, K.H. (1979). Exercise and aging. In R. Hutton (Ed.), *Exercise and sport science reviews* (Vol. 7) (pp. 1-57). Philadelphia: Franklin Institute Press.

# 10

## Personal Investment in Exercise Among Middle-Aged and Older Adults

JOAN L. DUDA

MARLENE K. TAPPE

## ABSTRACT

This chapter establishes the significance of determining the motivational orientations of middle-aged and older adults toward exercise and proposes the Theory of Personal Investment (Maehr & Braskamp, 1986) as a framework for studying these orientations. The theoretical premise of this cognitive motivational theory is that the subjective "meaning" of a situation is the critical determinant of an individual's personal investment of his or her resources into the situation. Meaning is comprised of three interrelated components: Personal incentives, sense of self, and perceived options. These major components and their related constructs are delineated and considered in regard to their application to exercise involvement among the elderly. Recent research which supports the tenets of the Theory of Personal Investment is highlighted. The chapter concludes with suggestions for future studies on the meaning of exercise among those in the later years of life.

## INTRODUCTION

The understanding of what motivates older adults to engage in physical activity is an important realm of inquiry for exercise scientists, health psychologists, gerontologists, and practitioners alike. In this chapter the significance of determining the motivation for participating in exercise or the meaning of physical activity among elderly adults is addressed. A recent theoretical perspective on motivation, i.e. the Theory of Personal Investment developed by Maehr and Braskamp (1986) is proposed as a framework for determining the motivational perspective of those in the later years of life toward exercise. This theory is described and the theoretical constructs critical to the determination of personal investment are defined in reference to the exercise domain. Recent research which supports the application of the Theory of Personal Investment to the study of physical activity among older adults is discussed. The chapter concludes with suggestions for future research on the motivational determinants of exercise behavior among the elderly.

## PHYSICAL AND PSYCHOLOGICAL BENEFITS OF EXERCISE IN LATER LIFE

A considerable body of literature has suggested that regular involvement in exercise has positive physical and psychological consequences for adults in the later years of life. The physiological benefits of physical activity among the elderly have been well documented (Bove, 1983; Shephard, 1986; Smith & Serfass, 1981), and studies have indicated that older adults can improve their physical capacity with exercise training (Davidson & Murphy, 1986). In general, this research suggests that the need for regular exercise continues with chronological aging and that the physical decline associated with aging is, in part, a function of muscular disuse (Smith & Gilligan, 1986). Moreover, past investigations have found a significant correlation between participation in physical activity and ratings of physical health among the elderly (Breslow & Enstrom, 1980; Franks, Lee, & Fullerton, 1983; Howze et al., 1986; McPherson, 1986).

Gerontological research has also indicated that there are psychological benefits from exercise for elderly participants (El-Naggar & Ismail, 1986; Griest et al., 1979; Jasnoski et al., 1981; McPherson, 1986; Ostrow, 1984; Price & Luther, 1980; Young, 1979). Specifically, involvement in physical activity has been linked to stress reduction, greater life satisfaction and self confidence, improved cognitive functioning, more positive perceptions of health, and overall improved mood states among older adults.

## EXERCISE AND THE ELDERLY

Given these reported benefits of exercise, it is interesting and important to point out that there is a reduction in physical activity level and intensity with age (Boothby, Tungatt, & Townsend, 1981; Curtis & White, 1984; McPherson, 1983; Prohaska et al., 1985; Rudman, 1986). This decreased involvement in exercise among older adults is not due to age-related physiological change alone (Spreitzer & Snyder, 1983). In fact, research (Harootyan, 1982) has indicated that more than half of elderly Americans have no health and/or medical limitations on their physical activity. Recently, an emphasis has been placed on the social and psychological factors which can explain the sedentary lifestyles of the elderly (McPherson, 1986).

Reasons suggested for this lack of involvement in physical activity include stereotypes concerning the appropriateness of physical activity for older adults (Ostrow & Dzewaltowski, 1986; Ostrow, Jones, & Spiker, 1981); lack of access to facilities and programs (Maloney, Fallon,

& Wittenberg, 1984); limited child socialization experiences; lack of present role models; concerns regarding personal limitations to participating in exercise (Maloney, Fallon, & Wittenberg, 1984); beliefs that exercise is harmful or at least not disease preventive (Maloney, Fallon, & Wittenberg, 1984; Prohaska et al., 1985); overestimation of the conditioning value of the exercise elderly people are currently involved in (Harris, 1979; Wiswell, 1980); and a low level of knowledge regarding appropriate exercise programs (Maloney, Fallon, & Wittenberg, 1984).

At the present time, research (Heckler, 1985; Hersey, Probst, & Portnoy, 1982; National Cancer Institute, 1984; Prohaska et al., 1985) is indicating that older adults are expressing significantly greater interest and concern regarding health issues than are younger adults. A recent report from the Office of Disease Prevention and Health Promotion (Maloney, Fallon, & Wittenberg, 1984) asserts that not only are the elderly interested in learning about maintaining and promoting their health, they are more willing to make lifestyle changes to be healthier. An evaluation study by Hersey, Klibanhoff, and Probst (1983), for example, revealed that participants aged 65 and older in a public education program showed greater knowledge and behavioral changes than participants from younger age groups. Specifically, in respect to exercise, evidence exists which suggests (Harris, 1979; Howze et al., 1986; Maloney, Fallon, & Wittenberg, 1984) that the elderly are becoming more aware of the link between physical activity and health status. A recent study by Heitmann (1986) revealed that health motives were the most salient incentives of older adults participating in physical activity programs. Further, research has indicated that physically active older adults tend to be more interested in their health (McPherson, 1986).

Given the benefits of regular physical activity for older populations and the fact that the elderly tend to adopt a sedentary lifestyle while becoming more concerned with their health status, there is a need to determine the meaning of exercise as an experience in itself and as a contributor to mental and physical health among the elderly. Such information would provide us with more insight into their degree of involvement in exercise, choice of physical activity, and continued participation. Further, an understanding of the meaning of physical activity to older adults will allow us to begin optimizing the likelihood of elderly participation in exercise. In a report of the U.S. Department of Health and Human Services (1980, p. 32), an objective was set that by 1990, "50% of adults 65 years and older should be engaging in appropriate physical activity (e.g., regular walking, swimming or other aerobic activity)". To reach this goal, it would appear that we need to develop and design exercise programs for the elderly which are sensitive to social and psychological dimensions as well as age-related differences in physiological capacity (Davidson & Murphy, 1986; Shepherd, 1986).

# APPROACHES TO EXAMINING MOTIVATION
# IN EXERCISE CONTEXTS

The examination of the motivational factors linked to involvement in physical activity among the elderly necessitates that we go beyond previous person approaches to predicting participation and adherence in exercise programs. Exemplified in the work of Dishman (Dishman & Gettman, 1980; Dishman & Ickes, 1981), perspectives which focus on the person examine whether there is anything about the individual's personality, physical characteristics, previous experience, and other factors that would lead to a prediction of his/her exercise behavior. In general, an individual difference perspective on physical activity tells us who does or does not engage in exercise. This approach does not provide insight, however, into *why* an individual participates or does not participate in exercise and/or which exercise environments would be more attractive to the person. One practical limitation of a person factor approach to exercise behavior, of course, is that this perspective does not readily suggest any intervention strategies for enhancing exercise involvement.

The determination of the meaning of exercise by older adults would also require that we move past a situational approach to understanding physical activity patterns. In general, previous exercise-related studies which focus on the situation have suggested that contextual factors such as program and facility accessibility (Andrew et al., 1981; Haskell, 1985); choice of activity and structured goal setting (Thompson and Wankel, 1980); structured self-monitoring (Oldridge and Jones, 1983); the intensity of the exercise program (Pollock et al., 1977); the quality of leadership and the amount of encouragement from program leaders (Durbeck et al., 1972; Martin & Dubbert, 1982); and whether the program allows people to exercise alone or in groups (Dishman, 1984) are important determinants of participation and persistence in exercise programs. In respect to the issue of exercise among the elderly, the situational perspective is limited in that it is assumed that all people (regardless of age, experience, physical capacity, etc.) would respond to an exercise environment in the same way.

It would seem that the most effective approach to determining exercise behavior among the elderly would be an *interactionist perspective,* which emphasizes the complex interplay between the characteristics of the person *and* the situation in which he/she is acting (Dishman, 1984). It is reasonable to assume that the meaning of physical activity in the lives of older adults would depend on age-related differences in self perceptions and the perceived value of exercise (Person Factors), and the extent to which physical activities are deemed available, appropriate and appealing for those in the later years of life (Situational Factors).

An interactionist perspective considers that participation in physical activity would be dependent on the person's actual and perceived physical capacity *in relation* to the actual and perceived physical demands of the exercise environment. Thus, if an elderly person perceives his/her physical competence to be lacking and the neighborhood exercise program to be too challenging, he/she would probably decide not to participate. An interactionist approach would also consider the possibility that exercise participation would correspond to the congruence between the participant's exercise goals *and* the incentives perceived to be available in the exercise setting. Drawing from an interactional framework, one might hypothesize that if an older adult values social experiences in leisure activities, and his/her exercise class does not provide the opportunity for social interaction, that person would be likely to drop out. The same would not be predicted for the elderly participant in the class who is motivated to exercise because of the fitness benefits.

An interactionist perspective holds that variations in exercise behavior would be a function of the degree to which an individual identifies himself/herself as an active person *as well as* the social support he/she receives for exercise. Thus, one might predict that if an older adult perceived himself/herself to be physically self efficacious and believed exercise to be critical to his/her sense of self and health status, then that person might engage in physical activity regardless of the degree of environmental support for an active lifestyle. Participation in exercise might also be predicted, however, in the case of an older adult who does not view exercise in the same light but has physically active friends or family and their social support.

## THE THEORY OF PERSONAL INVESTMENT

An interactionist perspective on behavior is exemplified in the theory of Personal Investment (Maehr, 1984; Maehr & Braskamp, 1986). In the case of exercise and aging, this theoretical perspective would assume that older adults are not more or less motivated to engage in exercise. Rather, one would argue that the elderly might be motivated in different ways because of age-related person characteristics in physical and other life domains.

Personal Investment Theory was developed by Maehr and his colleagues in an attempt to integrate the essential propositions and models from past and present research into a comprehensive approach for the study of motivation and behavior. This cognitive motivational theory proposes that the subjective perceptions or *meaning* of a situation is the critical determinant of a person's personal investment of his or her resources into the situation. That is, personal investment could be considered a course of action taken based upon choices made in reference to the meaning of the situation at hand (Maehr & Braskamp, 1986).

## Components of Personal Investment Meaning

Specifically, as depicted in Figure 10-1, Maehr and his associates (Maehr, 1984; Maehr & Braskamp, 1986) proposed that meaning is comprised of three interrelated facets: *personal incentives, sense of self,* and *perceived options.* Each of these facets are represented in some form in the literature on motivation theory and research. Further, these constructs are cognitive in nature as they are categories of thoughts, perceptions, and beliefs which are assumed to be critical mediators of present and future behavior in a particular context. In the theory of Personal Investment, personal incentives and sense of self variables are held to be characteristics of the person while perceived options are specific to the situation at hand.

**Personal Incentives:** The motivational focus of the activity is referred to as *personal incentives* (Maehr, 1984). According to Maehr and Braskamp (1986), there are four broad categories of incentives or motivational orientations which are assumed to be operative in guiding an indi-

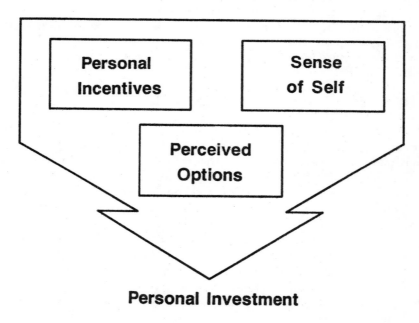

FIGURE 10.1. *The components of meaning. (Adapted from Maehr, 1984.)*

vidual's personal investment in most situations: task incentives, ego or self incentives, social incentives, and extrinsic rewards. In general, task incentives reflect an orientation to mastery, skill improvement, and/or becoming involved in an activity for it's own sake. Ego incentives relate to an individual's orientation to competition and power. Competition is the desire to do well in reference to a socially defined standard of excellence, particularly a standard based on the performance of others. This motivational orientation could be considered social comparison-oriented while task incentives tend to be self-referenced in nature. Power incentives, on the other hand, are distinguished by a person's desire to control the activities of others.

According to Maehr and Braskamp (1986), social incentives are exemplified by goals focused on affiliation and social solidarity. The desire to please others and be altruistic are also classified as social incentives.

The fourth category of personal incentives proposed by Maehr and Braskamp (1986) is that of extrinsic rewards. These incentives typically reflect a goal orientation based on financial reward and/or social recognition (fame, status.)

Importantly, the theory of Personal Investment (Maehr, 1984; Maehr & Braskamp, 1986) assumes that variations in personal incentives would relate to person factors such as age. In general, Maehr and Braskamp cite research (Edward & Wine, 1963; Klein, 1977; Neugarten, 1977) and offer evidence in the workplace (Wigfield & Braskamp, 1985) to suggest that competition and social recognition incentives are less salient and affiliation and task incentives are more important to the elderly, when compared with young and middle-aged adults. Congruent with the arguments of Maehr and Kleiber (1981), it is acknowledged that increasing age, and in particular, retirement, might result in the need to meet ego and extrinsic incentives in other life domains such as physical activity. In general, Maehr and Braskamp (1986) point out that there is no overall decline in incentive level with increasing age. Rather, they suggest that older people tend to redistribute their personal investment toward different incentives in different situations.

In support of the tenants of the theory of Personal Investment (Maehr and Braskamp, 1986), research has indicated that task, ego, social, and extrinsic reward incentives are manifested in physical activities. Further, studies conducted in exercise settings have revealed other incentives which capture the possible physical and mental benefits of exercise behavior (fitness, health, and stress reduction). Importantly, there is evidence to suggest that the varied personal incentives which appear to be operant in exercise settings provide us with insight into the meaning of exercise among older adults. Relevant research and an illustration of each of these incentives in the exercise domain is now highlighted.

*Task incentives:* Within the context of exercise, an individual who is task oriented would tend to focus on his or her personal improvements in physical skill and capacity and/or the intrinsic enjoyment of the exercise experience itself. Recent research has suggested that task incentives are salient in the exercise domain. Work by Pemberton & Roberts (1985) has indicated that task incentives (such as meeting one's personal exercise goal) are valued among young and older adults involved in a regular exercise program. Beran (1986) has noted that the desire to excel is evident among elderly women involved in structured exercise. In a study of older men and women, Steinkamp and Kelly (1986) reported that the emphasis placed on incentives reflecting personal challenge related positively to involvement in leisure activity. Research has found that task incentives are prevalent in physical contexts and relate to the intensity of participation and persistence among young adult recreational sport participants (Duda, 1987, 1988, in press).

*Ego incentives:* It appears that the ego incentive which is primarily operant in the exercise domain is that of competition. In an exercise setting, a person oriented to a competition incentive would tend to socially compare his/her performance and capacity with others (e.g., Am I stronger than others?; Do I have more endurance?; Can I beat others on the basis of my physical skills and physiological capabilities?), and to prefer competitive activities over those that are more cooperative or individualized in nature.

Given the present literature, it seems that the emphasis placed on competition in physical activity varies more as a function of gender than chronological age. In general, studies have indicated that the incentive of competition is consistently more salient among males than among females in physical activity settings, regardless of their age [Duda, 1986a, 1986b, 1988; Gill, 1986]. This gender difference has emerged in research examining personal incentives in the exercise domain among young, middle-aged, and older adults. Beran (1986), however, has noted that there are some women (regardless of age) who continue to compare their abilities with others and express a desire to compete in exercise programs.

*Social incentives:* In the exercise context, the social or affiliation incentive is primarily expressed when a person partakes in a physical activity in order to be involved with other people. It has been suggested that social affiliation is an important reason for participating in physical activity among older adults and women in general. Mobily (1981) found that elderly patients in nursing homes engaged in physical activity for social contact. We observed that young, middle-aged, and older women tended to emphasize affiliation exercise incentives more than men in the same age groups. (Please refer to Chapter 11.)

*Extrinsic rewards.* As suggested by the work of Pemberton and Roberts

(1985), social recognition is the reward incentive that is usually operant in respect to exercise behavior. People often participate in physical activities to gain attention or approval from significant others. At times, it may be the outcome of exercise (improved physical appearance) which yields social recognition, and thus motivates one to engage in physical activity. In other cases, individuals may be motivated to participate in exercise so that others notice that they are physically active.

Steinkamp and Kelly (1986) found the emphasis on social recognition incentives to be linked to involvement in leisure activities among older men and women. In our study of men and women involved in exercise specifically, we found that the social recognition received for participation in physical activity was particularly salient for young women and middle-aged and older men.

*Health, coping with stress, and improvement of physical capacity or fitness incentive:* Specific to the domain of exercise, research has indicated that there are other incentives operating which give meaning to physical activity behaviors. As suggested by the work of Heitmann (1986) and others (Mobily, 1981; Sidney & Shepherd, 1976) on older adults, *physical health and fitness benefits* and the possibility that exercise can help in *managing or coping with stress* can also be salient exercise incentives.

Noland and Feldman (1985) indicated that the emphasis placed on the fitness aspects of regular exercise by women (25 to 65 years of age) positively relates to exercise adherence. Research by Sidney and Shepherd (1976) has found the health and fitness attributes of exercise to be rated most important by the elderly.

In our study of exercise program participants 25 to 81 years of age, middle-aged and older adults emphasized the possible health benefits as an incentive for exercise more than young adults. The mean emphasis placed on the personal incentives of health benefits, fitness benefits, coping with stress, task mastery, affiliation, competition, and social recognition among the participants 40 years and older in this study (n = 80) can be seen in Figure 10-2.

Drawing from the tenets of the theory of Personal Investment, we have been developing the Personal Incentives for Exercise Questionnaire which can be utilized with young and older adult samples (Duda & Tappe, 1987). At the present time in this research, the multidimensional nature of exercise goals has been demonstrated, and seven valid and reliable personal incentive scales have emerged.

**Sense of Self:** The second facet of meaning proposed by Maehr and his associates (Maehr, 1984; Maehr & Braskamp, 1986) is *sense of self.* Sense of self is the individual's collection of thoughts, perceptions, beliefs, and feelings related to who he/she is. In his 1984 work, Maehr delineated four aspects of sense of self, namely *sense of competence, self-reliance, goal directedness,* and *social identity* (see Figure 10-3).

# Personal Investment Profiles

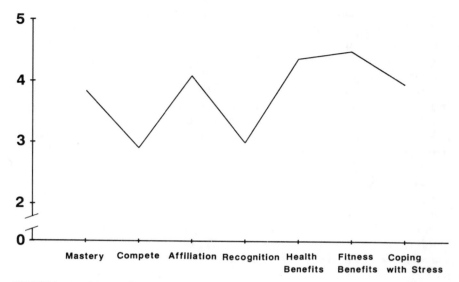

**FIGURE 10.2.** *Mean rankings for middle-age and older adults on each of the seven Personal Incentives for Exercise Questionnaire subscales.*

*Sense of competence*: An individual's sense of competence is his/her subjective judgment of his/her ability to do something successfully (Harter, 1980). According to Maehr (1984), a sense of competence is a powerful determinant of one's personal investment in that it leads the individual to select activities which are self-enhancing. Sonstroem (1978) has proposed that one's self perceptions of physical competence affect one's general self esteem, and in turn relate to participation in exercise.

In regard to the older adult specifically, it has been suggested that one of the important reasons why elderly people do not engage in exercise is that they tend to underestimate their physical capabilities (Conrad, 1976; Wiswell, 1980). In a study of 135 men and women (ages 17 to 64 years) who took part in a physical fitness evaluation program, Thorton and his colleagues reported an age-related decline in perceived physical ability (Thorton et al., 1987). Given that an age-related decline in *actual* physical ability was also observed among these subjects, the authors suggested that older adults might be judging their personal level of physical ability relative to the standards of young adults *or* their own ability when younger. Among young, middle-aged, and older adults who were regular participants in an exercise program, however, we found no significant age-group differences in perceptions of physical competence, fitness, and strength. Importantly, in this study of exercise participants, levels of per-

*AGING AND MOTOR BEHAVIOR*

# SENSE OF SELF

**Competence**
 **-Physical Self Efficacy**
 **-Health Status**

**Self-Reliance**
 **-Fitness Locus of Control**

**Goal Directedness**
 **-Self Motivation**

**Identity**
 **-Activity Level of Significant Others**
 **-Preceived Support from Significant Others**

FIGURE 10.3. *Components of sense of self according to Maehr and Braskamp (1986).*

ceived physical ability significantly predicted present life satisfaction among those program members 40 years and older (see Tappe & Duda, 1987). Dzewaltowski (1986) has also found perceived physical self efficacy to correspond to perceived future life satisfaction among the elderly.

*Self-Reliance:* According to Maehr (1984), self-reliance is an individual's perceptions regarding the origins of his/her destiny, as originally proposed by deCharms (1968). In terms of physical activity, self reliance would be reflected in the degree to which an individual views his/her level of exercise and fitness to be under his/her own control, or determined by external factors such as fate or significant others. A recent study by O'Brien (1981) found that a sense of personal control in leisure activities predicted life satisfaction among Australian retirees. Langlie (1977) found that a strong sense of personal control of one's health status is predictive of engagement in preventive health behaviors such as exercise. Noland and Feldman (1985) reported that scores on an internal exercise locus of control scale was positively related to exercise behavior among middle-aged and older women. In contrast, the chance and powerful others scales showed a strong negative relationship to exercise participation. Perceived self control over one's physical health status was found to be related to physical activity level in a study of young and older adults involved in fitness programs (Gottlieb and Baker, 1986).

*Goal Directedness:* In the theory of Personal Investment, the construct of goal directedness is defined as the individual's tendency to set goals and arrange his/her behavior accordingly (Maehr, 1984; Maehr & Braskamp, 1986). In their research focused on the occupational domain, Maehr and Braskamp (1986) observed that employees above the age of 54 years were lower in goal directedness than younger co-workers. Heinzelmann and Bagley (1970) observed that individuals who tend to set specific long-term health and exercise goals were more likely to adhere to an exercise regime. The concept of goal directedness is very similar to the personality trait of self motivation which has been found to significantly predict adherence in exercise programs among young and older adults (Dishman & Gettman, 1980; Dishman & Ickes, 1981).

*Social Identity*: Social identity is defined as an individual's perception of his/her association with certain groups and holding of selected others as significant. Although this dimension of sense of self has not been substantiated in Maehr's research in the occupational domain (Maehr, 1984; Maehr & Braskamp, 1986), Langlie (1977) found that social membership is an important predictor of an individual's likelihood to engage in exercise. Other studies have indicated that social support for exercise and identification with significant others who are active are critical to exercise adherence among healthy populations and cardiac patients (Andrews et al., 1981; Bjurstrom & Alexiou, 1978; Heinzelmann & Bagley, 1970). Research by Gottleib and Baker (1986) on young and older adults involved in exercise programs revealed that the level of physical activity of both male and female participants correlated with the degree of exercise involvement of their male friends. Whether or not one's female friends were physically active correlated with the exercise behavior of the women participants only.

**Perceived Options:** The final construct of meaning delineated by Maehr and his colleagues (Maehr, 1984; Maehr & Braskamp, 1984) is that of *perceived options*. Perceived options refer to the behavioral alternatives that an individual perceives to be available in a given situation. Not only must a significant number of these alternatives be present and perceived, they must also be acceptable to the individual. In the context of exercise and fitness for example, this construct is exemplified in the perceived barriers to regular exercise. (See Figure 10-4.) The unavailability of programs geared specifically to the elderly and lack of proximity to exercise facilities are critical barriers to exercise participation among older adults (Maloney et al., 1984). Other barriers include lack of time, family responsibilities, as well as concerns regarding the appropriateness of physical activity and personal limitations to participate in exercise (Maloney, Fallon, & Wittenberg, 1984; Ostrow, Jones, & Spiker, 1981; Prohaska et al., 1985).

The construct of perceived options also relates to an individual's perception that a given exercise program allows him/her to meet his/her program goals and personal incentives. In a recent study of the perceived

# PERCEIVED OPTIONS

# IN EXERCISE

## Perceived Barriers
## to Exercise

## Perceived Program
## Opportunities

FIGURE 10.4. *Components of perceived options in reference to exercise.*

options held by members of five different exercise programs, Pemberton (1986) found a link between this factor and exercise adherence. Specifically, those participants who perceived that their present fitness program provided them with the opportunity to realize their personal incentives were more likely to continue involvement in the program.

## Behavioral Indices of Motivation

According to Maehr (Maehr, 1984; Maehr & Braskamp, 1986), personal investment or motivation can be inferred from a variety of behavioral indices. In the exercise context these indices include choice of activity, persistence, intensity of activity level, and performance level.

**Choice:** The first of these indices, *choice* or direction, refers to the apparent choice that is made among a set of behavioral alternatives. Choice is not a simple behavioral observation; rather, in reality, it is an inference made when a person elects to do one thing when other possibilities are available to him or her. In research on the meaning of exercise among older adults, for example, choice might be inferred by distinguishing between those older adults who chose to attend a noon hour exercise program, instead of joining a friend for lunch (i.e., participants vs. nonparticipants). Choice can also be inferred from observing that, within a communty exercise program, an elderly adult prefers a specific exercise class such as aquacize rather than aerobics (i.e., specific form or type of exercise activity).

**Persistence:** The second behavioral pattern from which motivational or personal investment inferences can be made is *persistence*. Persistence refers to the behavioral patterns where an individual continues to attend to a behavior for an extended period of time. That is, the person repeatedly chooses the same behavioral alternatives while simultaneously rejecting other alternatives. Among older adults, persistence can be operationalized in respect to class attendance and/or years of involvement in regular physical activity.

**Intensity:** The third behavior pattern operant in an exercise context which infers motivation is *intensity* or activity level. Intensity refers to the amount of energy expended, and is a primary indicator of the exertion of physical effort. This index refers not only to the physiological intensity to which someone partakes in a particular physical activity, but also to the overall level of involvement in physical activity. It is important to point out, however, that especially among the elderly, the behavioral index of intensity is a less reliable indicator of motivation or personal investment as it is more likely to be influenced by physiological factors (level of strength, cardiovascular endurance, and physical health status) than the other indices.

**Performance:** The final behavioral pattern from which motivation can be inferred is performance. Good performance infers high levels of motivation in situations where variations in performance cannot be explained by other factors such as competence or skill. This may be exemplified by two older adults who are nearly identical in age, health and physical abilities but one of the individuals consistently outperforms the other during the exercise session. Performance, however, cannot be considered a pure measure of motivation, as the other indices of motivation (choice, persistence, and activity level) can be reflected in performance level. Furthermore, within the domain of exercise there are difficulties in determining physical performance among the elderly, with respect to measures of physiological and physical capacity (Shepherd, 1986; Smith & Serfass, 1981).

Each of the preceding indices may be considered descriptions of behavioral patterns indicative of motivation. The Theory of Personal Investment (Maehr & Braskamp, 1986) attempts to delineate the unifying principles which underlie these differing patterns of behavior. The metaphor of personal investment is viewed as an appropriate term for capturing the underlying *meaning* of the preceding patterns of behavior. Personal investment implies the distribution or investment of an individual's resources such as time, talent, and energy into particular situations such as physical activity. Specifically, the theory proposes that the investment of an individual's resources, his/her pattern of behavior, is determined by one's personal perception of the *"meaning"* of the situation in which he/she is acting.

## AN APPLICATION OF THE THEORY OF PERSONAL INVESTMENT TO EXERCISE BEHAVIOR AMONG THE ELDERLY

In a recent study of 47 older adults (50 to 81 years of age) who were regular participants in an organized exercise program, we examined the relationship of personal exercise incentives, sense of self variables, and perceived options to self-reported behavioral investment in physical activity, (Duda & Tappe, 1988). The emphasis each participant placed on the goals of mastery, competition, affiliation, social recognition, coping with stress, health benefits, and fitness benefits were determined with the Personal Incentives for Exercise Questionnaire. Perceptions of sense of self were assessed by examining the program members' level of physical self efficacy (perceived competence), fitness locus of control (self reliance), level of self motivation (goal directedness), and the perceived fitness level and social support provided by significant others (social identity). Consistent with Maehr and Braskamp's (1986) research in the occupational domain, perceived options were defined as the degree to which the participants believed they had the opportunity to meet each of the seven personal incentives in the exercise program.

Variables reflecting each of the three dimensions of meaning significantly predicted the participants' level of physical activity (intensity) and accounted for 39.5% of the variance. The older adults who exhibited a higher level of weekly exercise had higher perceived physical self efficacy and self motivation. They were also more likely to perceive their physical fitness status to be under their personal control. Levels of physical activity were best predicted by the personal incentives for exercise. Specifically, the program members who had a higher level of involvement in regular exercise were more likely to exercise for social recognition and fitness benefits.

Variables reflecting the third component of meaning, namely perceived options, also predicted exercise intensity. In particular, those older adults who reported a higher level of physical activity were more likely to perceive a congruence between their affiliative goals and the social opportunities presented in the exercise program.

Personal incentives, sense of self variables, and perceived options also significantly predicted the program members' expected level of physical activity in six months (37.5 % variance accounted for). The older adults who expected to maintain their regular involvement in exercise tended to stress mastery, affiliation, and fitness incentives. Further, they were more likely to perceive that their present physical health status was good, and less likely to view that their fitness level is controlled by chance or external factors. Finally, the older adults who believed that they would continue their exercise involvement tended to perceive a congruence between the importance they placed on mastery, health benefits, and fitness benefits in physical activities and the opportunities to meet those incentives in the exercise program.

Before these specific findings are given much consideration in the design of exercise programs for the elderly, of course, it is critical that our research be replicated with large and diverse samples of middle-aged and older adults. In general, however, this preliminary work supports the application of the Theory of Personal Investment (Maehr & Braskamp, 1986) to the study of exercise behavior among these age groups. Although much more research needs to be done on physical activity in the lives of the elderly, it appears that this interactional theory of motivation provides us with insight into variations in behavioral investment in the physical domain.

## CONCLUSION AND SUGGESTIONS FOR FUTURE RESEARCH

Despite the fact that research has clearly demonstrated the physiological and psychological benefits of exercise among older adults, there tends to be a marked decrease in participation in physical activity through the lifespan. To help us begin to understand these observed age-related changes in exercise patterns, there is a clear need to examine the motivational orientation of adults toward exercise and to determine how the meaning of exercise changes as people grow older. In this chapter, we suggest that the Personal Investment Theory (Maehr & Braskamp, 1986) provides a comprehensive approach to assessing variations in motivational perspectives in regard to exercise behavior. Drawing from this theoretical perspective, there are many interesting directions for future research on physical activity among elderly populations.

In our initial research on the meaning of physical activity among middle-aged and older adults, we have examined the personal incentives, sense of self, and perceived options among individuals who were personally invested in a structured exercise program. To better elucidate the impact of situational characteristics on personal investment in exercise, it would be intriguing to examine the three facets of meaning and behavioral patterns manifested by elderly participants across diverse exercise programs. Moreover, in future studies, it is important not to forget the elderly who engage in regular exercise but have made different choices in regard to the type of participation. That is, what is the meaning of exercise among the elderly who participate in physical activity informally? Would there be differences in the personal incentives, sense of self, and perceived options, for example, of an older adult who jogs three days per week around the neighborhood when compared to the perceptions of his/her same age counterpart who attends an aerobics class on similar days?

Future research also needs to begin to determine the meaning of exercise in the lives of inactive older adults. Such research, however, must be sensitive to whether the elderly in question are sedentary because of voluntary disengagement from physical activity or physical disabilities, physical illness, and/or mental health problems. It would be reasonable to assume that inactivity due to social psychological reasons or physical capacity and health factors would dramatically effect an individual's sense of self and perceived options for personal investment.

It is essential for future studies on the personal investment of older adults in physical activity to not simply group the elderly into categories based on their behavioral patterns alone (high active, low active, inactive). Besides functional capacity differences, we sometimes forget that older people also differ as a function of gender, race, ethnicity, and socio-economic class. Besides the practical significance of considering that there might be group differences in the meaning and personal investment in exercise, such "cross-cultural" work can provide us with more information on the diverse meanings that exist in regard to physical activity. Perhaps there are other exercise incentives, aspects of one's sense of self, and perceived options which have not yet been considered in exercise motivation research based on the Theory of Personal Investment (Maehr & Braskamp, 1986).

In conclusion, if we would hope that a broader segment of the elderly population can have the opportunity to reap the physiological and psychological benefits of regular physical activity, we must begin to understand what exercise means to older people. According to the theoretical perspective of Maehr and Braskamp (1986), this understanding would entail an awareness of their exercise goals, their sense of self as physical human beings, and their beliefs on whether physical activity is a viable, attractive behavioral alternative in their lives.

## REFERENCES

Andrew, G.M., Oldridge, N.B., Parker, J.O., Cunningham, D.S., Rechnitzer, P.A., Jones, N.L., et al. (1981). Reasons for dropout from exercise programs in post-coronary patients. *Medicine and Science in Sports and Exercise, 13,* 164-168.

Beran, J. (1986). Exercise and the elderly: Observation on a functioning program. In B. McPherson (Ed.), *Sport and aging.* (pp. 117-123). Champaign, IL: Human Kinetics.

Bjurstrom, L.A. & Alexious, N.G. (1978). A program of heart disease intervention for public employees. *Journal of Occupational Medicine, 20,* 521-531.

Boothby, J., Tungatt, M., & Townsend, A. (1981). Ceasing participation in sports activity: Reported reasons and their implications. *Journal of Leisure Research, 13,* 1-14.

Bove, A.A. (1983). Exercise in the elderly. In A.A. Bove & D.T. Lowenthal (Eds.), *Exercise medicine.* New York: Academic Press.

Breslow, L. & Enstrom, J.E. (1980). Persistence of health habits and their relationship to mortality. *Preventive Medicine, 9,* 469-483.

Conrad, C.C. (1976). When you're young at heart. *Aging, 258,* 11-13.

Curtis, J. & White, P. (1984). Age and sport participation: Decline in participation with age or increased specialization with age. In N. Theberge & P. Donnelly (Eds.), *Sport and the sociological imagination.* Fort Worth, TX: Texas Christian University Press.

Davidson, D. & Murphy, C. (1986). Exercise training in elderly persons. Do women benefit as much as men? In B. McPherson (Ed.), *Sport and aging* (pp. 273-278). Champaign, IL: Human Kinetics.

deCharms, R. (1968). *Personal behavior.* New York: Academic Press.

Dishman, R.K. (1984) Motivation and exercise adherence. In J. Silva & R. Weinberg (Eds.), *Psychological foundations of sport.* Champaign, IL: Human Kinetics.

Dishman, R.K. & Gettman, L.R. (1980). Psychobiologic influences on exercise adherence. *Journal of Sport Psychology, 2,* 295-310.

Dishman, R.K. & Ickes, W. (1981). Self-motivation and adherence to therapeutic exercise. *Journal of Behavioral Medicine, 4,* 421-438.

Duda, J.L. (1986a). A cross-cultural analysis of achievement motivation in sport and the classroom. In L. VanderVelden & J. Humphrey (Eds.), *Current selected research in the psychology and sociology of sport.* NY: AMS Press.

Duda, J.L. (1986b). Perceptions of sport success and failure among white, black, and Hispanic adolescents. In J. Watkins, T. Reilly, & L. Burwitz (Eds.), *Sport Science* (pp. 214-222). London: E. & F.N. Spon.

Duda, J.L. (1987). Toward a developmental theory of children's motivation in sport. *Journal of Sport Psychology, 9,* 130-145.

Duda, J.L. (in press). Goal perspectives and behavior in sport and exercise settings. In C. Ames & M. Maehr (Eds.), *Advances in Motivation and Achievement - Vol. 6,* Greenwich, CT: JAI Press.

Duda, J.L. (1988). The relationship between goal perspectives and persistence and intensity among recreational sport participants. *Leisure Sciences, 10,* 95-106.

Duda, J.L., & Tappe, M.K. (1987, September). Personal investment in exercise: The development of the Personal Incentives for Exercise Questionnaire. Paper presented at the Annual Meetings of the Association for the Advancement of Applied Sport Psychology, Newport Beach, CA.

Durbeck, D.C., Heizelmann, F., Schachter, J., Haskell, W.L., Payne, G.H., Moxley, R.T., Nemiroff, M., Limoncelli, D.D., Arnoldi, L.B., & Fox, S.M. (1972). The National Aeronautics and Space Administration - U.S. Public Health Service Health Education and Enhancement Program: Summary of results. *American Journal of Cardiology, 36,* 784-790.

Dzewaltowski, D.A. (1986, April). Physical self-efficacy and well being in older adult exercisers. Paper presented at the Annual Meetings of the American Alliance for Health, Physical Education, Recreation and Dance, Cincinnati, Ohio.

Edward, A.E., & Wine, D.B. (1963). Personality changes with age: Their dependency on concomitant intellectual decline. *Journal of Gerontology, 18,* 182-184.

El-Naggar, A.M. & Ismail, A.H. (1986). Cognitive processing, emotional health, and regular exercise in middle-aged men. In B. McPherson (Ed.), *Sport and aging* (pp. 205-209). Champaign, IL: Human Kinetics.

Franks, P., Lee, P.R. Fullerton, J.E.(1983). *Lifetime fitness and exercise for older people.* San Francisco: University of California, Aging Health Policy Center.

Gill, D.L. (1986). Competitiveness among females and males in physical activity classes. *Sex Roles, 15,* 233-247.

Gottlieb, N.H., & Baker, J.A. (1986). The relative influence of health beliefs, parental and peer behaviors and exercise program on smoking, alcohol use, and physical activity. *Soc. Sci. Med., 22,* 915-927.

Griest, J.H., Klein, M.H., Eischens, R.R., Faris, J., Gurman, A.S., & Morgan, W.P. (1979). Running as treatment for depression. *Comprehensive Psychology, 20,* 41-54.

Harootyan, R. (1982). The participation of older people in sports. In R. Pankin (Ed.), *Social approaches to sport.* East Brunswick, NJ: Associated University Press.

Harris, L. (1979). *The Perrier Study: Fitness in America.* Greenwich, CT: Perrier-Great Waters of France, Inc.

Harter, S.A. (1980). A model of instrinsic mastery motivation in children: Individual differences and developmental change. In W.A. Collins (Ed.), *Minnesota symposium in child psychology* (Vol. 14). Hillsdale, NJ: Earlbaum.

Haskell, W.L. (1985). Exercise programs for health promotion. In J.C. Rosen & L.J. Solomon (Eds.), *Prevention in health psychology.* Hanover: University Press of New England.

Heckler, M.M. (1985). Health promotion for older Americans. *Public Health Reports, 100,* 225-230.

Heinzelmann, F. & Bagley, R.W. (1970). Response to physical activity programs and their effects on health behavior. *Public Health Reports, 85,* 905-911.

Heitmann, H.H. (1986). Motives of older adults for participating in physical activity programs. In B. McPherson (Ed.), *Sport and aging* (pp. 199-204). Champaign, IL: Human Kinetics.

Hersey, J.C., Klibanoff, L.S. & Probst, J.C. (1983). *An evaluation of "Friends can be good medicine": Long term impacts of the pilot project and a study of the statewide project.* California Department of Mental Health (Contract No. 82-73052). Kappa Systems, Inc.

Hersey, J.C., Probst, J.C. & Portnoy, B. (1982). *Evaluation of a national health promotion campaign.* Washington, DC: Office of Disease Prevention and Health Promotion.

Howze, E.H., DiGilio, D.A., Bennett, J.P. & Smith, M.L. (1986). Health education and physical fitness for older adults. In B. McPherson (Ed.), *Sport and aging* (pp. 153-156). Champaign, IL: Human Kinetics.

Jasnoski, N., Holmes, D., Oloman, S., & Agular, C. (1981). Exercise changes in aerobic capacity and changes in self perception: An experimental investigation. *Journal of Research in Personality, 15,* 460-466.

Klein, R. (1972). Age, sex, and task difficulty as predictors of social conformity. *Journal of Gerontology, 27,* 229-236.

Langlie, J.K. (1977). Social network, health beliefs, and preventive health behavior. *Journal of Health and Social Behavior, 18,* 244-260.

Maehr, M.L. (1984). Meaning and motivation. In R. Ames and C. Ames (Eds.), *Research on motivation in education (Vol. 1).* (pp. 115-144) New York: Academic Press.

Maehr, M.L. & Braskamp, L.A. (1986). *The motivation factor: A theory of personal investment.* Lexington, MA: Lexington Press.

Maehr, M.L. & Kleiber, D.A. (1981). The graying of achievement motivation. *American Psychologist, 36,* 787-793.

Maloney, S.K., Fallon, B. & Wittenberg, C.K. (1984). *Aging and health promotion: Market research for public education, executive summary* (Contract No. 282-83-0105). Washington, DC: Public Health Service, Office of Disease Prevention and Health Promotion.

Martin J.E. & Dubbert, P.M. (1982). Exercise applications and promotion in behavioral medicine: Current status and future directions. *Journal of Clinical and Consulting Psychology, 50,* 1004-1017.

McPherson, B.D. (1983). *Aging as a social process. An introduction to individual and population aging.* Toronto: Butterworths.

McPherson, B.D. (1986). Sport, health, well-being, and aging: Some conceptual and methodological issues and conclusions for sport scientists. In B. McPherson (Ed.), *Sport and aging.* (pp. 3-23). Champaign, IL: Human Kinetics.

Mobily, K.E. (1981). Attitudes of institutionalized elderly Iowans toward physical activity. *Therapeutic Recreation Journal, 15,* 30-40.

National Cancer Institute, (1984). *Cancer prevention awareness survey.* (NIH Publication No. 84-2677). Bethesda, MD: National Institutes of Health.

Neugarten, B.L. (1977). Personality and aging. In J.E. Birren & K.W. Schaie (Eds.), *Handbook of the psychology of aging* (pp. 626-649). New York: Van Nostrand Reinhold.

Noland, M.P. & Feldman, R.L. (1985). An empirical investigation of leisure exercise behavior in adult women. *Health Education, 16*(5), 29-34.

O'Brien, G.E. (1981). Locus of control, previous occupation, and satisfaction with retirement. *Australian Journal of Psychology, 33,* 305-318.

Oldridge, N. & Jones, N. (1983). Improving patient compliance in cardiac exercise rehabilitation: Effects of written agreement and self-monitoring. *Journal of Cardiac Rehabilitation, 3,* 257-262.

Ostrow, A. (1984). *Physical activity and the older adult: Psychological perspectives.* Princeton, NJ: Princeton Book Co.

Ostrow, A. & Dzewaltowski, D. (1986). Older adults' perceptions of physical activity participation based on age-role and sex-role appropriateness. *Research Quarterly for Exercise and Sport, 57,* 167-169.

Ostrow, A., Jones, D. & Spiker, D. (1981). Age role expectations and sex role expectations for selected sport activities. *Research Quarterly for Exercise and Sport, 52,* 216-227

Pemberton, C. (1986). Motivational aspects of exercise adherence. Unpublished doctoral dissertation, University of Illinois at Urbana-Champaign.

Pemberton, C. & Roberts, G. (1985, May ). To jog or not to jog: The motivational goals of adult exercisers. Paper presented at the Annual Meetings of the North American Society for the Psychology of Sport and Physical Activity, Gulf Park, Miss., University of Southern Mississippi.

Pollock. M., Gettman, L., Milesis, C., Bah, M., Durstine, L. & Johnson, R. (1977). Effect of frequency and duration of training on attrition and incidence of injury. *Medicine and Science in Sports, 9,* 31-36.

Price, J.H. & Luther, S.L. (1980). Physical fitness: Its role in health for the elderly. *Journal of Gerontological Nursing, 6,* 517-521.

Prohaska, T.R., Leventhal, E.A., Leventhal, H. & Keller, M.L. (1985). Health practices and illness cognition in young, middle aged, and elderly adults. *Journal of Gerontology, 40,* 569-578.

Rudman, W. (1986). Life course socioeconomic transitions and sport involvement: A theory of restricted opportunity. In B. McPherson (Ed.), *Sport and aging* (pp. 25-35). Champaign, IL: Human Kinetics.

Shepherd, R.J. (1986). Physiological aspects of sport and physical activity in the middle and later years of life. In B. McPherson (Ed.), *Sport and aging* (pp. 221-232). Champaign, IL: Human Kinetics.

Sidney, K.H., & Shepherd, R.J. (1976). Attitudes toward health and physical activity in the elderly: Effects of a physical training program. *Medicine and Science in Sports, 8,* 246-252.

Smith, E.L. & Gilligan, C. (1986). Exercise, sport, and physical activity for the elderly: Principles and problems of programming. In B. McPherson (Ed.), *Sport and aging* (pp. 91-105). Champaign, IL: Human Kinetics.

Smith, E.L. & Serfass, P.E. (Eds.) (1981). *Exercise and aging: The scientific basis.* Hillside, NJ: Enslow Publishers.

Sonstroem, R.J. (1978). Physical estimation and attraction scales: Rationale and research. *Medicine and Science in Sports, 10,* 97-102.

Spreitzer, E. & Snyder, E. (1983). Correlates of participation in adult recreational sports, *Journal of Leisure Research, 15*(1), 28-38.

Steinkamp, M.W. & Kelly, J.R. (1986). Relationships among motivational orientation, level of leisure activity, and life satisfaction in older men and women. *The Journal of Psychology, 119,* 509-520.

Thompson, C.E., & Wankel, L. (1980). The effects of perceived activity choice upon frequency of exercise behavior. *J. of Applied Social Psychology, 10,* 436-443.

U.S. Department of Health and Human Services, Public Health Service. (1980). *Promoting health and preventing disease: Objectives for the nation.* Washington, DC: U.S. Government Printing Office.

Wigfield, A. & Braskamp, L.A. (1985). Age and personal investment in work, In D.A. Kleiber & M.L. Maehr (Eds.), *Advances in motivation and achievement - Vol. 4: Motivation and adulthood.* (pp. 297-333). Green-

*PERSONAL INVESTMENT IN EXERCISE*       **237**

wich, CT: JAI Press.

Wiswell, R.A. (1980). Relaxation, aging and exercise. In J.E. Birren & R.B. Sloane (Eds.); *Handbook of mental health and aging*. Englewood Cliffs, NJ: Prentice-Hall.

Young, R.L. (1979). The effect of regular exercise on cognitive functioning and personality. *British Journal of Sports Medicine, 13*, 111-117.

# 11

## Personal Investment in Exercise Among Adults: The Examination of Age and Gender-Related Differences in Motivational Orientation

Joan L. Duda

Marlene K. Tappe

### ABSTRACT

The purpose of this study was to examine whether the motivational orientations of physically active adults (age 25 to 81 years) vary as a function of gender and age. Motivational orientation was determined in accordance with the tenets of Personal Investment Theory which holds that the subjective meaning of a situation is the critical determinant of an individual's investment of his or her resources into the situation. This meaning is comprised of three interrelated facets: personal incentives, sense of self, and perceived behavioral options.

The first two of these facets were assessed by a questionnaire administered to 144 regular participants in structured exercise programs. Discriminant analyses indicated that groups defined by age and gender could be distinguished on their personal incentives for exercise and the sense of self subscales. ANOVAs revealed that males engaged in exercise for competition more than females and perceived themselves to be higher in physical self efficacy. Females placed more emphasis on fitness benefits as an exercise incentive, perceived greater social support for exercise, and were more likely to attribute their fitness status to chance than males. The salience of the health benefits of exercise increased with age. Significant interactions with age emerged on the incentives of social recognition and coping with stress.

### INTRODUCTION

Gender and age-related differences in the intensity and frequency of exercise involvement have been well documented. In general, activity level tends to decrease with increasing age (Boothby, Tungatt, & Townsend, 1981; Curtis & White, 1984; McPherson, 1983; Prohashka et al., 1985). Further, from adolescence through adulthood, males are likely to be more physically active than females (Rudman, 1986).

The Theory of Personal Investment (Maehr & Braskamp, 1986) is an approach which can be utilized as a framework for determining how motivational perspectives toward exercise vary according to characteristics of the participant. This theory proposes that there are important social psychological factors which correspond to variations in behavior in specific contexts such as physical activity *and* that these factors differ in relation to the age and gender of the individual.

Specifically, this theory suggests that the subjective perception or *meaning* of a situation is the critical mediator of an individual's personal investment or behavioral choices in that situation. Maehr and Braskamp (1986) hold that the meaning of a particular context is comprised of three interrelated components: *personal incentives, sense of self,* and *perceived options.* The first two components are person-related factors and are assumed to vary as a function of group membership (e.g., gender, age, culture). Perceived options, on the other hand, are situation-specific.

## Personal Incentives

Personal incentives refer to the motivational focus of an activity (Maehr, 1984). Included among the personal incentives proposed to be operant in exercise contexts are the desire to: 1) try one's best and demonstrate skill improvement (mastery), 2) compete and socially compare one's abilities with others (competition), 3) exercise and socially interact with others (affiliation), 4) receive support and recognition for one's involvement and accomplishments in physical activity (social recognition), 5) avoid disease and/or maintain one's health through exercise (health benefits), 6) increase one's level of physical capacity (fitness), and 7) cope with and relieve stress (coping with stress).

Maehr and his colleagues (Maehr & Braskamp, 1986; Maehr & Kleiber, 1986) have argued that variations in the emphasis placed on different personal incentive are age-related. Research has indicated that the importance of more extrinsic incentives, such as competition and social recognition, tends to decrease with age while mastery and affiliation incentives become more important as one grows older (Edward & Wine, 1963; Klein, 1972; Neugarten, 1977; Wigfield & Braskamp, 1985). Within the exercise domain specifically, it has also been suggested that older adults tend to emphasize the health and fitness benefits of physical activity more than younger adults (Beran, 1986; Heitmann, 1986; Mobily, 1981; Sidney & Shepherd, 1976; Spreitzer & Snyder, 1983).

It has also been proposed that personal incentives vary as a function of gender (Maehr & Braskamp, 1986; Maehr & Nicholls, 1980; Steinkamp & Maehr, 1984). In general, the literature has suggested that women tend to emphasize affiliation and task mastery incentives more than men. Males, on the other hand, are more likely to place importance on competition incentives than females (Alper, 1979; Harnisch & Maehr, 1985; Spence & Helmreich, 1978; Steinkamp & Maehr, 1984). In sport and exercise settings specifically, the gender difference in orientations to competitive goals has consistently emerged regardless of the age of the subjects (see Duda, 1986a, 1986b, in press (a); Gill, 1986).

## Sense of Self

The second set of characteristics of the person which influence meaning are perceptions related to sense of self (Maehr & Braskamp, 1986). Sense of self perceptions include sense of competence, self-reliance, goal directedness, and social identity.

Sense of competence is the individual's subjective judgment of his/her ability to do something successfully. Since Maehr (1984) argued that people tend to participate in activities in which they feel efficacious, perceptions of competence are held to be an important mediator of behavior. In support of Maehr's contentions in the exercise domain, perceived ability has been found to predict exercise adoption (Dishman, 1986) and declining physical ability through lack of fitness and/or disability has been linked to the cessation of exercise involvement (Boothby et al., 1981).

It has been suggested that one of the major reasons why older adults reduce their level of physical activity is because they perceive their physical competence to be low (Boothby et al., 1981; Conrad, 1976; Wiswell, 1980). Research (Thorton et al., 1987) has indicated that positive perceptions of physical ability are associated with increased levels of aerobic activity and measures of physical fitness among older adults. Research has also revealed that females tend to view themselves as less able than men (Lenny, 1977). Importantly, this gender difference has emerged in the physical domain (Corbin, 1981).

Self-reliance is the individual's perceptions regarding his/her sense of personal control (deCharms, 1968). Although perceptions of high internal control have been linked to exercise involvement among women (Noland & Feldman, 1985), females are more likely to demonstrate a pattern of externality and tend to attribute successful outcomes to chance more than men (Lopez & Staszkiewicz, 1985; McHugh, Frieze, & Hanusa, 1982; Strickland & Haley, 1980). In reference to possible age-related differences in self reliance, research has suggested that older adults are more likely to perceive that they have less personal control over their physical health status than younger adults (Bausell, 1986).

Goal directedness is the individual's tendency to set goals and arrange their behavior in accordance with these goals. In Maehr and Braskamp's research (1986) in the occupational domain, older adults tended to be less goal directed than younger employees. No gender differences emerged in their analyses.

Although the tendency to set goals and persevere in respect to goal accomplishment has been positively linked to exercise adherence (Dishman & Ickes, 1981; Heinzelmann & Bagley, 1970), the possibility that goal directedness might vary as a function of age has not been addressed in the exercise domain. There is evidence, however, to suggest that men and women do not significantly differ in the tendency to be self motivated to achieve one's goals in exercise programs (Ward & Morgan, 1984).

The construct of social identity is the individual's perception of association with certain groups and holding of selected others as significant. Research in the exercise domain has indicated that social support for one's participation and the physical activity level of significant others positively related to exercise involvement among adults (Andrew et al, 1981; Bjurstrom & Alexious, 1978; Gottleib & Baker, 1986; Heinzelmann & Bagley, 1970; Langlie, 1977). At the present time, little is known about possible gender and age-related differences in social identity within physical contexts among exercise participants (see Gottleib & Baker, 1986).

## Perceived Options

A situation-based characteristic which is held to influence meaning is the perceived options in a specific situation (Maehr & Braskamp, 1986). Perceived options refer to the behavioral alternatives and opportunities which are deemed possible in a particular context. Within physical activity, perceived options could be operationalized as the degree to which a person can achieve his/her exercise goals in a particular environment and/or the various barriers to participation which influence involvement in exercise. Little is known about the relationship between an exercise participant's motivational orientation and their perceptions of the exercise context, particularly in regard to how this relationship may vary according to the age and gender of the participant.

The purpose of this study was to examine whether the person-focused components of the Theory of Personal Investment (i.e., personal incentives and sense of self characteristics) vary as a function of age and gender in an exercise environment. Variations in the meaning of exercise were determined among adults who were personally invested in physical activity as reflected by their participation in an organized exercise program.

## METHOD

### Subjects

One hundred forty-five male and female adults who were involved in an organized exercise program in a midwestern community (population of 100,000) volunteered to participate in this study. All subjects were white and from a middle-class background.

The exercise program was primarily designed to improve/maintain the cardiovascular endurance of the participants although exercises to increase flexibility and muscular endurance were also included. The exercise program had been ongoing for at least one month before the assessments were taken.

Program participants who were approximately of college or high school age (i.e., 24 years or younger) were excluded from this study. The remaining subjects (males, $n=46$; females, $n=89$) were classified into the following groups based on age: young adults between 25 and 39 years of age ($n=45$), middle-aged adults betwen 40 and 60 ($n=34$), and elderly adults 61 years and older ($n=56$).

## PROCEDURE

All subjects anonymously completed a questionnaire during their leisure time at home which examined: a) relevant demographic and background information, b) personal incentives for exercise, c) sense of self, and d) perceived options with respect to exercise. This study focused on the results related to the participants' personal incentives and sense of self characteristics.

### Assessment of Personal Incentives

The incentives toward exercise were assessed through the use of the Personal Incentives for Exercise Questionnaire, or PIEQ (Duda & Tappe, 1987). The PIEQ (Version 2) utilizes 48, five-point likert-type items to assess seven categories of personal incentives related to the exercise context: mastery, competition, affiliation, social recognition, health benefits, coping with stress, and fitness benefits. The scales have been found to be reliable and valid as indicated by a stable factor structure across samples and factor analytic techniques. The Cronbach's alpha reliability coefficients for the seven scales ranged from .74 - .94 (Duda & Tappe, 1987).

### Assessments of Sense of Self

**Sense of Competence:** The subjects were requested to complete the 10-item Perceived Physical Ability subscale of the Physical Self-Efficacy Scale (Ryckman et al., 1982), which assessed their perceptions of general physical confidence. The scale demonstrated test-retest reliability ($r = .85$) and internal reliability (Cronbach's alpha coefficient = .85) as well as convergent and predictive validity (Ryckman et al., 1982). Perceived health status was also determined as an index of sense of physical competence by having subjects respond to the following questions: "How much do your health troubles stand in the way of your doing the things you want to do?" (Mancini & Quinn, 1981). Possible responses included "a great deal," "some," "not at all," and "I currently have no health problems" (rating 1-4, respectively).

**Self Reliance:** In general, results regarding Rotter's (1966) locus of control construct and Wallston and Wallston's (1978) health locus of control scale are inconclusive in terms of their predictive value for exercise adherence. In the present study, self reliance was measured by the situationally-specific Fitness Status Locus of Control Scale (Whitehead & Corbin, 1985). This instrument, which is similar in design to Wallston and Wallston's Health Locus of Control Scale, includes 11 items comprising three subscales. The first subscale assesses the degree to which one's physical fitness is perceived to be a function of personal control, the second assesses the degree to which one's physical fitness is perceived to be a function of a significant other influence, and the third assesses the degree to which fitness level is believed to be associated with chance occurrences. The instrument has demonstrated validity through factor analysis, and reliability through Cronbach's alpha and test-retest reliability analyses.

**Goal Directedness:** Goal directedness was determined by having subjects respond to a 10-item abbreviated version of Dishman's Self Motivation Questionnaire (Dishman & Ickes, 1981). This instrument assessed an individual's general tendency to set his or her own goals and persevere in respect to goal accomplishment. The instrument has demonstrated test-retest reliability ($r$ = .92) and internal consistency (Cronbach's alpha coefficient = .91) as well as construct and discriminant validity (Dishman & Ickes).

**Social Identity:** Sense of social identity in respect to involvement in exercise was measured in two ways. First, on a 9-point likert-type scale, participants were asked to indicate the present physical activity level of their close friends, loved one (i.e., husband/wife, boyfriend/girlfriend), and children. To determine overall Fitness Level of Significant Others, scores were summed. Second, subjects were requested to rate on an identical scale the perceived degree of support for their fitness activities provided by friends, loved one, children, fellow exercise program members, and exercise leader. The scores on each item were summed to determine the overall Social Support from Significant Others measure.

## RESULTS

### Incentives

Subjects were classified into one of six groups as a function of their gender and age (i.e., 25 - 39 years, 40 - 60 years, 61 years or older). A stepwise (Wilks' Method) discriminant analysis was performed to determine whether male and female young, middle-aged, and elderly adults could be distinguished on the basis of their personal incentives for exercise. Two significant functions emerged, $X^2(25) = 57.1$, $p < .001$ and $X^2(16) = 31.1$, $p < .02$, which accounted for 77.1% of the variance between groups. As can be seen in Table 11-1, the groups were significantly

**TABLE 11.1.** *Discriminant Analysis on Personal Incentives for Groups Defined by Gender and Age.*

| Variables | | Step | Wilks' Lambda | p | Std. Canonical Discriminant Function Coefficients | |
| Entered | Removed | | | | FN. 1 | FN. 2 |
| --- | --- | --- | --- | --- | --- | --- |
| Competition | | 1 | .839 | .008 | | |
| Coping with Stress | | 2 | .745 | .004 | | .140 |
| Health Benefits | | 3 | .685 | .004 | | .896 |
| Fitness | | 4 | .585 | .001 | −.703 | |
| Recognition | | 5 | .532 | .001 | 1.023 | |
| Affiliation | | 6 | .497 | .001 | −.561 | .436 |
| | Competition | 5 | .521 | .001 | | |
| Percent of Variance | | | | | 47.3 | 29.8 |

discriminated in terms of whether they exercise for health benefits, fitness reasons, affiliation, recognition received from others, and/or mental relaxation. The personal incentives of Fitness and Affiliation negatively loaded and Recognition positively loaded on the first discriminant function. Since this function reflected a de-emphasis on some of the intrinsically enjoyable aspects of exercise (i.e., increasing one's physical capacity, interacting with friends) and a strong emphasis on a more extrinsic facet (Maehr & Braskamp, 1986) of physical activity (i.e., receiving recognition and praise), it was labelled Extrinsic Incentives.

The incentives of Coping with Stress, Health, and Affiliation all had positive weights on the second function. As this function reflected an orientation to the positive physical, mental, and social health consequences of exercise involvement, it was labelled Wellness Incentives.

Pairwise F tests for the Mahalonobis distance between groups in reference to each of the dimensions revealed that young men were significantly lower on the Wellness Incentives dimension than middle-aged and elderly men and women. Middle-aged and elderly men were significantly higher on the Extrinsic Incentive Dimension than middle-aged and elderly women.

The observed means and standard deviations of each exercise incentive for male and female young, middle-aged and elderly adults are presented in Table 11-2. As can be seen, fitness and health incentives were the most salient for all the participants.

Two-way ANOVAs were conducted to determine whether the emphasis placed on each exercise incentive varied as a function of gender and age group. There was a significant main effect for Gender on the salience of social recognition in exercise, $F(1,102) = 4.61, p < .04$. This main effect was superceded by a significant Gender X Age group interaction, $F(2,102) = 4.81, p < .01$. As illustrated in Figure 11-1, middle-aged and elderly males engaged in exercise more because of social recognition

**TABLE 11.2.** *Means (and standard deviations) for Exercise Incentives Across Gender and Age Groups.*

| Incentive | Young | Adult Males Middle-aged | Elderly | Young | Adult Females Middle-aged | Elderly |
|---|---|---|---|---|---|---|
| Recognition | 2.93(.59) | 3.30(.56) | 3.38(.78) | 3.30(.66) | 2.57(.52) | 2.88(.81) |
| Competition | 3.50(.49) | 3.17(.83) | 3.16(.63) | 3.30(.89) | 2.38(.91) | 2.75(.92) |
| Affiliation | 3.48(.62) | 4.08(.53) | 4.07(.74) | 4.13(.55) | 4.14(.41) | 4.12(.57) |
| Mastery | 3.79(.38) | 3.99(.56) | 3.94(.43) | 4.12(.61) | 3.88(.65) | 3.81(.83) |
| Health | 3.81(.63) | 4.23(.52) | 4.42(.44) | 4.12(.53) | 4.34(.53) | 4.33(.57) |
| Fitness | 4.30(.39) | 4.11(.64) | 4.34(.53) | 4.39(.43) | 4.43(.53) | 4.55(.50) |
| Coping with stress | 3.28(1.1) | 3.95(.56) | 4.01(.72) | 4.06(.53) | 4.17(.63) | 3.90(.62) |

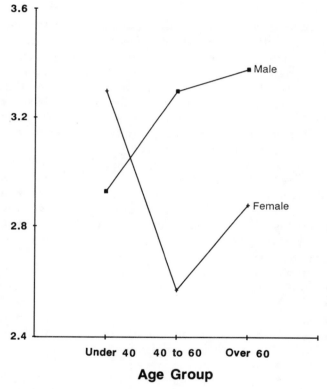

**FIGURE 11.1.** *Gender X Age interaction on Social Recognition incentives.*

than females of the same age groups. Among younger adults, females emphasized the recognition incentive more than males. Exercising because of the recognition one receives was less important to young adult

*AGING AND MOTOR BEHAVIOR*

males than his older counterparts. The reverse was true for the female subjects.

Results revealed a significant difference between males and females in the emphasis placed on competition, $F(1,102) = 6.76, p < .02$, and fitness benefits, $F(1,114) = 4.51, p < .04$, when involved in physical activity. Males engaged in exercise more for the competition than females while females exercised more for fitness reasons than male adults. There was also a trend for females to emphasize affiliation incentives in exercise more than males, $F(1,102) = 3.66, p < .06$.

A significant age main effect emerged in respect to the salience of the health incentives, $F(2,114) = 3.86, p < .03$. As can be seen in Figure 11-2, middle-aged and elderly adults tended to engage in exercise more for the positive consequences on health status than young adults.

The relevance of engaging in exercise for the purpose of coping with stress varied as a function of age and gender, $F(2,114) = 4.00, p < .03$. As depicted in Figure 11-3, young adult women emphasized this exercise

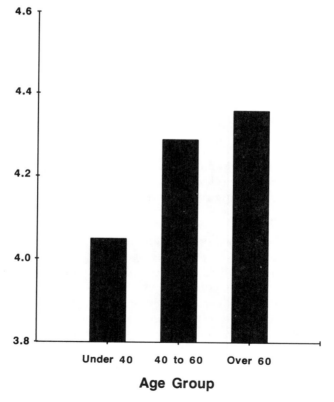

**FIGURE 11.2.** *Mean emphasis placed on the Health Benefits Incentives for the three age groups.*

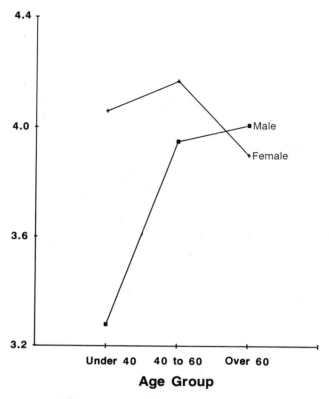

**FIGURE 11.3.** *Gender X Age interaction on Coping with Stress incentives.*

incentive more than young adult men. Middle-aged and elderly males and females indicated that the relaxation benefits of exercise was a more salient reason for participating than young adult males.

## Sense of Self Variables

A stepwise (Wilks' Method) discriminant analysis was performed to determine whether groups defined by age and gender could be distinguished on the basis of their sense of self. Two significant functions emerged, $X^2(30)$ 52.7, $p < .003$ and $X^2(20) = 33.2$, $p < .05$, which accounted for 76.7% of the variance between groups. As can be seen in Table 11-3, the groups were significantly discriminated by the domain-specific variables reflecting the subject's sense of competence, self reliance, and social identity. Physically Self Efficacy weighed negatively and the Locus of Control - Other subscale and Significant Other's Social Support variable loaded positively on the first function This function was labelled Low Competence/High Support. The Significant Other's Fitness Level variable and Locus of Control - Internal subscale loaded positively

**TABLE 11.3.** *Discriminant Analysis on Sense of Self Variables for Groups Defined by Gender and Age.*

| Variables | Step | Wilks' Lambda | P | Std. Canonical Discriminant Function Coefficients FN. 1 | FN. 2 |
|---|---|---|---|---|---|
| Physical Self Efficacy | 1 | .746 | .009 | -.946 | |
| Locus of Control-Luck | 2 | .594 | .003 | | -.851 |
| Significant Others' Fitness Level | 3 | .499 | .002 | | .766 |
| Locus of Control-Internal | 4 | .421 | .002 | | .666 |
| Locus of Control-Other | 5 | .363 | .002 | .133 | |
| Significant Others' Social Support | 6 | .319 | .002 | .462 | |
| Percent of Variance | | | | 44.8 | 31.9 |

and the Locus of Control - Luck subscale received a negative weight on the second function. This function was labelled Internal/Fitness Oriented.

Pairwise F tests for the Mahalonobis distance between groups in reference to each of the dimensions indicated that young and middle-aged men were significantly lower than the three groups of women and elderly men on the Low Competence/High Support dimension. Elderly women were significantly lower on the Internal/Fitness Oriented dimension in comparison to the other five groups.

The observed means and standard deviations of each sense of self variable for male and female young, middle-aged and elderly adults are presented in Table 11-4.

Two-way ANOVAs were conducted to determine whether the sense of self variables varied as a function of age and gender. There was a significant main effect for gender on Physical Self Efficacy, $F(1,93) = 6.82$, $p < .01$, perceived Social Support, $F(1,93) = 5.17$, $p < .03$, and Fitness Locus of Control - Luck, $F(1,106) = 5.11$, $p < .03$. Women tended to view themselves to be less physically able, perceive greater significant other support for their involvement in exercise, and believe that one's fitness status is primarily a result of fate or chance occurrences. No significant age main effects or interactions emerged.

## DISCUSSION

In his 1986 review paper on the topic of exercise compliance, Dishman proposed that (p. 137) "we cannot hope to understand why some people stop exercising, or never begin at all, if we can't explain why others exercise faithfully." The present study focused on the determination

**TABLE 11.4.** *Means (and standard deviations) for Sense of Self Variables Across Gender and Age Groups.*

| Incentive | Young | Adult Males Middle-aged | Elderly | Young | Adult Females Middle-aged | Elderly |
|---|---|---|---|---|---|---|
| Physical Self Efficacy | 49.21(6.78) | 44.59(6.17) | 41.26(6.81) | 43.96(8.33) | 36.21(9.24) | 39.52(8.47) |
| Self Motivation | 169.6(15.12) | 162.0(22.52) | 154.0(18.80) | 162.8(44.48) | 158.0(22.56) | 157.2(17.28) |
| Locus of Control-Internal | 4.08(.53) | 4.15(.47) | 4.39(.42) | 4.26(.53) | 4.55(.47) | 4.43(.96) |
| Locus of Control-Other | 2.53(.84) | 3.08(1.18) | 3.37(1.19) | 3.16(.98) | 2.45(.94) | 2.90(1.39) |
| Locus of Control-Luck | 1.78(.96) | 1.69(.44) | 1.63(.62) | 1.89(.62) | 1.73(.74) | 2.25(1.38) |
| Significant Others' Fitness Level | 5.14(1.08) | 5.08(1.12) | 5.11(1.53) | 6.00(1.31) | 5.35(1.62) | 7.95(1.14) |
| Significant Others' Social Support | 6.83(.92) | 6.86(1.68) | 7.69(1.18) | 7.56(.88) | 8.00(1.02) | 7.95(1.14) |
| Perceived Health Status | 3.22(.55) | 3.00(.71) | 3.09(.93) | 3.48(.87) | 2.94(.98) | 2.92(.83) |

of motivational factors which are held to mediate exercise behavior among a sample of regular exercise program participants. This research was based on the Theory of Personal Investment (Maehr & Braskamp, 1986) which provides a comprehensive approach to assessing variations in motivational perspectives in regard to exercise involvement. Importantly, present results supported the tenets of this theory which hold that the meaning of specific domains such as physical activity is dependent on group membership. It was found that the meaning of exercise among physically active subjects was related to the age and gender of the participants. Specifically, young, middle-aged, and elderly men and women could be distinguished on the basis of their personal exercise incentives and sense of self characteristics.

## Personal Incentives

Discriminant analyses and analyses of variance indicated that groups significantly varied in their exercise goals. Congruent with past studies (Beran, 1986; Heitmann, 1986; Mobily, 1981; Sidney & Shepherd, 1976), older adults (40 years of age and older) tended to exercise more for the health benefits than younger adults. Moreover, in contrast to young men, middle-aged and elderly men and women were more likely to emphasize Wellness incentives as the focus of their exercise involvement. That is, older adults tended to place more importance on the possible physical health benefits as well as mental (i.e., stress management) and social health consequences (i.e., affiliation) of regular physical activity. Thus, consistent with past work, the older adults in this study tended to view exercise as a health-related behavior (Howze et al., 1976; Maloney et al., 1984) as well as an important means of coping with life stresses (Antonovsky, 1980) and meeting affiliation needs (Mobily, 1981).

A significant Gender X Age Group interaction emerged with respect to the Coping with Stress personal exercise incentive Specifically, young men placed less emphasis on this exercise incentive than young women and middle-aged and elderly men and women. The finding that older men and women tended to place importance on this psychological benefit of exercise is consistent with the work of Danielson and Wanzel (1977) on exercise program dropouts. As stated above, it appears that older adults are more likely to view exercise as a health behavior and it has been found that health practices in general which focus on reducing stress tend to increase with age (Prohaska et al., 1985).

The result that women, regardless of age, tended to view stress reduction as an important incentive for exercise involvement is also consistent with past research (Danielson & Wanzel, 1977). Although the present study did not determine why physical activity tends to have this meaning to women, an examination of the items which are included on the Coping with Stress subscale might provide some insight into this finding (see Duda & Tappe, 1987). Specifically, factor analyses of the PIEQ revealed that the tension reducing aspects of exercise (e.g., "After exercise I tend to feel more calm") seem to relate to the opportunity which exercise provides for having private time (e.g., "I exercise because it provides me with an opportunity to be alone with my thoughts," or "I enjoy exercise because of the sense of solitude"). It might be the case that for women, involvement in an exercise program may be one of those rare times in the week (Shaw, 1985) when they can get away from family and work responsibilities and enjoy a personal leisure experience. The fact that a significant gender difference emerged among young adults only (i.e., the life period when child care demands are at their greatest) supports this interpretation.

Significant gender effects also emerged on the importance placed on the Competition and Fitness incentives. In accord with past research in the physical domain (Duda, 1986a, 1986b, 1988; Gill, 1986), males seem to focus on engaging in challenging, competitive activities and comparing with others in the exercise context more than females. Women, on the other hand, found the improvement in fitness status which is associated with regular exercise more salient than males. It could be suggested that the Fitness incentive is more intrinsic and self-referenced while the Competition incentive can be considered an extrinsic goal which is other-referenced (Nicholls, 1984).

Present results also revealed a significant Gender X Age Group interaction on the importance placed on the more extrinsic incentive of Social Recognition. Young women and middle-aged and older men tended to be concerned that others were aware and acknowledged their participation. Future research needs to examine the reasons why certain exercise participants are dependent on the approval and feedback of others, and why this dependency seems to fluctuate as a function of life stage among men and women.

In general, drawing from the age group and gender differences which emerged in personal incentives, it appears that exercise has different meanings to young, middle-aged and elderly men and women. These variations in incentives are important to consider as research has found a link between goal orientations and behavior (Duda, in press; Maehr & Braskamp 1986; Nicholls, 1984). In the exercise domain specifically, Danielson and Wanzel (1977) reported that exercise program participants who obtained their program objectives demonstrated greater adherence. Thus, although fitness and health incentives were found to be important to all ages, the present results would suggest designing programs for older adults which promote social interaction, emphasize the health benefits of physical activity, and allow for tension reduction. Further, if we are interested in structuring exercise programs which are meaningful and attractive to women in general, present findings would suggest that the exercise program leaders downplay competition between participants and stress the personal fitness benefits accrued through physical activity.

## Sense of Self

In the present study of adult exercise program participants, ANOVAs revealed no significant age group main effects on the sense of self variables. That is, young, middle-aged, and elderly men and women did not significantly differ in self reliance, goal directedness, or social identity in respect to the physical domain. Further, consistent with past research which has found a correspondence between exercise involvement and ratings of physical health (Breslow & Enstrom, 1980; Franks, Lee, & Fullarton, 1983; Howze et al., 1986), older and younger physically active adults in the present study did not differ in perceived physical self efficacy and health status.

In contrast to the research of Maehr and Braskamp (1986) in occupational settings, the sense of self variables in this investigation varied more as a function of gender than age. Women tended to perceive themselves to be lower in physical self efficacy and were more likely to perceive that their fitness status was related to chance occurrences than men. As suggested in past research (Maehr & Braskamp, 1986; Duda, in press) low perceived competence and the belief that one's level of fitness is externally controlled would not be predictive of intense, continued involvement in exercise.

Female exercise participants, however, tended to also perceive that they had more social support for their exercise involvement than male participants. Drawing from past studies which have revealed a positive relationship between social support and engagement in physical activity (Andrew et al., 1981; Gottlieb & Baker, 1986; Heinzelmann & Bagley, 1970; Langlie, 1977), it could be suggested that it is the social identity dimension of sense of self which gives exercise meaning and leads to personal investment among young and older women. This proposition is supported in the study of Danielson and Wanzel (1977) on exercise adherence. Specifically, they observed that women were more likely than men to attend a fitness program if they were accompanied by a companion.

The observed group differences in sense of self also suggest strategies for enhancing personal investment in exercise. For example, among those groups who are likely to perceive their physical competence to be low, goal setting or self monitoring can be employed to increase physical self efficacy. Informational lectures or counseling (Long & Haney, 1985) which accentuate the link between an individual's exercise behaviors and changes in physical capacity and health status can be a supplement to structured physical workouts among participants who tend to perceive that fitness status is not under their control. If social support for exercise involvement is deemed important to exercise participants and appears to be lacking, then program leaders should put special effort into creating a supportive class environment (see Wankel, 1984 for strategies to increase social support).

## CONCLUSION

Although the physiological and psychological benefits of regular exercise are available to men and women of all ages (Ostrow, 1984; Shepherd, 1986; Smith & Serfass, 1981), age and gender are strong predictors of participation in physical activity. The Theory of Personal Investment (Maehr & Braskamp, 1986) suggests that such variations in involvement correspond to age and gender-related differences in the meaning of exercise.

Because of the limited scope of the present sample, it is not suggested that the observed variations in meaning are reflective of young, middle-aged, and elderly physically active men and women *in general*. However, present data do indicate that age- and gender-related differences in why people exercise and how they perceive themselves and process the exercise experience exist. Consequently, if we desire to predict whether an adult would personally invest himself/herself in physical activity, it seems critical to be cognizant that the meaning of exercise does not tend to be the same for men and women of different ages. Further, if we would like to design and implement effective exercise programs for older adults, an awareness of the observed age and gender-related differences in personal incentives and sense of self is critical.

### REFERENCES

Alper, T.G. (1979). Achievement motivation in college women: A-now-you-see-it-now-you-don't phenomenon. *American Psychologist, 29*, 194-203.

Andrew, G.M., Oldridge, N.B., Parker, J.O., Cunningham, D.S., Rechnitzer, P.A., Jones, N.L., Buck, C., Caranagh, T., Shephard, R.J., & Sutton, J.R. (1981). Reasons for dropout from exercise programs in post-coronary patients. *Medicine and Science in Sports and Exercise, 13*, 164-168.

Antonovsky, A. (1980). *Health, stress and coping.* San Francisco: Jossey Bass.

Bausell, R.B. (1986). Health seeking behavior among the elderly. *The Gerontologist, 26*, 556-559.

Beran, J. (1986). Exercise and the elderly: Observation on a functioning program. In B. McPherson (Ed.), *Sport and aging.* (pp. 117-123). Champaign, IL: Human Kinetics.

Bjurstrom, L.A. & Alexious, N.G. (1978). A program of heart disease intervention for public employees. *Journal of Occupational Medicine, 20*, 521-531.

Boothby, J., Tungatt, M., & Townsend, A. (1981). Ceasing participation in sports activity: Reported reasons and their implications. *Journal of Leisure Research, 13*, 1-14.

Breslow, L. & Enstrom, J.E. (1980). Persistence of health habits and their relationship to mortality. *Preventive Medicine, 9*, 469-483.

Conrad, C.C. (1976). When you're young at heart. *Aging, 258*, 11-13.

Corbin, C.B. (1981). Sex of subject, sex of opponent, and opponent's ability as factors affecting self-confidence in a competitive situation. *Journal of Sport Psychology, 4*, 265-270.

Curtis, J. & White, P. (1984). Age and sport participation: Decline in participation with age or increased specialization with age. In N. Theberge & P. Donnelly (Eds.), *Sport and the sociological imagination.* Fort Worth, TX: Texas Christian University Press.

Danielson, R., & Wanzel, R. (1977). Exercise objectives of fitness program dropouts. In D. Landers & R. Christina (Eds.), *Psychology of Motor Behavior and Sport* (pp. 310-320). Champaign, IL: Human Kinetics.

deCharms, R. (1968). *Personal behavior.* New York: Academic Press.

Dishman, R.K. (1986). Exercise compliance: A new view for public health. *Physician and Sportsmedicine, 14,* 127-145.

Dishman, R.K. & Ickes, W. (1981). Self-motivation and adherence to therapeutic exercise. *Journal of Behavioral Medicine, 4,* 421-438.

Duda, J.L. (1986). A cross-cultural analysis of achievement motivation in sport and the classroom. In L. VanderVelden & J. Humphrey (eds.), *Current Selected research in the psychology and sociology of sport* (pp. 115-134). NY: AMS Press (a).

Duda, J.L. (1986). Perceptions of sport success and failure among white, black, and Hispanic adolescents. In J. Watkins, T. Reilly, & L. Burwitz (Eds.), *Sport Science* (pp. 214-222). London: E. & F.N. Spon (b).

Duda, J.L. (1988). The relationship between goal perspectives and persistence and intensity among recreational sport participants. *Leisure Sciences 10,* 95-106.

Duda, J.L. (in press). Goal perspectives and behavior in sport and exercise settings. In C. Ames & M. Maehr (Eds.), *Advances in Motivation and Achievement - Vol. 6.* Greenwich, CT: JAI Press.

Duda, J.L., & Tappe, M.K. (1987, September). Personal investment in exercise: The development of the Personal Incentives for Exercise Questionnaire. Paper presented at the Annual Meetings of the Association for the Advancement of Applied Sport Psychology, Newport Beach, CA (a).

Duda, J.L., & Tappe, M.K. (1988). Predictors of personal investment in physical activity among middle-aged and older adults. *Perceptual and Motor Skills, 66,* 543-549.

Edward, A.E., & Wine, D.B. (1963). Personality changes with age: Their dependency on concomitant intellectual decline. *Journal of Gerontology, 18,* 182-184.

Franks, P., Lee, P.R., Fullarton, J.E. (1983). *Lifetime fitness and exercise for older people.* San Francisco: University of California, Aging Health Policy Center.

Gill, D.L. (1986). Competitiveness among female and males in physical activity classes. *Sex Roles, 15,* 233-247.

Gottleib, N.J., & Baker, J.A. (1986). The relative influence of health beliefs, parental and peer behaviors and exercise program on smoking, alcohol use, and physical activity. *Social Science and Medicine, 22,* 915-927.

Harnisch, D., & Maehr, M.L. (1985). Gender differences in motivation and achievement: A personal investment perspective. Unpublished manuscript.

Heinzelmann, F. & Bagley, R.W. (1970). Response to physical activity programs and their effects on health behavior. *Public Health Reports, 85,* 905-911.

Heitmann, H.H. (1986). Motives of older adults for participating in physical activity programs. In B. McPherson (Ed.), *Sport and aging* (pp. 199-204). Champaign, IL: Human Kinetics.

Howze, E.H., DiGilio, D.A., Bennett, J.P. & Smith, M.L. (1986). Health education and physical fitness for older adults. In B. McPherson (Ed.), *Sport and aging* (pp. 153-156). Champaign, IL: Human Kinetics.

Klein, R. (1972). Age, sex, and task difficulty as predictors of social conformity. *Journal of Gerontology, 27,* 229-236.

Langlie, J.K. (1977). Social network, health beliefs, and preventive health behavior. *Journal of Health and Social Behavior, 18,* 244-260.

Lenney, E. (1977). Women's self confidence in achievement situations. *Psychological Bulletin, 84,* 1-13.

Long, B.C., & Haney, C.J. (1986). Enhancing physical ability in sedentary women: Information, locus of control, and attitudes. *Journal of Sport Psychology, 8,* 8-24.

Lopez, L.C., & Staszkiewicz, M.J. (1985). Sex differences in internality-externality. *Psychological Reports, 57,* 1159-1164.

Maehr, M.L. (1984). Meaning and motivation. In R. Ames and C. Ames (Eds.), *Research on motivation in education (Vol. 1).* (pp. 115-144) New York: Academic Press.

Maehr, M.L. & Braskamp, L.A. (1986). *The motivation factor: A theory of personal investment.* Lexington, MA: Lexington Press.

Maehr, M.L. & Kleiber, D.A. (1981). The graying of achievement motivation. *American Psychologist, 36,* 787-793.

Maehr, M.L. , & Nicholls, J.G. (1980). Culture and achievement motivation: A second look. In N. Warren (Ed.), *Studies in cross-cultural psychology (Vol. 3).* (pp. 221-267) New York: Academic Press.

Maloney, S.K., Fallon, B. & Wittenberg, C.K. (1984). *Aging and health promotion: Market research for public education, executive summary* (Contract No. 282-83-0105). Washington, DC: Public Health Service, Office of Disease Prevention and Health Promotion.

Mancini, J.A., & Quinn, W.H. (1981). Dimensions of health and their importance for morale in old age: A multivariate examination. *Journal of Community Health, 7,* 118-128.

McHugh, M.C., Frieze, I.H., & Hanusa, B.H. (1982). Attributions and sex differences in achievement: Problems and new perspectives. *Sex Roles, 8,* 467-479.

McPherson, B.D. (1983). *Aging as a social process: An introduction to individual and population aging.* Toronto: Butterworths.

Mobily, K.E. (1981). Attitudes of institutionalized elderly Iowans toward physical activity. *Therapeutic Recreation Journal, 15,* 30-40.

Neugarten, B.L. (1977). Personality and aging. In J.E. Birren & K.W. Schaie (Eds.), *Handbook of the psychology of aging* (pp. 626-649). New York: Van Nostrand Reinhold.

Nicholls, J.G. (1984). Conceptions of ability and achievement motivation. In R. Ames & C. Ames (Eds.), *Research on motivation in education: Student motivation. Vol. 1.* New York: Academic Press.

Noland, M.P. & Feldman, R.L. (1985). An empirical investigation of leisure exercise behavior in adult women. *Health Education, 16*(5), 29-34.

Ostrow, A. (1984). *Physical activity and the older adult: Psychological perspectives.* Princeton, NJ: Princeton Book Co.

Price, J.H. & Luther, S.L. (1980). Physical fitness: Its role in health for the elderly. *Journal of Gerontological Nursing, 6,* 517-521.

Prohaska, T.R., Leventhal, E.A. Leventhal, H. & Keller, M.L. (1985). Health practices and illness cognition in young, middle aged, and elderly adults. *Journal of Gerontology, 40,* 569-578.

Rotter, J.B. (1966). Generalized expectancies for internal versus external control of reinforcement. *Journal of Consulting and Clincial Psychology, 43,* 56-67.

Rudman, W. (1986). Life course socioeconomic transitions and sport involvement: A theory of restricted opportunity. In B. McPherson (Ed.), *Sports and aging* (pp. 25-35). Champaign, IL: Human Kinetics.

Ryckman, R., Robbins, M., Thorton, B., & Cantrell, P. (1982). Development and validation of a physical self-efficacy scale. *Journal of Personality and Social Psychology, 42,* 891-900.

Shaw, S.M. (1985). Gender and leisure: Inequality in the distribution of leisure time. *Journal of Leisure Research, 17,* 266-282.

Sidney, K.H., & Shepherd, R.J. (1976). Attitudes toward health and physical activity in the elderly: Effects of a physical training program. *Medicine and Science in Sports, 8,* 246-252.

Smith, E.L. & Serfass, P.E. (Eds.) (1981). *Exercise and aging: The scientific basis.* Hillside, NJ: Enslow Publishers.

Spence, J.T., & Helmreich, R.L. (1978). *Masculinity and femininity.* Austin: University of Texas Press.

Spreitzer, E. & Snyder, E. (1983). Correlates of participation in adult recreational sports. *Journal of Leisure Research, 15*(1), 28-38.

Steinkamp, M., & Maehr, M.L. (1984). *Advances in motivation and achievement - Vol. 2: Women in Science.* Greenwich, CT: JAI Press.

Strickland, B.R., & Haley, W.E. (1980). Sex differences on the Rotter I-E Scale. *Journal of Personality and Social Psychology, 39,* 930-939.

Wallston, B., & Wallston, K. (1978). Locus of control and health: A review of the literature. *Health Education Monographs, 6,* 107-117.

Wankel, L.M. (1984). Decision-making and social support strategies for increasing exercise involvement. *Journal of Cardiac Rehabilitation, 4,* 124-135.

Ward, A., & Morgan, W.P. (1984). Adherence patterns of healthy men and women enrolled in an adult exercise program. *Journal of Cardiac Rehabilitation, 4,* 143-152.

Whitehead, J., & Corbin, C. (1985, May). Multidimensional locus of control scales for physical fitness behavior. Paper presented at the Annual Meetings of the North American Society for the Psychology of Sport and Physical Activity, University of Southern Mississippi, Gulf Park, Miss.

Wigfield, A. & Braskamp, L.A. (1985). Age and personal investment in work, In D.A. Kleiber & M.L. Maehr (Eds.), *Advances in motivation and achievement - Vol. 4: Motivation and adulthood.* (pp. 297-333). Greenwich, CT: JAI Press.

Wiswell, R.A. (1980). Relaxation, aging and exercise. In J.E. Birren, & R.B. Sloane (Eds.), *Handbook of mental health and aging.* Englewood Cliffs, NJ: Prentice-Hall.

# 12

# A Social Cognitive Theory of Older Adult Exercise Motivation

David A. Dzewaltowski

## ABSTRACT

Although scientists have investigated the psychological and physical benefits of exercise for older adults, there has been a lack of research investigating the factors that influence exercise participation and adherence. Also, numerous research studies on other age groups have not been fruitful due to a lack of a unified theoretical framework. It is proposed that social cognitive theory (Bandura, 1986) may be the appropriate framework to study older adult exercise motivation. Social cognitive theory focuses on the mechanisms in which behavioral change operates. The central predictor of behavior is self-efficacy or individuals' confidence that they can complete a task. Another factor influencing exercise motivation is outcome expectations. Older adults may be confident that they can complete an exercise program (i.e., self-efficacy) but doubt that exercise will lead to a desired outcome (e.g., improved stamina).

In addition, the value that older adults place on the exercise outcomes may mediate involvement. Social cognitive theory also postulates that individuals self-evaluate how they stand with respect to an outcome or goal. The individuals' self-evaluated dissatisfaction may then serve as the motivator for future exercise behavior. Thus, future research should establish whether these mechanisms moderate older adults exercise motivation. Then intervention programs can be developed to target the important mechanisms affecting exercise participation and adherence.

## INTRODUCTION

Science has made great strides in documenting the benefits of physical activity. Physical activity has been associated with increased physical and psychological well-being in older adults (Ostrow, 1984; Piscopo, 1985; Shephard, 1978). While this documentation should be encouraging for researchers and health care professionals, this may be an overly optimistic perception. Although the benefits of physical activity are well documented, the number of older adults who participate in physical activity is low. A recent review estimated that only 10 to 20 percent of those over 65 years of age participated in appropriate physical activity (Powell et al., 1986). Appropriate physical activity was defined as that which leads to moderate-to-high levels of cardiorespiratory fitness. This corresponds to the Public Health Service Guidelines as the rhythmic contraction of large muscle groups, a minimal intensity of 60 percent of maximal aerobic capacity, a frequency of three or more sessions per week, and a duration of 20 or more minutes (Powell et al., 1986).

Adherence to exercise programs for the older adult is also poor. Unfortunately, this statement must be based on results from exercise adherence research frequently conducted on middle aged men. When older adults are studied, they are usually included within a group of middle age individuals who are recovering from a coronary heart attack or some type of physical impairment. Martin and Dubbert (1985) reviewed several studies, including all age groups, and found that a majority of individuals will drop out of an exercise program within the first few months. Even those who were participating in cardiac rehabilitation programs showed dropout rates as high as 87 percent (Oldridge, 1984). For example, Gale et al. (1984) examined adherence of healthy men and women to an exercise program that met in the mornings three times a week for 6 months. The results indicated that only 42 percent of the individuals attended over 50 percent of the sessions.

To date, the factors that influence exercise participation and adherence in older adults have not been examined from a theoretical framework. Research on exercise participation and adherence in other age groups, while more numerous, has also suffered from a lack of a unifying theory. The purpose of this paper is to propose a theoretical framework in which older adult exercise participation and adherence may be examined. This paper will begin with a definition of exercise participation and adherence. Then, a unifying theoretical framework will be proposed (social cognitive theory). This framework will be applied to exercise motivation and the issues facing future research and interventions on the older adult population will be discussed.

## EXERCISE MOTIVATION DEFINED

The question of older adults' involvement in exercise has been addressed from two directions. Researchers have asked, "why don't older adults participate in exercise?" This has been examined by the work of Ostrow and colleagues (Ostrow, & Dzewaltowski, 1986; Ostrow, Jones, & Spiker, 1981; Ostrow, Keener, & Perry, 1986-1987). Complementary to this question, researchers have investigated why individuals adhere to or dropout from exercise programs (Martin & Dubbert, 1985). Note, the terms "compliance" and "adherence" have both been used to represent the second question. For the purposes of this chapter, these two questions will be classified as exercise motivation. Most older adults have had unstructured exercise program sometime in their lives. Many older adults have participated in exercise programs for short periods only to stop participating. Moreover, Ostrow (1984) reviewed data indicating that individuals become less active with age. Therefore, the distinction between these two questions is not clear and the mechanisms mediating exercise participation and adherence may be similar. Adopting the term "exercise motivation" focuses the study of these two questions on the motivational mechanisms of the individual. Also, focusing on these mechanisms may be a more direct route to developing intervention programs.

To examine exercise motivation from this perspective, inferences must be made from behavior patterns. The exercise literature has measured participation and adherence in many different ways. Those examining adherence to exercise programs have defined adherence as the number of classes attended, the percent of classes attended, program dropout, attendance during the last two weeks of the program, and so forth (Martin & Dubbert, 1985). Also, the exercise participation literature has not been consistent in the distinction between an exerciser and nonexerciser. The definitions have been so diverse that it has been difficult to establish if there has been any change in the number of exercisers within the last 20 years (Stephens, Jacobs, & White, 1985). Researchers should define an exerciser with respect to the Public Health Service Guidelines for exercise behavior that were discussed earlier. Then there will be a correspondence between the behavior necessary to improve fitness and the behavioral indicator of exercise motivation.

The lack of consistent behavioral definitions has hindered the assimilation of research results. Maehr (1984) identified five behavior patterns that may be useful in making motivational inferences: continuing motivation, direction, persistence, activity, and performance. Each of these variables apply to the exercise environment.

*Continuing motivation* was defined as returning to a previously encountered task or task area on one's own, without any external constraints to do so. This definition corresponds to the traditional manner in which exercise adherence and participation has been examined (i.e., attendance). Alternatively, *direction* is a term for choice of activity. Exercise programs often offer only one type of physical exercise. If older adults cannot participate in that type of exercise dropout will occur. Researchers make motivational inferences from this behavior change, when actually the dropout may have occurred due many other reasons such as a physical injury or limitation. If the research study or exercise program includes alternate physical activities, motivated individuals may continue to exercise. For example, older adults who have injured a foot from walking could direct their motivation toward a swimming program. The swimming program might allow older adults to continue with exercise and, depending on the injury, provide therapy to the injured area. Thus, allowing for the choice of type of physical activity within an exercise study may control for some of the dropout that occurs due to reasons other than motivation.

Concentrating on the same task without a break has been labeled *persistence.* This is analogous to duration in the exercise period. Older adults who fail to exercise long enough (i.e., persistence) and frequently enough (i.e., continued motivation) to elicit fitness improvement may lose motivation. Thus, by recording these behaviors, greater explanation can be gained for program dropout. Another useful indicator is *activity.* Those who study exercise motivation should also take into account the overall level of activity of the older adult. The older adult may vary in the amount of involvement in all activities, and a lack of exercise motivation may be due to a lack of motivation for some or all activities. The final indicator is *performance.* If the difference in performance cannot be attributed to variations in skill or fitness level, then motivation may be inferred. An analogous term used in the exercise environment is intensity. However, caution should be adopted in the interpretation of intensity, because older adults have been shown to overestimate their perceived exertion (Bar-Or, 1977).

To describe these varied behavior patterns Maehr (1984) has used the term "personal investment." It is a useful term in studying exercise motivation (see the preceding Chapters by Duda and Tappe) because it recognizes that there are many ways a person can direct one's resources. Clearly, when trying to make motivational inferences, the assessment of multiple indicators of behavior is necessary.

## SOCIAL COGNITIVE THEORY

Exercise motivation has been examined from several different perspectives with adult populations. The lack of a unifying conceptual framework has limited the usefulness of past research on exercise participation and adherence. If older adult exercise motivation research adopts a unified theoretical framework, it may be able to bypass the lack of integration that has occurred with research on other age groups. Several models have been applied to explain exercise behavior such as interactional (e.g., Dishman, 1982, 1984), attitudinal (e.g., Godin & Shephard, 1986, Sonstroem, 1978), and social learning (Long & Haney, 1986; McCready & Long, 1985). Dishman's (1984) interactional model provides organization to person and situation variables that predict exercise adherence. While this model has assisted in organizing the research base, it has failed to address any cognitive or affective processes that may mediate these variables.

The attitudinal models have examined cognitive and affective variables; however, they have failed to predict a large amount of variance in exercise behavior. In addition, the attitudinal models have not addressed social learning principles. Thus, each model proposes constructs that may be important for a theory of exercise motivation. None of these models, however, integrate these constructs in a parsimonious model. Bandura (1986) proposed a theoretical framework that encompassed many aspects included in other models. It is proposed that the application of Bandura's social cognitive theory (1986) to the exercise environment will provide a unified conceptual framework to examine exercise motivation. Moreover, the model includes mechanisms which may explain how exercise motivation may uniquely operate in the older adult population.

Bandura (1986) has relabeled social learning theory as social cognitive theory to separate it from other theories that fall under the social learning heading (e.g., Rotter, 1954). The social component of the term proposes that much of human thought and action has social origins. The cognitive component illustrates the importance of human thought to motivation, affect, and action (Bandura, 1986). This section will describe social cognitive theory. First, assumptions of the theory will be discussed. The role of self-efficacy expectations in adherence to health behaviors and exercise motivation will be examined. Then Bandura's recent research on self-efficacy, self-evaluation and self-set goals will be reviewed. Finally, research which has attempted to use outcome expectations to enhance prediction of behavior will be summarized.

## Assumptions

Social cognitive theory separates itself from other social psychological approaches in that it recognizes that behavior, cognitive and other personal factors, and environmental events interact in a triadic reciprocal fashion (see Figure 12-1). The person, situation and behavior all serve as causes and effects. This contrasts with dispositional approaches which see behavior primarily being caused by personal factors (e.g., traits, instincts, drives), or situational positions which view behavior as primarily a function of environmental factors (Endler & Magnusson, 1976).

The assumption of *reciprocal causation* is really an optimistic view of the life span developmental process. It proposed that change is always possible. Consistencies in older adults' behavior patterns are not assumed to be due to relatively stable personality traits, but rather to older adults' consistent cognitive processes. This consistency in cognitive processes is fostered by older adults avoiding environments that are inconsistent with their cognitions. For example, older adults who have low confidence that they will adhere to an exercise program will not be likely to perform that behavior. Avoiding exercise will cause these older adults' confidence to stay the same or decrease, and this will lead to continued avoidance of exercise behavior. The personal factor of confidence as it relates to an interpretation of the exercise environment is interacting in this example.

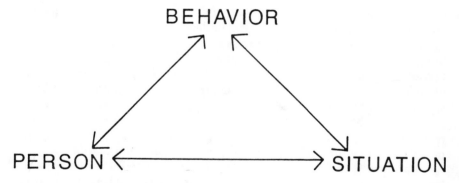

**FIGURE 12.1.** *Triadic reciprocal interaction among the person, situation, and behavior.*

However, if older adults decide to exercise it is likely to increase. The personal variable of confidence has interacted with the behavior and will lead older adults to be more likely to enter future exercise environments. Therefore, reciprocal determinism allows older adults to control their future behavior. However, there are limits in the system. These limits rest in the capabilities of human functioning.

For older adults, increases in exercise motivation are possible under this model. However, as will be discussed later, many biological and environmental factors may make it very difficult for older adults to achieve increases in exercise motivation.

## Outcome and Efficacy Expectations

Bandura (1986) postulated that human capabilities of symbolic and self-referent thought are mechanisms which guide human behavior. Through cognition, the capacity to represent future consequences serves as a motivator. From this perspective, future outcomes form expectations in the individual, termed *outcome expectations*, that behaving in a certain way will lead to future rewards or punishments. Subsequently, outcome expectations influence motivation and behavior.

A second system that affects behavioral change stems from humans' capability of self-referent thought. In exercise, self-referent perceptions of efficacy are most important. *Self-efficacy* can be thought of as a situational specific self-confidence and should not be confused with a global personality trait. Perceived self-efficacy is defined as "people's judgments of their capabilities to organize and execute courses of action required to attain designated types of performances" (Bandura, 1986, p. 391). It is more than an estimate of skill or competence; self-efficacy expectations include judgments of capabilities to organize and execute courses of action to attain specific performances.

Perceptions of self-efficacy are distinguished from outcome expectations. Self-efficacy is the perception of one's capability to accomplish a certain level of performance, whereas an outcome expectation is a judgment of the likely consequence such behavior will produce. In exercise one can be confident that they can exercise three times a week for eight weeks (i.e., efficacy expectation), but doubt that this exercise behavior will lead to the outcomes they desire (e.g., weight loss, improved stamina) (O'Leary, 1985). Researching under a different model, Sonstroem (1978) found support in the exercise environment for a similar construct (estimation). Sonstroem argued that before individuals participate in physical activity, they must feel capable of experiencing some success at the activity.

Kirsch (1985) contended that there are many problems with Bandura's definition of, and distinctions for, outcome expectations. According to Kirsch (1985), Bandura has defined outcome expectations in two ways. First, in Bandura's earlier writing (1977) outcome expectations and efficacy expectations were defined as independent causes of behavior:

> An outcome expectancy is defined as a person's estimate that a given behavior will lead to certain outcomes. An efficacy expectation is the conviction that one can successfully execute the behavior required to produce the outcomes. Outcome and efficacy expectations are differentiated, because individuals can believe that a particular course of action will produce certain outcomes, but if they entertain serious doubts about whether they can perform the necessary activities, such information does not influence their behavior (p. 193).

In this case outcome expectations are a belief about the general environment and not a belief about the effects of one's own behavior. Kirsch (1985) defined this type of outcome expectation as a perceived environmental contingency or a person's "knowledge of what leads to what" (Bandura, 1978, p. 238). Under these conditions, people drop out of exercise due to efficacy or an unresponsive environment. Kirsch (1985) contended that Bandura's second definition of outcome expectations is revealed by the statements "the outcomes one expects derive largely from judgments as to how well one can execute the requisite behavior" (Bandura, 1978, p. 241). Kirsch (1985) argued that this point suggests that outcome expectancies refer to people's beliefs about the consequences of their own behaviors rather than general environmental contingencies. He stated that this usage is consistent with Rotter's (1954) definition of expectancy as "the probability held by an individual that a particular reinforcement will occur as a function of a specific behavior on his part" (p. 107).

Subsequently, Kirsch has argued that Bandura's theory is similar to Rotter's expectancy construct and Bandura's self-efficacy construct was really old wine with new labels. The construct of self-efficacy is viewed as the expectancy of success, which is a function of perceived competence and perceived task difficulty. In addition, Kirsch viewed outcome expectations as the value term in Rotter's theory because outcome expectancies are the only determinant of reinforcement. Therefore, value for an activity and the expectation for reinforcement from an activity are functionally equivalent.

While Kirsch points are well taken, and aspects of social learning theory (the locus of control construct) have been suggested for use in the study of exercise motivation (e.g., Long & Haney, 1986), I believe that Bandura's distinction is different from prior theoretical perspectives and may provide more explanation.

Bandura's definitions of efficacy and outcome expectations may be most apparent in tasks not yet addressed by Bandura. In tasks such as paper wad basket shooting or coping with snakes, the performance of the behavior is closely tied to the outcome. Bandura argued that self-efficacy expectations are the central predictor of behavior for tasks in which efficacy is tied to the outcome. However, Bandura (1986) points out that for certain activities, the outcomes are neither inherent in the action nor tightly linked by social codes. In these tasks, outcome expectancies can be disjoined from self-efficacy judgments on performance from which they stem. For example, winning a gold medal in the Senior Olympics and the social recognition that goes along with that cannot be dissociated from the performance. Therefore, because the outcome is so highly dependent on self-efficacy judgments, Bandura argues that outcome expectations will not enhance the amount of behavior predicted over self-efficacy judgments. Thus, many studies have indicated that self-efficacy expectations predict much better than expected outcomes (Barling & Abel, 1983; Barling & Beattie, 1983; Godding & Glasgow, 1985; Lee, 1984a, 1984b; Manning & Wright, 1983; Williams & Watson, 1985).

Outcome expectations can be dissociated from self-efficacy judgments in activities where the behavior is loosely tied to the outcome, or when a certain level of performance over time is necessary to gain the outcome. O'Leary (1985) reviewed self-efficacy research and stated that efficacy expectations refer to ". . . judgments of their capabilities to execute certain levels of performance; outcome expectations are judgments of the likely consequences such behavior will produce. These may refer, for example, to a patients' belief that pursuing a particular medical procedure will prevent illness, reduce pain or increase physical strength" (O'Leary, 1985, p. 438). This dissociation of efficacy expectations from outcome expectations is clearly the case in exercise where the performance of the behavior is a different expectancy from the desired outcome (e.g., a weight loss, a muscle mass increase). However, for the behavior of exercise, outcome expectations are influenced by efficacy expectations.

For example, older adults who doubt they can stay with an exercise program with adequate frequency may have expectations of continual muscle soreness and fatigue that are not present for those who are more confident.

## Sources of Efficacy Information

From the social cognitive theory postulates, Bandura contended that there are four principal information sources or antecedents of efficacy: enactive experiences, vicarious experience, verbal persuasion, and physiological states. The older adult uses these information sources during self-referent thought to make self-ascriptions of efficacy. These categories may suggest how many of Dishman's (1984) person and situation variables influence self-efficacy, and, thus, effect exercise behavior.

*Enactive experiences* give older adults the strongest source of efficacy information. Through performance accomplishments or failures, a corresponding raising or lowering of efficacy expectations occurs (Bandura, Adams, & Beyer, 1977; Feltz, Landers, & Raeder, 1979). Older adults who have not exercised for years are likely to have low efficacy with respect to staying with an exercise program. By participating in a swimming program, for example, older adults raised their swim self-efficacy (Hogan and Santomier, 1984). This increase in swim efficacy may lead to increased swimming participation by the older adults.

The *vicarious experience* of observing a model also provides information for self appraisals of efficacy (McAuley, 1985). Observing others maintain an exercise program for eight weeks may increase the observer's perceptions of his or her own ability to exercise. For the older adult, however, the availability of successful models who exercise is limited.

A weaker source of efficacy information is *verbal persuasion*. Encouragement from individuals may cause older adults to raise their own assessment of their abilities. Compared to young adults, the social encouragement or acceptability of older adults participating in physical activity may be suspect (Ostrow, 1984). Therefore, older adults who have the inclination to exercise may have their efficacy lowered by warning statements about the dangers of exercising at their age.

Finally, *physiological states* can affect efficacy. Fatigue and heavy breathing as well as increased heart rate and sweating may lower perceptions of confidence to complete the task. This may be a major contributor to older adults' low levels of self-efficacy while exercising because they have been shown to overestimate their perceived exertion (Bar-Or, 1977).

## Self-Efficacy and Adherence to Preventive Health Behaviors

There is a large amount of research examining self-efficacy's role in affecting approach/avoidance, and persistence on tasks. Bandura's early research on snake phobics and agoraphobics indicated that the level of behavioral change was more closely related to self-efficacy than to performance attainments during the treatment (Bandura & Adams, 1977). Recent support has been found for the importance of self-efficacy in the compliance and adherence to preventive health behaviors.

Researchers have examined perceived self-regulatory efficacy in smoking behavior. In a review it was found that "self-efficacy to abstain is a better predictor of relapse than physiological dependence, coping history, motivation to quit, confidence in the treatment rationale, and expectancies concerning the rewards of smoking" (O'Leary, 1985, p. 442).

The support for self-efficacy mediating the preventive behaviors leading to weight loss has also been documented. Chambliss and Murray (1979) manipulated 61 overweight women's self-efficacy. During the first two weeks of the treatment all the women received bottles containing 14 brightly colored capsules. The women were told the pills aided weight reduction when in reality they were a lactose placebo. The placebo was reinforced by weekly meetings in which physicians took painless mouth swabs to measure "metabolic changes". All the subjects also participated in a standard weight reduction program including moderate diet, mild exercise, and behavioral techniques such as slow chewing and self-reward. After the two-week period subjects lost an average of 1.8 pounds.

The women were then placed into three treatment groups. An equal number of external and internal locus of control subjects were placed in each treatment condition. Subjects in the self-efficacy condition were given information to reattribute the weight loss to their own effort rather than the medication. Subjects in the drug efficacy condition were not debriefed but were encouraged to attribute weight loss to the drug. Subjects in the control condition were given no information concerning the source of success at weight loss. All the women were asked to continue for two weeks while the medication placebo was discontinued. The subjects were weighed weekly and continued to monitor their diet and exercise. The results indicated that, for those who were internal in locus of control (e.g., the belief that one is in control of the reinforcements one receives from the performance of behavior) there was greater weight loss in the self-efficacy increase group; alternatively, the externals (e.g., belief that control of reinforcement is external to one's behavior) responded better with weight loss attributed to medication. Though the use of locus of control in the understanding of weight loss was supported, the study did not assess outcome expectations. It is possible those who did not believe that the diet and exercise program led to weight loss were external in locus in control. Therefore, there may have been no effect for the external group in the efficacy manipulation because the outcome expectancy of weight loss from diet and exercise was not present.

Bernier and Avard (1986) showed further support for self-efficacy theory with 62 volunteer overweight women. Bernier and Avard examined pretreatment, posttreatment, and follow-up assessments of subjects' self-efficacy toward their ability to execute the cognitive-behavioral strategies in the treatment package, and also a situational measure indicating how capable they felt they were in coping with risk situations associated with eating. All subjects received the same treatment consisting of information on nutrition and exercise, and the presentation and rehearsal of 10 cognitive-behavioral self-control strategies. The strategies included "(a) stopping and thinking before any eating episodes, (b) attempting to identify hunger and satiety cues, (c) identifying and disputing dysfunctional thoughts associated with eating, (d) identifying and preparing for 'risk situations' associated with eating, (e) setting short-term, flexible goals relating to eating behavior, (f) emitting self-reinforcing statements, (g) imagining and cognitively rehearsing alternate strategies in order to deal with risk situations, and (h) delaying eating in risk situations" (p. 323). Results indicated support for self-efficacy theory because weight change was associated with personal efficacy during the follow-up interval. Efficacy expectations predicted outcome during the six-week and six-month follow-up interval where posttreatment weight loss was unrelated to later weight loss. Individuals who dropped out of the treatment phase had substantially lower levels of personal efficacy than nondropouts. Notably, there was no relationship between level of self-efficacy and amount of weight loss during the treatment.

**Exercise Motivation.** Researchers have begun to examine the role of self-efficacy in the exercise environment. This research has examined motivation toward exercise across time, the effect of self-efficacy on fitness gains and participation, and the role of self-efficacy in preventing dropout.

Ewart et al. (1983) found that efficacy expectations for treadmill exercise tolerance increased after a group of heart attack victims were trained to exercise on a treadmill. In a follow-up study, the increase in efficacy expectations from experiencing a treadmill stress test was linked to heart attack recovery (Taylor et al., 1985). The authors examined the effect of wives' perceptions of their husbands' physical and cardiac capabilities on heart attack recovery, and the use of an exercise test to alter these perceptions. Three weeks after a clinically uncomplicated acute myocardial infarction, patients and wives rated their confidence in the physical and cardiac capabilities of the patient. The husbands then underwent treadmill testing in which the degree of wives' involvement was manipulated. Three groups were formed. The 10 wives in the first group sat in the waiting room during the treadmill test, 10 wives observed their husband during the test, and 10 wives observed and then walked for three minutes on the treadmill at their husbands' peak treadmill workload. After the treadmill test the couples were counseled on the patient's abilities to perform various physical activities. Patients exhibited a significant increase in efficacy expectations of their cardiac and physical capabilities after the treadmill test. Wives' expectations of their husbands' physical and cardiac efficacy were significantly lower than their husbands'. Wives who walked on the treadmill experienced a sharp increase in their efficacy expectations toward their husbands' physical and cardiac abilities and were more congruent with their husbands' self-perceptions than were the other groups. Husbands' maximum workload and heart rate at 11 and 26 weeks were significantly predicted by treadmill performance at the third week. However, the strongest predictor of 11- and 26-week performance was wives' and patients' efficacy expectations at three weeks toward the patients' physical and cardiac capabilities. These results support the contention that efficacy expectations can be positively influenced and that efficacy expectations mediate one's participation in exercise rehabilitation.

Further support for self-efficacy's role in the improvement of fitness was found by Ewart and colleagues with a circuit weight training program in men with coronary artery disease (Ewart et al., 1986). In this study, self-efficacy expectations of 40 men with coronary artery disease participating in 10 weeks of circuit weight training (CWT) or volleyball were assessed pre and post of the program. Participation in the CWT program led to greater strength gains and was associated with greater gains in self-efficacy. The contention that self-efficacy expectations mediate the participation in physical activities was supported. The results indicated that pre-training self-efficacy judgments predicted post-test strength gains after baseline strength and type of training, and frequency of participation in the exercise sessions were controlled for statistically.

Support was found for the self-efficacy construct in a comprehensive three month study on exercise adherence of chronic obstructive pulmonary disease patients (Atkins et al., 1984; Kaplan, Atkins & Reinsch, 1984). The patients were randomly assigned to one of five experimental treatment groups: behavior modification, cognitive modification, cognitive-behavior modification; attentional control, and no-treatment control. During the first three months of the program, the three treatment groups showed significantly greater increases in activity than the control groups. These changes were mediated by changes in perceived self-efficacy for walking. Specifically, the greater the self-efficacy toward walking, the greater the activity level, regardless of the nature of the intervention program.

In addition, self-efficacy changes for other behaviors were measured (i.e., general exertion, climbing, lifting, pushing, tension, anger) as well as health locus of control. The results indicated that as the efficacy expectation becomes more similar to the target behavior, in this case walking, more variance is accounted for in the dependent measures of exercise tolerance, health status, expiratory volume, and vital capacity. Locus of control, not surprisingly, was superior in predicting behavior over pushing, tension, and anger efficacy measures, but did not predict behavior as well as efficacy responses toward the tasks of lifting, climbing, and general exertion. This supports the contention that locus of control measures a generalized outcome expectation. A median split on the health locus of control scores indicated that those who had an internal locus had a greater relationship between self-efficacy and adherence. Moreover, the correlations became nonsignificant for the external subjects (i.e., $r = .33$ or less).

## Self-Evaluation, Goals and Self-Efficacy

In another line of research, Bandura and Cervone (1983, 1986) have examined self-efficacy in concert with other mechanisms of motivation within Bandura's social cognitive theory. In their first study they tested whether self-efficacy, self-evaluated dissatisfaction, and goals affected exercise motivation. Subjects exercised on a bicycle ergometer with either goals and performance feedback, goals alone, feedback alone, or without either treatment. When the subjects were exposed to performance information and a goal there was a motivational impact; however, no changes were found when feedback or goals were applied independently. When both factors were applied, Bandura contended that a self-evaluation process occurs. The individuals compare their performance against a standard, in this case their goals, and evaluated whether they were satisfied or dissatisfied with their performance. This study supported Bandura's prediction that one's dissatisfaction (self-evaluation against goal standard) and efficacy predicted the level of motivation change.

In their follow-up study, they examined the three cognitive mechanisms of self-efficacy, self-evaluated dissatisfaction, and self-set goals. All the subjects exercised for five minutes on a bicycle ergometer. The subjects then picked their goal for improvement on the next exercise trial from a bag of goal cards. Unknown to the subjects, each individual received a goal of 50 percent improvement. Then the subjects exercised for five minutes and received bogus performance feedback. The bogus feedback indicated either a 24 percent, 36 percent, 46 percent, or 54 percent improvement. At this time, subjects indicated their satisfaction or dissatisfaction on a 25 interval scale with their performance based on the bogus feedback. This self-evaluation of the past performance was proposed to serve as a motivator for future performance. Also, subjects reported their strength of self-efficacy for attaining the original goal of a 50 percent increase in performance during a subsequent session. Self-set goals were measured by asking the subjects what level of attainment they were aiming for in the next session. Then the individuals exercised on a bicycle ergometer for five minutes and their performance was used as an indicator of motivation.

Bandura's prediction was supported because self-efficacy predicted persistence (motivation) on the exercise task across all discrepancy conditions. Self-evaluation was an influential motivation only when performance was moderately or greatly below the standard (e.g., dissatisfaction). Self-set goals contributed to persistence at all discrepancy levels except when performance attainments were much poorer than the standard. In concert, the motivational mechanisms indicated that optimal motivation is achieved with a strong self-efficacy for goal attainment, with the highest goal possible that still maintains self-efficacy, and with more dissatisfaction with substandard attainments.

Clearly, future research on self-efficacy should examine the other mechanisms of social cognitive theory such as self-set goals and self-evaluated dissatisfaction. In addition, Bandura (1986) suggested that the associations between the cognitive mechanisms are not linear. Performances that fall far below standards lead to dissatisfactions that may cause individuals to give up their goals because of a decreasing self-efficacy. Thus, the interactions between these mechanisms should be examined.

## Research on Outcome Expectations

For certain behaviors, self-efficacy and outcome expectations are not inherently related. This is especially true for some health behaviors. Older adults can have high confidence in their ability to take a medication three times a day, but not believe the medication leads to an improvement in the condition; thus, adherence to the medication regime may be curtailed. To date, this issue has not been examined with respect to exercise. Other studies have shown, however, a lack of additional predictive utility by assessing outcome expectations (Barling & Abel, 1983; Barling & Beattie, 1983; Godding & Glasgow, 1985; Lee, 1984a, 1984b; Manning & Wright, 1983; Williams & Watson, 1985).

Researchers have examined the use of outcome expectations in enhancing the prediction of a preventive health behavior. In two studies, Godding and Glasgow (1985) tested the usefulness of self-efficacy and outcome expectation measures in predicting smoking status. In the first study, chronic smokers involved in a treatment program were assessed on psychological and physiological measures. While there was no relationship with outcome expectancies and the smoking measures, significant correlations were found between self-efficacy and nicotine content, amount of each cigarette smoked, and carbon monoxide levels. In study two, self-efficacy assessed after the treatment program was able to predict smoking behavior at a six month follow-up. Multiple regression indicated that outcome expectancies did not add any variance to the prediction over and above self-efficacy expectations for any of the smoking measures.

Indirectly, support has been shown for the use of outcome expectations in predicting exercise motivation. Fishbein and Ajzen's (1975) theory of reasoned action definition of the indirect assessment of an attitude is similar to Bandura's definition of an outcome expectation.

Fishbein and Ajzen's theory of reasoned action has been applied to many preventive health behaviors including exercise motivation (Godin & Shephard, 1986). Attitudes are defined by the theory of reasoned action as a multiplicative function of the information that a person has about the attitude object and an evaluation of that information. Therefore, attitude is measured indirectly by assessing the salient beliefs that a person has about the action, in terms of the perceived probability that an action will lead to a certain outcome, and the evaluation of that outcome. Thus, an indirect measure of attitude is a summation of the beliefs and the evaluation of the beliefs (i.e., Aact = $\Sigma$ (B × E) ). The definition of Bandura's outcome expectations construct is very similar to Fishbein and Ajzen's definition of a belief. Also, Fishbein and Ajzen's use of a value term seems necessary to account for individual differences in perceptions of outcomes. A value term would account for the multiple goals that individuals may have in the exercice environment (e.g., Kenyon, 1968; Pemberton, 1986).

Recently, Maddux and colleagues (Maddux, Norton, & Stoltenberg, 1986) examined self-efficacy in concert with outcome expectancy and outcome value. Outcome value has been largely ignored in self-efficacy research. Perhaps this is due to the outcome of the behavior being highly valued in many of the behaviors studied, for example snake-phobic patients losing their fears of coping with snakes (Maddux, Norton, & Stoltenberg, 1986). Exercise behavior is somewhat unique in that the outcomes can be both positive and negative. Individuals may be positive toward the increase in vigor but feel negative about the time demands of the behavior. Manning and Wright (1983) have argued for including outcome value or importance as a variable in self-efficacy research. Bandura (1986) has also suggested that some of the variation in behavior can be attributed to values. He stated, "the higher the incentive value people attach to certain outcomes, the more effort they will expend if they judge themselves capable of obtaining them" (p. 357). Thus, if people have high self-efficacy toward the behavior, they will be motivated toward the behavior if they value the outcomes associated wtih the behavior. Recent research has suggested that self-efficacy expectancy, outcome expectancy, and outcome value all may be important predictors of intentions (Maddux, Norton, & Stoltenberg, 1986).

To this point, the reviewed literature has established the importance of several cognitive and affective constructs in the prediction of exercise motivation. Bandura made a distinction between self-efficacy expectations and outcome expectations. In addition, Bandura suggested that the value which individuals place on the outcome expectations influences motivation. Also, Bandura pointed out the importance of the self-evaluation process. Older adults set goals, and the attainment or unattainment of these goals leads older adults to be satisfied or dissatisfied. It is the personal dissatisfactions from the self-evaluation process that serve as motivators. Bandura (1986) pointed out that goals enhance motivation through this self-reactive influence, rather than through the goals themselves. "The motivational effects do not derive from the goals themselves but rather from the fact that people respond evaluatively to their own behavior" (p. 469).

## SOCIAL COGNITIVE THEORY APPLIED TO EXERCISE MOTIVATION

Researchers have yet to apply the constructs of social cognitive theory in the examination of motivation to participate in an exercise program. Exercise is a unique behavior because many of the rewards associated with exercise are not inherently tied to the behavior. Therefore, it is necessary to modify Bandura's cognitive mechanisms so that they are applicable for examining exercise motivation.

First, self-efficacy is defined as the individual's judgment of his or her capabilities to complete courses of action required to attain designated types of performances. In the examination of exercise motivation, efficacy can be thought of as an individual's confidence that he or she can continue with an exercise program. Research on self-efficacy and smoking behavior has shown that an individual's efficacy toward coping with situations that are conducive to smoking is a better predictor of abstaining from smoking than just assessing one's efficacy toward not smoking (O'Leary, 1985). Thus, a measure of self-efficacy in the exercise environment should examine the individual's efficacy toward coping with difficult situations and still adhering to an exercise program (e.g., exercising with time demands, exercising with family responsibilities).

Self-efficacy is postulated to be the central predictor of behavior. If individuals have low-efficacy they will not approach the behavior because they do not believe they can attain the desired outcomes. The reinforcers or outcomes of the behavior also serve as incentive for the individual to participate in the behavior. In exercise, individuals may differ in their expectations and value for each possible outcome. To take into account the uniqueness of the exercise environment, outcome expectations should be examined in concert with evaluations of the expected outcomes. This may be accomplished by creating a multiplicative function between the individual's subjective probability that the outcome will occur and an evaluation of the outcome. Therefore, this function summed across all the salient positive and negative outcomes of exercise, designated as $\Sigma(OE \times E)$, would apply Bandura's incentive mechanism of outcome expectations and value to the exercise setting. Note that this is analogous to Fishbein and Ajzen's (1975) definition of the indirect measurement of attitude.

In addition, Bandura postulated that individuals are motivated if they are dissatisfied with their performance when compared to some standard of reference. In exercise motivation, individuals evaluate themselves based on their standing on the multiple outcomes of exercise. For example, if individuals are satisfied with their current fitness level, they may not be as motivated to exercise as those who are dissatisfied. Thus, to determine one's self-evaluated dissatisfaction, the exerciser's evaluation of his or her standing on all the outcomes of exercise must be examined. Therefore, the self-evaluated dissatisfaction (D) mechanism in an exercise context may be assessed by a summary score of the individuals' satisfaction or dissatisfaction with the multiple outcomes of exercise.

An individual's multiple self-set goals might also be an important variable influencing exercise behavior. However, according to Bandura, the self-evaluated satisfaction or dissatisfaction of goal attainment rather than the goal itself serves as the motivator. In the exercise setting it is difficult to create a variable that would summarize the multiple goals that individuals may have. For example, a goal of 20 pounds of weight loss cannot be compared to an increase in fitness level by 10 percent.

Therefore, the application of Bandura's theory to examine exercise motivation would include the cognitive mechanisms of self-efficacy toward the act of adhering to an exercise program (SE), a summation of the outcome expectations from exercise multipled by their evaluations $(\Sigma(OE \times E))$, and individual's self-evaluations as to whether they are satisfied or dissatisfied with their current levels on these outcomes (D). (See Figure 12-2.)

Also, Bandura pointed out that these constructs may interact. While self-efficacy is central to the approach and avoidance of a behavior, individuals who have high self-efficacy and low $\Sigma(OE \times E)$ will not have a large incentive to participate in exercise behavior. Conversely, if the individuals became more positive in their perceptions of the rewards associated with exercise, they would be motivated to participate.

In addition, high efficacious individuals may not be motivated to exercise if they are already satisfied with their level on the outcomes of exercise. If the individuals became dissatisfied with their weight and fitness level, however, motivation would increase. Alternatively, exercise motivation will not be as strong if individuals are dissatisfied with their present weight and they do not perceive exercise as a mode to attain their

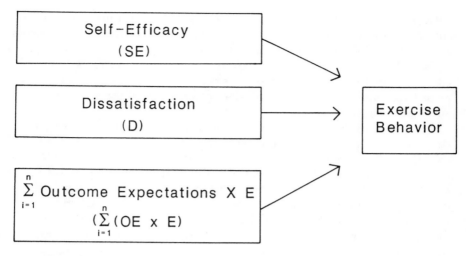

**FIGURE 12.2.** *The motivational mechanisms effecting exercise behavior.*

ideal weight. Finally, if one is high on efficacy and not dissatisfied with the outcomes of exercise, then motivation is not optimal.

In sum, self-efficacy (SE), $\Sigma(\text{OE} \times \text{E})$, and self-evaluated dissatisfaction (D) all moderate exercise participation. In addition, they all interact to increase the incentive to exercise. Optimal motivation may occur when the individual has high self-efficacy, high self-evaluated dissatisfaction with exercise outcomes, and believes in and values the multiple outcomes of exercise. Thus, researchers should examine the proposed interactions between the social cognitive theory constructs as well as their main effects.

## FUTURE DIRECTIONS FOR OLDER ADULT RESEARCH

To this point, the mechanisms that may mediate motivation toward exercise behavior have been proposed. Social cognitive theory assumes that reciprocal causation exists between the person, situation, and behavior. The assumption of reciprocal causation is an optimistic view of change throughout the lifespan. However, for older adults, biological and societal factors may uniquely influence the mechanisms which mediate exercise motivation and constrain behavioral change. The following section will illustrate how motivational mechanisms may limit older adult exercise participation and adherence. Suggestions for future research to document these illustrations will be proposed. In addition, possible intervention techniques to enhance older adult exercise motivation will be suggested.

Self-efficacy, $\Sigma(\text{OE} \times \text{E})$, and self-evaluated dissatisfaction all interact to effect exercise motivation. Self-efficacy is the central or most important predictor of exercise motivation. Individuals use information to form self-efficacy expectancies. Unfortunately for the older adult population, opportunities to gain information to increase self-efficacy expectations toward performing exercise behaviors are few.

Increases in self-efficacy are found with performance accomplishments. Therefore, how older adults evaluate success and failure may be very important. If older adults perceive success based on performing as well as when they were younger, the opportunities for success are limited due to the biological constraints of aging on physical performance. Also, older adults will not have many opportunities to perceive success if they compare their performance to others. Exercise locations are often occupied by younger and more physically fit individuals. Thus, if older adults socially evaluate their performance in this environment, they will certainly perceive failure and have perceptions of low efficacy.

It may be possible to increase performance accomplishments and perceptions of success by structuring the older adult exercise environment. Older adults should evaluate their performance based on their current fitness levels. By having older adults set realistic personal goals because success is determined by personal improvement, performance accomplishments may become more prominant. Also, if perceptions of personal task improvement are made salient in the environment, older adults will be less likely to evaluate success by social comparison. Therefore, information should be provided so older adults can determine whether they achieved personal improvement. Also, it may be a negative influence on older adults' exercise motivation if they exercise with individuals with superior fitness levels. Isolating older adults with individuals of similar fitness levels will lower the opportunity for social comparison with more successful individuals. Thus, because the possibility of perceiving competitive failure has been reduced, self-efficacy perceptions may be maintained.

Vicarious experiences may offer older adults information for self-efficacy improvement. However, the number of older adult models who exercise are few. Furthermore, older adults may feel less confident when viewing the abilities of younger adult models. We may find greater motivation toward exercise if older adults are exposed to models who are similar in age. If exercise programs are conducted by older adult instructors an increase in perceptions of efficacy by the participants may be experienced. Also, by viewing successful older adults, such as master Olympians, a greater awareness of the possibilities for exercise improvement within their age group may be provided to the new exerciser. Researchers should begin to examine the effects of age and fitness level of the exercise instructor on older adults' perceptions of self-efficacy toward exercise behaviors.

## SOCIAL COGNITIVE THEORY

The social environment may also influence older adult self-efficacy perceptions. Verbal persuasion has been found to be a source of efficacy information. Exercise motivation may increase if older adults are encouraged that they can perform and adhere to exercise tasks. The strength of this efficacy information source may be a function of who is providing the encouragement. While persuasion from salient others, such as a spouse, may raise efficacy expectations, encouragement of this type from exercise leaders may not be effective. It may be more important for the instructor to reinforce behavior and provide information to older adults' on their improvements in health status.

Finally, older adults sensory perceptions will influence self-efficacy perceptions. Feelings such as fatigue and pain may lower the older adults self-confidence. Research results, that have already been reviewed, indicated that older adults may overestimate their intensity of exercise. The exercise adherence literature suggests that cognitive strategies such as disassociation from the sensations of exercise may improve motivation (Dishman, 1984). However, this may not be an appropriate strategy for older adults because of the greater health risks associated with overexertion. Older adults may have to be trained to monitor their exercise behavior, and to differentiate between sensations related to coronary distress and the normal fatigue associated with physical activity. Also, if older adults are prescribed exercise for ailments, such as chronic lower back pain and arthritis, it may be beneficial to dissociate from the chronic pain and associate or tune into sensory signals of exercise intensity.

Older adults' motivation is influenced by the outcomes they expect to receive from exercise. These outcome expectations may be positive (e.g., improved vigor, muscle tone) and/or negative (e.g., fatigue, pain). Furthermore, the performance of exercise behaviors may elicit multiple outcome expectations. As stated earlier, this mechanism has been operationally defined as a multiplicative function between the outcome expectation and a positive or negative affective evaluation of the outcome (i.e., $\Sigma(OE \times E)$.

Older adults' outcome expectations are influenced by judgments of self-efficacy as well as other sources of information. Older adults perceive outcomes based on the adequacy of their exercise performance. If they doubt that they will adhere to an exercise program, then they will also not expect to receive many of the possible exercise outcomes. Therefore, the incentive created by outcome expectations to exercise will only become prominant when self-efficacy reaches a level where these outcomes seem attainable. Perceptions of efficacy would completely predict outcome expectations if the outcomes were directly tied to the performance of the behavior. However, for exercise behavior, outcome expectations are influenced by a number of other information sources.

When examining exercise motivation, the sources of information that older adults use to form outcome expectations may be similar to those used to make judgments of self-efficacy. Experiencing an outcome from performing a task is a strong source of outcome expectation information. However, older adults may have the expectation that fitness and other improvements in health status should occur soon after beginning an exercise program. If this expectation for reward does not occur, then older adults may lower their outcome expectations and lose motivation. To enhance motivation it may be necessary to inform older adults of the time period necessary to obtain rewards from exercising. This temporal factor influencing outcome expectations is an issue that has yet to be addressed in the research literature.

To maintain outcome expectations it may be very important to give feedback on any improvements in expected outcomes to the older adult exercisers. For example, older adults who are exercising to decrease their percentage of body fat should be given feedback that exercise is having a positive effect. This may be very important with respect to body fat because the increase in muscle mass that occurs with exercise causes an increase in body weight. Vicariously observing outcomes occur in others is an information source for forming expectations. Individuals perceiving older adult models attaining the outcomes of exercise may be a strong influence on outcome expectations. To significantly influence outcome expectations, the older adult must see *improvement* demonstrated. Individuals who are low in exercise motivation may perceive that physically fit older adults have been that way their whole lives. Unless the older adult perceives change, the positive influence on outcome expectations from vicarious experiences may not occur due to the individual perceiving he/she is "too old" to change.

Another influence on outcome expectations may come from verbal persuasion. The persuasive communication research on influencing beliefs may be directly applicable here. Although beyond the scope of this chapter, researchers and professionals may want to examine this literature. For a extended review, see Petty and Cacioppo (1986).

To this point, the effect of outcome expectations on older adults' exercise motivation has been discussed without respect to the values that are placed on these outcomes. It must be emphasized that outcome expectations that may be perceived as negative (i.e., fatigue, muscle soreness) are influenced by the same information sources as the positive outcomes.

Therefore, older adults can be confident that they can adhere to an exercise program and believe that they will receive a valued outcome; however, if they are not dissatisfied with their standing on those outcomes they will not be motivated. Goals can influence motivation. However, goals are hypothesized by social cognitive theory to only raise motivation through the self-evaluation process. Older adults are motivated to attain a goal if they are dissatisfied with their present state. Older adults may not begin an exercise program unless they are dissatisfied with their level on one of the many outcomes that occur from participation in an exercise program. Therefore, it may be necessary to make older adults aware of their levels on the outcomes of exercise to create dissatisfaction. For example, if older adults have gradually lost their motor capabilities, information about this may serve to create a dissatisfaction and thus increase motivation to exercise. Osteoperosis diagnosis may also be another example. Older adults may be satisfied with their health status and have no motivation to exercise until they learn about their level of bone density. Thus, the dissatisfaction with health status serves to motivate older adults to exercise. Unfortunately, one of the greatest information sources is a heart attack or some type of traumatic health event in older adults' lives. These events may motivate individuals to exercise because it provides information that creates dissatisfaction within the individual.

Note, that the self-evaluation mechanism may operate differently in those that are maintaining their current exercise level. It may be that these older adults are satisfied with their current outcome levels but are exercising to maintain this satisfaction. In other words, it may be the expectation of future dissatisfaction if the exercise program is curtailed that fosters continued exercise motivation.

The psychological and physical benefits of exercise for older adults are becoming clear. The task of the future is to understand how to increase exercise participation and adherence in older adults. Examining the mechanisms of self efficacy, $\Sigma(OE \times E)$, and self-evaluated dissatisfaction may be the best direction to achieving an understanding of exercise motivation. Then intervention programs can be designed to maximize change in these mechanisms and create improvements in exercise motivation within the older adult population.

## SUMMARY

Social cognitive theory was proposed as a framework for the examination of exercise motivation among older adults. Because of the assumption of triadic reciprocal causation, social cognitive theory is an optimist view of the aging process. The person, behavior, and situation all are hypothesized to interact allowing for change to occur across the lifespan. Three mechanisms were focused as important mediators of behavioral change.

Self-efficacy, or individuals confidence that they can complete a task, may be the first most important mechanism. Older adults who lack self-efficacy toward exercise tasks will drop out of exercise programs. To increase self-efficacy it is necessary to provide the older adult with positive exercise experiences. These experiences should provide information to the older adult in the form of positive enactive and vicarious experiences, verbal persuasion, and sensory perceptions.

The second mechanism affecting behavior is outcome expectations. Outcome expectations influence older adults by providing incentives to perform exercise. In the exercise environment, the outcomes of exercise may be perceived as both positive and negative. Therefore, the value older adults place on the outcome is important. It was suggested that a multiplicative function $\Sigma(OE \times E)$ takes into account older adults' differences in expectations about the outcomes received from exercise (i.e., OE) and the value (i.e., E) that they place on these outcomes.

The third mechanism discussed was self-evaluated dissatisfaction. Older adults will not be motivated to exercise unless they are disssatisfied with their standing on one of the many outcomes of exercise. For example, older adults who lack muscular strength become dissatisfied and this serves to motivate them to exercise. Then if exercise increases older adults strength level, satisfaction occurs. Those who maintain an exercise program continue exercising not because they are dissatisfied, but rather because they have the expectation of becoming dissatisfied if they drop out.

Thus, self-efficacy, $\Sigma(OE \times E)$ and self-evaluated dissatisfaction all influence exercise participation. Also, these mechanisms interact to increase the incentive to exercise. Older adults have optimal motivation when they perceive high self-efficacy, high self-evaluated dissatisfaction with exercise outcomes, and believe in and value the multiple outcomes of exercise.

More importantly, societal and biological constraints operate on these mechanisms to limit exercise motivation within the older adult age group. It was recommended that future researchers document the effect of these mechanisms on exercise motivation. Then, intervention programs can be refined to influence these mechanisms and increase exercise behavior among older adults.

## REFERENCES

Atkins, C.J., Kaplan, R.M., Timms, R.M., Reinsch, S., & Lofback, K. (1984). Behavioral exercise programs in the management of chronic obstructive pulmonary disease. *Journal of Consulting and Clinical Psychology, 52*, 591-603.

Bandura, A. (1977). Self-efficacy: Toward a unifying theory of behavioral change. *Psychological Review, 84*, 191-215.

Bandura, A. (1978). Reflections on self-efficacy. In S. Rachman (Ed.), *Advances in behaviour research and therapy* (Vol. 1) (pp. 237-269). Oxford, Pergamon.

Bandura, A. (1986). *Social foundations of thought and action.* Englewood Cliffs, NJ: Prentice-Hall.

Bandura, A., & Adams, N.E. (1977). Analysis of self-efficacy theory of behavioral change. *Cognitive Therapy and Research, 1*, 287-308.

Bandura, A., Adams, N.E., & Beyer, J. (1977). Cognitive processes mediating behavioral change. *Journal of Personality and Social Psychology, 35*, 125-139.

Bandura, A., & Cervone, D. (1983). Self-evaluative and self-efficacy mechanisms governing the motivational effects of goal systems. *Journal of Personality and Social Psychology, 45*, 1017-1028.

Bandura, A., & Cervone, D. (1986). Differential engagement of self-reactive influences in cognitive motivation. *Organizational Behaviors and Human Decision Processes, 38*, 92-113.

Barling, J., & Abel, M. (1983). Self-efficacy beliefs and performance. *Cognitive Therapy and Research, 7*, 265-272.

Barling, J., & Beattie, R. (1983). Self-efficacy beliefs and sales performance. *Journal of Organizational Behavior Management, 5*, 41-51.

Bar-Or, O. (1977). Age-related changes in exercise perception. In G. Borg (Ed.), *Physical work and effort*. New York: Pergamon Press.

Bernier, M., & Avard, J. (1986). Self-efficacy, outcome, and attrition in a weight-reduction program. *Cognitive therapy and research, 10*, 319-338.

Chambliss, C.A., & Murray, E.J. (1979) Efficacy attribution, locus of control, and weight loss. *Cognitive Therapy and Research, 3*, 349-353.

Dishman, R.K. (1982). Compliance/adherence in health-related exercise. *Health Psychology, 3*, 237-267.

Dishman, R.K. (1984). Motivation and exercise adherence. In J.M. Silva III, & R.S. Weinberg ( Eds.) *Psychological foundations of sport* (pp. 420-434). Champaign, IL: Human Kinetics.

Endler, H.S., & Magnusson, D. (1976). Toward a interactional psychology of personality. *Psychology Bulletin, 83*, 956-975.

Ewart, C.K., Stewart, K.J., Gillilan, R.E., & Kelemen, M.H. (1986). Self-efficacy mediates strength gains during circuit weight training in men with coronary artery disease. *Medicine and Science in Sports and Exercise, 18*, 531-540.

Ewart, C.K., Taylor, C.B., Reese, L.B., & DeBusk, R.F. (1983). Effects of early postmyocardial infarction exercise testing on self-perception and subsequent physical activity. *American Journal of Cardiology, 51*, 1076-1080.

Feltz, D.L., Landers, D.M., & Raeder, U. (1979). Enhancing self-efficacy in high avoidance motor tasks: A comparison of modeling techniques. *Journal of Sport Psychology, 1*, 112-122.

Fishbein, M., & Ajzen, I. (1975). *Belief, attitude, intention, and behavior: An introduction to theory and research*. Reading, MA: Addison-Wesley.

Gale, J.B., Eckhoff, W.T., Mogel, S.F., & Rodnick, J.E. (1984). Factors related to adherence to an exercise program for healthy adults. *Medicine and Science in Sports and Exercise, 16*, 544-549.

Godding, P.R., & Glasgow, R.E. (1985). Self-efficacy and outcome expectancy as predictors of controlled smoking status. *Cognitive Therapy and Research, 9*, 591-593.

Godin, G., & Shephard, R.J. (1986). Psychosocial factors influencing intentions to exercise of young students from grades 7 to 9. *Research Quarterly for Exercise and Sport, 57*, 41-52.

Hogan, P.I., & Santomier, J.P. (1984). Effect of mastering swim skills on older adults' self-efficacy. *Research Quarterly for Exercise and Sport, 55*, 294-296.

Kaplan, R.M., Atkins, C., & Reinsch, S. (1984). Specific efficacy expectations mediate exercise compliance in patients with COPD. *Health Psychology, 3*, 223-242.

Kenyon, G.S. (1968). Six scales for assessing attitudes toward physical activity. *Research Quarterly, 39*, 566-574

Kirsch, I. (1985). Self-efficacy and expectancy: Old wine with new labels. *Journal of Personality and Social Psychology, 49*, 824-830.

Lee, C. (1984a). Accuracy of efficacy and outcome expectations in predicting performance in a simulated assertiveness task. *Cognitive Therapy and Research, 8*, 37-48.

Lee, C. (1984b). Efficacy expectations and outcome expectations as predictors of performance in a snake-handling task. *Cognitive Therapy and Research, 8*, 509-516.

Long, B.D, & Haney, C.J. (1986). Enhancing physical activity in sedentary women: Information, locus of control, and attitudes. *Journal of Sport Psychology, 8*, 8-24.

Maddux, J.E., Norton, L.W., & Stoltenberg, C.D. (1986). Self-efficacy expectancy, outcome expectancy, and outcome value: Relative effects on behavioral intentions. *Journal of Personality and Social Psychology, 51*, 783-789.

Maehr, M.L. (1984). Meaning and motivation: Toward a theory of personal investment. In R.E. Ames & C. Ames (Eds.) *Research on motivation in education: Student motivation* (Vol. 1) (pp. 115-144). Orlando, FL: Academic Press.

McAuley, E. (1985). Modeling and self-efficacy: A test of Bandura's model. *Journal of Sport Psychology, 7*, 283-295.

McCready, M., & Long, B.C. (1975). Locus of control, attitudes toward physical activity, and exercise adherence. *Journal of Sport Psychology, 7*, 346-359.

Manning, M.M., & Wright, T.L. (1983). Self-efficacy expectancies, outcome expectancies, and the persistence of pain control in childbirth. *Journal of Personality and Social Psychology, 45*, 421-431.

Martin, J.E., & Dubbert, P.M. (1985). Adherence to exercise. *Exercise and Sport Sciences Reviews, 13*, 137-167.

Oldridge, N.B. (1984). Compliance and dropout in cardiac exercise rehabilitation. *Journal of Cardiac Rehabilitation, 4*, 166-177.

O'Leary, A. (1985). Self-efficacy and health. *Behavioral Research Therapy, 23*, 437-451.

Ostrow, A.C. (1984). *Physical activity and the older adult: Psychological perspectives*. Princeton, NJ: Princeton Book Company.

Ostrow, A.C., & Dzewaltowski, D.A. (1986). Older adults' perceptions of physical activity participation based on age-role and sex-role appropriateness. *Research Quarterly for Exercise and Sport, 57,* 167-169.

Ostrow, A.C., Jones, D.C., & Spiker, D.D. (1981). Age role expectations and sex role expectations for selected sport activities. *Research Quarterly for Exercise and Sport, 52,* 216-227.

Ostrow, A.C., Keener, R.E., & Perry, S.A. (1986-1987). The age grading of physical activity among children. *International Journal of Aging and Human Development. 24,* 103-113.

Pemberton, C.L. (1986, June). Motivation and exercise adherence. Paper presented at the North American Society for the Psychology of Sport and Physical Activity Conference, Scottsdale, AZ.

Petty, R.E., & Cacioppo, J.T. (1986). *Communication and persuasion: Central and peripheral routes to attitude change.* New York: Springer/Verlag.

Piscopo, J. (1985). *Fitness and aging.* New York: John Wiley & Sons.

Powell, K.E., Spain, K.G., Christenson, G.M., & Mollenkamp, M.P. (1986). The status of the 1990 objectives for physical fitness and exercise. *Public Health Reports, 101,* 15-21.

Rotter, J.B. (1954). *Social learning and clinical psychology.* New York: Prentice-Hall.

Shephard, R.J. (1978). *Physical activity and aging.* Chicago: Yearbook Medical Pub.

Sidney, K.H., & Shephard, R.J. (1977). Perception of exertion in the elderly, effects of aging, mode of exercise, and physical training. *Perceptual and Motor Skills, 44,* 999-1010.

Sonstroem, R.J. (1978). Physical estimation and attraction scales: Rationale and research. *Medicine and Science in Sports, 10,* 97-102.

Stephens, T., Jacobs, D.R., & White, C.C. (1985). A descriptive epidemiology of leisure-time physical activity. *Public Health Reports, 100,* 147-158.

Taylor, C.B., Bandura, A., Ewart, C.K., Miller, N.H., & DeBusk, R.F. (1985). Exercise testing to enhance wives' confidence in their husbands' cardiac capability soon after clinically uncomplicated acute myocardial infarction. *American Journal of Cardiology, 55,* 635-638.

Williams, S.L., & Watson, N. (1985). Perceived danger and perceived self-efficacy as cognitive mediators of acrophobic behavior. *Behavior Therapy, 16,* 136-146.

# Part VI
# Aging and Motor Skill Enhancement

## INTRODUCTION

In recent years, there has been a proliferation of physical activity programs for the older adult. The vast majority of these programs have been exercise programs emphasizing cardio-respiratory fitness, muscular strength and endurance, and range-of-motion enhancement among the elderly. Most of these programs have not been data-based; i.e., they have lacked adequate scientific documentation as to their effectiveness, particularly in terms of claims for mental health improvements among elderly participants. (Refer to Chapters 6 and 8 for more details.) In fact, most exercise programs are not structured systematically to effect positive psychological change in the elderly.

It is rather surprising (and disappointing) to note how few physical activities programs emphasize motor skill acquisition and development among the elderly. For example, *A National Directory of Physical Fitness Programs for Older Adults* (Lyon, 1981) lists few, if any, programs devoted exclusively to motor skills enhancement among the elderly. It is as if professionals have endorsed subtly the adage "You can't teach old dogs new tricks."

In one of the only known intergenerational motor development programs in the country, Carson and Ostrow (1986) reported on the success of a grandparent-grandchild motor skills enhancement program termed KinderSkills. For a number of years, KinderSkills has focused on the enhancement of motor skill among preschool children using the child's parent as a teaching mentor. Weekly for ten weeks each semester, parents are actively involved in structuring, supervising, and evaluating their child's progress in acquiring basic motor skills such as catching, striking, balance, throwing, kicking, and jumping. These skills are developed in the gymnasium and in an aquatic environment.

As an offshoot to the program, Carson and Ostrow (1986) reported on the utilization of the child's grandparent as a teaching mentor. Three specific objectives of this intergenerational program emerged: 1) to improve the efficiency of movement patterns in preschool children, 2) to improve the instructional behaviors of the grandparents, and 3) to improve the efficiency of movement patterns of grandparents as a result of their improved modeling techniques. From a psychosocial perspective, it was felt that a program of this nature would enable young children to see their grandparents as physically active role models. This experience was designed to counter the pre-school child's perspective that participation in physical activity is less appropriate as people grow old (Ostrow, Keener, and Perry, 1986-87).

In developing motor skill acquisition programs for older adults, it is important to be sensitive to changes in sensory and psychomotor function that occur with advancing age. For example, declines in visual acuity (Kalish, 1982) and auditory acuity (Colavita, 1978), and the inability of older people to process complex information rapidly particularly when a task is not self-paced (Welford, 1980), impact the types of instructional delivery systems employed in a motor skills program.

In the chapter that follows, Anshel utilizes an information processing framework to outline a number of instructional strategies relevant to enhancing motor skill among older adults. The reader is cautioned to remember that older people are more diverse than similar and that, with increasing age, greater *interindividual* and *intraindividual* differences emerge on most motor performance parameters related to skill acquisition. Thus, the older person's functional capacity (as well as chronological age) must be considered when programming motor skill activities.

# REFERENCES

Carson, L.M. & Ostrow, A.C. (1986). KinderSkills: An intergenerational motor development program. *Journal of Physical Education, Recreation, & Dance, 57*, 45-48.

Colavita, F.B. (1978). *Sensory changes in the elderly.* Springfield, IL: Charles C. Thomas.

Kalish, R.A. (1982). *Late adulthood: Perspectives on human development.* Monterey, CA: Brooks/Cole.

Lyon, L. (1981). *A National Directory of Physical Fitness Programs for Older Adults.* Reston, VA: American Alliance for Health, Physical Education, Recreation, & Dance.

Ostrow, A.C., Keener, R.A., & Perry, S.A. (1986-87). The age grading of physical activity among children. *International Journal of Aging and Human Development, 24*, 103-113.

Welford, A.T. (1980). Motor skill and aging. In C.H. Nadeau, W.R. Halliwell, K.M. Newell, & G.C. Roberts (Eds.), *Psychology of motor behavior and sport-1979* (pp. 253-68). Champaign, IL: Human Kinetics.

# 13

## An Information Processing Approach for Teaching Motor Skills to the Elderly

Mark H. Anshel

## ABSTRACT

Although there are marked individual differences on the affect of aging on learning and performing motor skills, there is widespread agreement that the human organism processes information less efficiently with advanced age. Due primarily to deficits in the central nervous system, our ability to take in, deal with, and appropriately respond to information decreases with the aging process. Significant decrements have been found specifically with motor tasks that are characterized as externally-paced (in which the speed and direction of the stimulus and response is not under the performer's control), rapid (in which speed rather than accuracy is a primary component), complex (entails more than one component and/or the use of different sense modalities performed almost simultaneously), requiring rapid decision-making and multiple responses.

The likely causes of poorer performance with age are based on limitations in the ability to: (a) discriminate between relevant from irrelevant input, (b) quickly identify and categorize input into meaningful and familiar information, (c) quickly rehearse a large quantity of information in short-term memory for storage in permanent (long-term) memory, or pass it on to the decision mechanism, (d) make rapid decisions based on available information, (e) make a series of motor responses autonomously (in the virtual absence of cognitions), and (f) interpret and use information about the response in subsequent trials.

The purposes of this chapter are to identify the likely causes of these limitations in cognitive processing and to suggest guidelines for providing the elderly with quality instruction to facilitate the learning, remembering, and performing of motor skills. The objective of this chapter is to demonstrate that, despite limitations in cognitive and motor performance that is inherent in aging, the elderly are quite capable of contributing to society and to the maintenance of their own well-being when provided with the appropriate environment in which to function.

## INTRODUCTION

As the average age of our population continues to climb, the care and well-being of the elderly will be of increasing importance. Improvement in health through advancements in medical research will bring a longer life expectancy to the older members of our society. But merely living longer is not enough. Logically, these individuals should continue to lead productive, satisfying lives. Government, in an attempt to reduce ever-increasing costs in health care is concerned with improving the person's quality of life rather than merely prolonging it. This includes, as scientists and health care workers have already found, maintaining a physically and mentally active life style. It is apparent that educators, medical practitioners, and recreation leaders will carry the burden of providing older citizens with the opportunity to meet their needs. The federal government, for example, recognizes the potential contributions of older members of the work force by prohibiting mandatory retirement in federal jobs. And an increasing percentage of the population will be spending more and more time in recreational pursuits. What this all means is that the needs of older persons to learn and perform physical skills, for a variety of physiological and psychological reasons, will continue to grow.

The purposes of this chapter are: (a) to discuss the unique needs of the elderly as learners and performers of motor skills, and (b) to describe the use of instructional techniques in teaching motor skills that meet these needs. To understand the psychological factors which underlie motor skill acquisition and retention, an information processing model will be used to detect how a person deals with information and the changes that occur with age. Once we can identify the effect of aging on a person's ability to process information, guidelines can be offered on the teaching of motor/sports skills which utilize the individual's strengths and minimize his/her weaknesses. Thus, the chapter will be divided into two sections: (1) identifying the manner in which the processing of information is uniquely affected by aging, and (2) guidelines for teaching motor skills which meet the particular needs of the elderly performer. Due to the availability of information processing models in the human performance literature, it will not be included in this chapter (see Marteniuk, 1976; Schmidt, 1982; and Singer, 1980 for thorough reviews of information processing in the psychomotor area).

Before continuing, three issues need to be addressed in order to keep the aging process in perspective. First, it's important to remember that *each person ages differently.* Some age sooner than others or have certain limitations that are unique to that individual. This chapter is concerned with tendencies of aging that may or may not be experienced by an older person. Second, the term "elderly" is defined differently among research scientists. Is there a difference in a person's ability to learn and perform motor tasks at age 65 years as compared to ages 75 or 80? Apparently there is. Butler and Lewis (1977) categorized the elderly as young-old (ages 65 to 74) and old-old (age 75 and older). It is widely held that the salient deficits in performing motor skills, when compared to younger persons, are far more prevalent at the old-old stage (see Spirduso, 1987, and Welford, 1977, for reviews of the literature). For example, Haaland et al. (1987) compared five age groups (ages 17 to 25 yrs., 64 to 69, 70 to 74, 75 to 79, and 80 to 87), all in good health, on performing a card sorting task. They found that the oldest group, ages 80 to 87, made significantly more errors than the other participants. All other groups were statistically similar. In addition, scientists have found that the effect of aging on performing motor tasks differs markedly among individuals who remain physically active in contrast to their inactive counterparts (Ostrow, 1984; Spirduso, 1975; Spirduso & Clifford, 1978; Young, 1979). Perhaps, then, age per se is not the most important criterion for defining, and having expectations of, the elderly.

The third issue is crucial to any attempt at analyzing the effect of aging on performing cognitive and motor tasks—the role of physical activity in the way an older person thinks and performs. Reviewing the literature on the effects of physical activity on performing motor skills goes beyond the purposes of this chapter. Nevertheless, it is important to recognize that despite the normal deficits that occur with age in performing physical and cognitive tasks, a program of vigorous exercise has been shown to slow the aging process (see Shephard, 1978 and McPherson, 1986 for literature reviews), although additional longitudinal research is needed to confirm this belief. This is also true in terms of the person's information processing capability - to perceive an event, decide what to do about it, and then carry out the action decided upon (Spirduso, 1987; Spirduso & Clifford, 1978). The next section will review how the processing of information for learning and performing motor skills changes with advanced age.

## Information-processing and Aging

It is becoming increasingly less popular in our aging society to inform an elderly person about deficits in the way a person thinks and performs physical tasks simply due to the aging process. As one elder told me after a conference presentation. "This old gal is doing just fine." Indeed, the older person who maintains a physically and mentally active life may "age" less quickly and, in some tasks such as reaction/movement time (Spirduso, 1975; Spirduso & Clifford, 1978) and coincidence-anticipation (Haywood, 1980) perform equal to or better than others much younger who are less active. Undoubtedly, the above respondent *was* doing "just fine." But the aging process does result in slower, less efficient motor performance under certain conditions. The following is an analysis of where this slowing occurs and under which conditions, based on the manner in which we process information.

**Sense organs.** Aging affects the detection of both visual and auditory cues. Elders are less able to visually focus on the relevant environmental cues (Welford, 1977). Because of visual limitations with aging, older people are more dependent on auditory input to obtain information as the basis for making decisions and responding. However, although audition tends to be stronger in the elderly than vision (Brinley, 1965), higher pitched tones are more difficult to perceive. An increase in vocal amplitude raises the pitch of a person's voice making it more, not less, difficult to hear. In addition, older persons are aware of being addressed in a loud manner and are often embarrassed by it.

**Filter.** This is a primary area where the system begins to deteriorate with age. To understand the deficit in this segment of the processing system, imagine having a conversation while attending a football game with the crowd cheering all around you. You can hear the other person but with far more difficulty than if you communicated when the stadium was less populated. As our hearing begins to become less acute with age, we become more susceptible to "neural noise," i.e., random neural activity (Welford, 1977). According to Welford, this is particularly the case "where fine discriminations have to be made" (p. 453). The relationship between the ability to detect a signal and the interfering neural activity is called the *signal-to-noise ratio*. As Welford (1962) explained, "Various neurological changes in the brain and falls in the sensitivity of the sense organs, such as are known to occur in older people, would tend to lower the signal level, and . . . ambient 'noise' level tends to rise with age. . . . The signal-to-noise ratio would be lowered and the information transmission capacity thereby reduced" (p. 141).

Welford's contention that poor signal-to-noise ratio partly causes a deterioration of central processing has been challenged in the literature. Salthouse and Lichty (1985), in a test of the neural noise hypothesis, found, as predicted, that elders had longer choice reaction time scores as compared to younger performers. However, the age groups were similar in their ability to tolerate additional "noise" in stimulus display and stimulus distortion when, according to the neural noise hypothesis, elders should have been more negatively affected by interfering visual and auditory input than their younger counterparts. In a likely explanation of the Salthouse and Lichty (1985) findings, Cremer and Zeef (1987) distinguished between two types of noise: (a) the ratio of signal strength to random background as described earlier by Welford (1977), and (b) proximal noise, the consistency of the connections among neuronal units. Cremer and Zeef contended, in support of the neural noise hypothesis, that ". . . the (central nervous system) of older adults appears to differ from that of younger adults by an increase in a random type of noise and not by an increase in a proximal type of noise" (p. 518).

**Perception.** At the perceptual stage, the person is asked to identify, categorize, and transform incoming information into something that is meaningful and, if necessary, quickly store or retrieve it from the memory stores. Adamowicz (1976) referred to perception as the "registration phase" (p. 45). In perception, information is given meaning for further processing, e.g., decision-making, covert rehearsal in short-term memory (STM), or permanent storage in long-term memory (LTM). The ability to make sense out of the input is crucial before it can be acted upon and given an appropriate response. And it is at this point where the person uses selective attention strategies to determine which information is acted upon and which is ignored (Marteniuk, 1976). The filter mechanism dismisses most of the unnecessary and intrusive input. However, the processes of attending to only relevant information and avoiding distraction by irrelevant, redundant input, deteriorates with advanced age. Older performers find it increasingly difficult to divide their attention between, and respond to, two or more stimuli, especially when presented in very rapid succession (Craik, 1977). Thus, *under high attention-demanding conditions,* the aging process often decreases a person's ability to perceive information accurately and expeditiously.

There is a disproportionate rise in time to respond to a stimulus as the task becomes more difficult with older performers (Brinley, 1965). There are two probable causes for these slower reactions. The first concerns the person's immediate response to a stimulus-reaction time. The second cause is a function of limitations in short-term memory.

Reaction time (RT) has been described as that period of time from the presentation of a stimulus to the beginning of a muscular response. Older people show greater variability in their performance and tend to be statistically slower than younger persons in simple RT, i.e., making one response to a single stimulus (Spirduso, 1975). These differences are exacerbated under conditions of choice reaction time, i.e., having more than one signal or response alternative (Welford, 1977). Older persons need more time to make sense of incoming information when there is a rise in its amount and complexity as compared to younger performers (Clark, Lanphear, & Riddick, 1987). One possible explanation for this tendency is the poor signal-to-noise ratio mentioned earlier. New incoming information is melded with ongoing signals, thereby delaying a response until signal amplitude is sufficient to differentiate it clearly from background noise (Shephard & Sidney, 1979). The neural causes of this slowing go beyond the scope of this chapter, but these observations should be considered in providing motor skill instruction to older people.

**Short-term memory.** Short-term memory (STM) is especially important in learning motor skills. During skill acquisition, the individual tries to add each of the skill's parts together in a progressive manner until the whole movement assumes a form of its own (Marteniuk, 1976). One of the functions of STM is to take in and rehearse information for immediate use, usually for purposes of decision-making. Another function is to register and store information in long-term memory. Extensive reviews of the literature by Craik (1977) and Welford (1958, 1977) for cognitive and motor tasks, respectively, indicate that age-related decrements occur more conclusively for planning and decision-making than for storing input. Researchers contend that age deficits in STM are due primarily to less ability to *rapidly* integrate and rehearse new data, especially of a complex nature. For example, Rabbitt (1965) asked subjects to sort cards according to letters printed on them. He found that older subjects performed more poorly than younger subjects when additional, irrelevant letters on the cards were added. However, the limitation in processing and performance speed dissipates in closed motor tasks when the speed of incoming information is relatively slower (Anshel, 1980). The task in Anshel's study consisted of limb reproduction—locating and moving slowly toward the criterion target based on verbal information about performance accuracy on previous attempts. Although younger subjects executed the movement more accurately, both age groups performed similarly after a one-minute rest. This suggests that elders might perform and remember a motor skill more efficiently when they are allowed more time to process and store task-related information at their own speed as compared to tasks requiring more speed.

In summary, then, greater susceptibility to irrelevant, interfering stimuli, a preoccupation with monitoring the previous response, difficulty in focusing attention to the proper cues—an attentional deficit, and decreased visual and auditory acuity partially explain age-related changes in STM. This is particularly the case with tasks which involved the processing of visual, as opposed to auditory stimuli (Craig, 1977).

**Long-term memory.** The permanent storage of information, similar to mastering a motor skill, is generally resistent to aging. In his literature review, Cratty (1973), in agreement with Anshel (1978, 1980) and Craig (1977), concluded that "long-term retention is less affected by old age than is short-term memory of immediately needed performance elements" (p. 242). And tasks which are highly motoric are more impervious to forgetting compared to more cognitive tasks, similar to the ability to ride a bicycle over many years, even without practice (Welford, 1968). Past studies in the verbal learning literature indicate that age decrements are more likely and more severe in tasks that involve recall than recognition (see Benham & Heston, this book, and Craig, 1977). Recognition procedures are relatively less cognitively demanding and relatively less difficult for retrieving information than recall procedures. This indicates that age decrements are at least partially due to failures of registration, not retrieval (Schonfield, Trueman, & Kline, 1972). Thus, it appears that any significant age-related loss in LTM is likely due to the failure to register and/or store the novel skill in LTM rather than the inability to retrieve it, although more related research in the psychomotor area is needed (Anshel, 1978; see Spirduso, 1987, for a review).

**Decision-making.** In addition to STM, perhaps the most salient performance deficit with aging occurs in the decision mechanism. Older people differ more from younger ones in the time taken to make decisions to initiate an action as described in the perception section. These differences are noted in choice reaction time tasks when the person is offered

*AGING AND MOTOR BEHAVIOR*

more than one stimulus and/or given more than one response alternative. Birren and Botwinick (1955) found that age groups differ as a function of the choice of which response to make. According to Singleton (1954), "The difference (with older subjects) in overall speed is not due to slower movements so much as to longer times spent at points where the movement direction must be altered" (p. 171). More recently, Clark et al. (1987) supported these earlier conclusions. However, they also found that training on decision-making tasks (in this study, seven weeks of playing videogames) markedly improved the speed of responding on a two-choice reaction time task among older adults.

The probable cause of slower decision-making capacity is that older persons spend more time (up to .5 sec) monitoring their previous response before switching attention to a new signal (Suominen-Troyer et al., 1986). This is particularly true in continuous-type tasks which require a rapid response. Thus, the processing of information from perception to decision-making is delayed (Clark et al., 1987).

**Motor programming.** The ability to perform a series of well-learned responses automatically is not dependent on age. People of all ages are capable of performing at, what Fitts and Posner (1967) call, the autonomous stage. But elders are less able to program a series of actions due to their preoccupation with monitoring their past actions (Welford, 1977). The elderly are more concerned with accuracy than speed. This is likely due to both neurological (lower signal-to-noise ratio) and social reasons (they may be more self-conscious than others about being perceived as incompetent). However, Spirduso (1987) concluded, based on her review of related literature, that "psychomotor speed seems to be maintained in individuals who are physically active, exercising several days a week" (p. 148). Older adults who exercise regularly display a greater capacity to program and carry out a series of movements more quickly than their inactive counterparts. More research on the motor programming capability of older adults is needed. However, based on past studies, programming a series of movements is less dependent on age per se than on the behavioral tendencies of older persons during the performance of these movements, but the evidence is less than conclusive (Spirduso, 1987). In general, the elderly prefer, and can more easily program, tasks which are relatively low in speed and complexity.

**Muscles.** Despite the obvious decreases in muscular strength and endurance that occur with age, differences in movement speed and accuracy between younger and older individuals are a function of changes in the central nervous system, not because of muscular deterioration. However, there is a slowing of sensory and motor fibers past the age of 50 years (Mayer, 1963). This means that although the ability of muscle fibers to contract is not significantly slower later in life, the speed at which signals translate perception into action does slow down. Why? According to Mayer, with aging (1) there is a degeneration of nerve fibers, (2) the oxygen supply to nerve cells slows with age which decreases cell metabolism, (3) the temperature of nerve branches become lower, and (4) the peripheral neuromuscular system becomes less sensitive. Welford (1984) suggested that despite some muscular and neuromuscular slowing with age, most of the decrement can be attributable to central mechanisms, specifically the signal-to-noise ratio within the central nervous system, or by the types of strategies used by the performer. As Cratty (1973) concluded, "differences in movement speed (as a function of age) seem to be caused by a lessening of the ability to integrate input to output in the central nervous system, rather than to movement capacities at the peripheral level" (p. 241).

**Using feedback.** Because the elderly monitor the accuracy and success of their responses more closely than younger performers, information feedback is a valuable asset in learning and performing motor skills. To compensate for this extra time, elders need - and take - longer to view input (Welford, 1984). This can work to the person's advantage in that feedback is frequently solicited in the form of knowledge of results (KR) and used for future performance attempts. But it can be disadvantageous in that the preoccupation with results limits the person's ability to use internal (kinesthetic) feedback, referred to as knowledge of performance (KP) (Singer, 1980). Therefore, instead of being cognizant of the sensations and correctness of movement execution, the person's attention is prematurely directed externally on the results; an important source of information to improve subsequent performance is neglected.

Ironically, there is evidence that elderly learners do not use information feedback as effectively as younger individuals. This is particularly true with continuous tasks when each signal or movement follows immediately after a response. For example, Brown (1961) found that older subjects failed to utilize important directions that ostensibly would have facilitated comprehension of a complex motor skill. One possible reason for not using feedback efficiently is again related to the tendency of older performers to monitor their previous response. This makes them less receptive to external input. This view is supported by research that shows that the elderly tend to make more errors of omission (exclude necessary skill components) than commission (make performance errors) (Welford, 1977).

## TEACHING MOTOR SKILLS TO THE ELDERLY

We know some of the information processing limitations that accompany the aging process. There are changes in the ability to take in, deal with, and respond to internal and external information with advanced age. These changes require certain considerations when teaching motor skills to an older person. The purposes of this section are to determine the *instructional strategies* for teaching motor skills to the elderly and the *optimal conditions* under which learning should occur. Instructional considerations will be linked with the unique needs of older learners given the changes in their ability to process information. It is important to note that in many cases, the teaching techniques are valid for all learners irrespective of age. However, the manner in which they are implemented are especially relevant to the elderly.

## Preparing For and Dealing With
## Sensory Input—Instructional Strategies

Teaching the older adult entails being sensitive to the affect of environmental conditions on their ability to take in, and selectively process, incoming information.

**Psychological readiness.** The learners should be psychologically prepared to engage in the skill acquisition process. This means establishing and maintaining the proper arousal level. Instructional strategies that foster the processing of input include: (a) maintaining eye contact with the learner, (b) speaking with adequate amplitude, (c) communicating at a relatively close distance to the learner, (d) informing the person about the importance of a particular technique or strategy in performing the skill successfully, and (e) addressing the learner by name. Each of these techniques better prepares the person to anticipate and deal with subsequent responses.

**Reducing verbal input.** Instructors of motor skills are very often guilty of being overly verbal in describing task demands and techniques. This overloads and slows the information processing system, particularly at the STM stage. Verbal cues in the form of a word or phrase both before and during task performance reduces the volume of input. For example, the instructor should verbalize only the basic information a person needs to know before learning and performing the task (Singer, (1980). It is important that verbal input be relatively brief, at a relatively reduced speed, and articulated in a clear and concise manner at normal amplitude to allow for information rehearsal and storage (Heitmann, 1982).

**The learning environment.** The physical surroundings should be void of factors which could interfere with the individual's ability to perceive input. Examples of interfering factors include unusually bright or poor lighting, inclement weather conditions, extraneous noise, and a low figure-ground discrimination, i.e., the manner in which a person selects and visually tracks objects from their backgrounds and the relative dependency on the object, or its surroundings, when making perceptual judgments (Cratty, 1973). *The elderly need stronger input cues than younger* *learners to overcome limitations in the functioning of sense organs* (Cremer & Zeef, 1987). Objects should have a color and/or shape that is distinct from their background. In short, keep the surrounding performance environment void of distractions and the objective of the task salient to the performer.

**Attentional strategy.** To help other learners deal with, what is perceived as, a barrage of rapid information, teach learners the appropriate attentional strategy. This entails indicating what input to ignore and what to integrate; where to look, what to listen for, and the type of sensations that should accompany performance. The best way to do this is to facilitate the person's attentional focus on the relevant cues based on the guidelines of Nideffer (1981).

Nideffer originated the concept of attentional style in which a person has a predisposition for directing his/her attention in a certain direction -internal versus external and narrow versus broad. A more important component of Nideffer's theory is that each skill has certain attentional requirements, and that performance success is partly based on attending to the proper task components. For example, shuffleboard requires a narrow, external attentional style as the performer focuses exclusively on the target for which he/she is aiming. Thinking about a response strategy before making the actual movement entails a broad, internal attentional focus. The teacher, then, should first determine the appropriate attentional needs for each task. Should the person focus externally on a single object such as working the brake system on a wheelchair? Or is an external, more broad style of vision more advantageous when the person, riding in a wheelchair, approaches a hallway corner and must anticipate colliding with another person? What are the attentional demands for a stroke victim attempting to eat, drink, or take medication? Where should the person focus when walking on a patch of ice, walking up or down stairs, or playing a game of ping-pong? Teachers have a role in helping older learners develop the ability to respond to the attentional demands of a task.

## Making Sense Out of Incoming Information

It is important to remember that actions which follow the perception of information can be performance-based, such as rapidly responding to a stimulus, or learning-based, for instance rehearsing information before it is stored in long-term memory or acted upon where it is used immediately for decision-making. Therefore, suggested guidelines for teaching motor skills to the elderly differ in accordance with the objective of the task, making rapid responses with relatively little cognitive activity (performance) or engaging in slower movements which allow for rehearsal and storage (learning).

## Instructional Strategies

Strategies that facilitate perception in the elderly to learn and perform motor skills are a function of: (1) anticipating incoming information, (2) pointing out the relevant features of the task and the environment in which it will be performed, and (3) consolidating these relevant features into meaningful and recognizable units. Singer (1980) and Marteniuk (1976) suggested using the following techniques to enhance the perceptual mechanism.

**Develop the proper sensory and motor set.** "Set" is a person's readiness to use appropriate sensory modalities to receive information (Brinley, 1965). When an athlete hears, "On your mark, get set, go!" his/her set should be focused on the starter pistol. This sense of auditory readiness is referred to as *sensory set*. However, sometimes it is more appropriate to focus one's attention internally on the physical response, just prior to lifting a heavy weight in power lifting, for instance. Attention that is directed to the movement in response to a particular stimulus is called *motor set*. When attention is directed toward the proper set, perceiving and reacting to the stimulus occurs more quickly. Proper set is important for tasks which demand very rapid and immediate responses.

**Develop anticipatory cognitive strategies.** What are the demands of the approaching task? What environmental considerations should be acknowledged prior to receiving the information? Successful baseball pitchers know that the ability to throw a curve ball accurately in a situation that requires a strike will greatly enhance their success because the batter is probably expecting a fast ball. Help the older performer deal with subsequent input by providing cues about response alternatives, e.g., "Watch out for 'such and such.' If 'this' happens, then do 'that' but if 'that' happens, be ready to do 'this.' " How should a person in a wheelchair physically react if he/she is suddenly required to turn the chair left or right? The ability to predict stimuli greatly improves the person's ability to deal with, and respond to it quickly and accurately.

**Analyze the features of the task and the environment.** Performance improves when skills are learned and executed in the proper context and situation. Instruction should consist of practicing how to deal with incoming stimuli or with producing skilled movements: (1) *in the proper sequence,* and (2) under conditions that *simulate the actual demands of the task.* Learning to operate a wheelchair, for example, might include making sudden stops and quick turns to the left or right, or descending steep embankments. Each hand has a certain task that should be executed in a particular manner. These skills should first be learned under simulated conditions and then performed under simulated conditions before skill mastery is assured.

But perhaps the most efficient way to deal with perception in old age is to provide an environment or situation for the older person that is compatible with certain processing limitations which were mentioned earlier. Examples include:

1. requiring or allowing longer viewing time of stimuli before a response,

2. reducing the speed and complexity of the incoming information,

3. allowing more time for the person to alter the direction of movement,

4. using cues that remind the person of previously learned tasks, e.g., "Remember when we did 'such and such' yesterday? Well, try to do the same thing but this time do 'this.' " According to the educational psychologist Robert Gagne (1977), one of the most effective ways to promote learning is to attach "old" learning (i.e., what a person has already mastered and retained) to "new" learning,

5. allowing more time to monitor the previous response before presenting a new stimulus. Remember that older people tend to be more concerned with accuracy than speed.

## Rehearsing and Storing Information—Instructional Strategies

Much activity occurs in short-term memory (STM) before, during, and after performing a motor task. The aging process reduces the ability of STM to take in and remember information that is, for the elderly, relatively complex, rapidly produced, and abundant. This tendency is exacerbated in tasks in which the person's attention is divided (Craik, 1977). There are several very clear recommendations in teaching motor skills based on these STM deficits.

(1) Have the older person engage in *self-paced tasks* instead of externally-paced activities. Having an environment in which the individual is able to regulate the speed of incoming information and outgoing responses is an important factor in performance success. The elderly are less successful in situations in which task demands are externally-imposed and require a series of rapid responses. This may be why recreational pursuits such as fishing, shuffleboard, dart-throwing, bowling, hunting, swimming, and card-playing are especially popular among older adults.

(2) Instruct, and allow the person to use *self-talk* as a self-induced mental strategy. This reinforces the objectives of STM processing (i.e., the registration and storage of input). For instance, while opening a child-proof bottle of medication, the person can self-verbalize the task demands, step-by-step, e.g., "Press down, turn to the right,

lift." While learning a dance step or regaining the use of the legs, the individual covertly articulates a series of lower limb movements such as "heel-toe-heel-toe, side-together-side-together."

(3) Researchers have found that a greater age-related deficit in STM occurs in the storage/encoding phase of learning rather than in the retrieval of permanently stored information. This means that the learner should try to store *meaningful cues* that can be subsequently used to retrieve information. For example, a strategy called labeling can be used to direct the person's limbs based on a clock face (Singer, 1980). Serving a tennis ball should entail swinging the racquet in a "12 o'clock" trajectory; hitting a drive, however, requires striking the ball at an angle of 3 o'clock. This strategy is particularly effective for the visually impaired individual who can associate visual images of the clock face with limb placement.

(4) Promote the use of *mental imagery* throughout the learning process. Evidence exists that a greater amount of information can be covertly rehearsed in STM if it is in imaginal, as compared to verbal, form (Paivio, 1971) (see Harris & Harris, 1984 or Orlick, 1986 for the proper use of imagery strategies). Mental imagery is also apparently a useful technique to facilitate the storage and recall of information in LTM.

## Permanent Memory

We never stop becoming surprised at an older persons' uncanny ability to recall events, feelings, and skills from decades ago. Anything that could be remembered from over 50 years ago had to have been quite important and given some thought over the years. Indeed, researchers have found that LTM is the cognitive process relatively less affected by age. For instance, Hulicka and Weiss (1965) found no age differences in recall after a 1-week interval for material that had been learned to criterion. Welford (1966), however, acknowledged that aging does affect LTM. Based on his review of the literature, he concluded:

> Although the knowledge and experience stored in memory obviously increase with age, there are signs that older people often have difficulty in getting at it when required. This difficulty probably accounts for the longer time taken by older people to identify objects - a slowing which, although not great in absolute terms, can nevertheless cause hesitation and confusion in the face of unexpected events (p. 5)

**Instructional Strategies.** It seems that the primary objective in teaching motor skills to the elderly is the efficient storage of it into LTM rather than how to retrieve it. However, as Welford (1966) suggested, retrieval can be a problem if elders are not given sufficient time to do so. The following suggestions to facilitate the storage and retrieval of information from LTM appear warranted:

(1) If older people need time to identify objects and find previously stored input, give it to them. Don't rush the person to recall information faster than is absolutely necessary.

(2) Even better, avoid placing an older person in the position where the rapid recall of information is required. Slower, stable environments are more compatible with the needs of older people.

(3) Researchers have found that a far more common memory deficit occurs in recalling information than recognizing it (see Craik, 1977, for a review). Thus, provide visual and auditory cues that allow the person to scan his/her LTM for that can help detect stored material.

(4) One technique that has been shown to improve recall/recognition in LTM is *mental imagery*. In his theory of dual-coding, Paivio (1971) asserted that information can be encoded and stored in two forms, verbal (linguistic) and nonverbal (imaginal). Consequently, input stored in both forms is more accessible than input stored in only one system.

(5) The principle of *encoding specificity* (cf. Gagné, 1977) indicates that recall from LTM is improved when the person uses the same cues when retrieving information that were used during its storage. As noted earlier, this reinforces Gagné's (1977) notion of attaching "new learning to old learning." The person should be asked to recall something from the past that they could already perform or had previously learned to meet new task demands. Example: "Remember when you did 'such and such'? Well, instead of 'that,' do 'this.' " This process is further facilitated when the person's emotions at the time of information storage and retrieval are consistent. If skill acquisition occurs in a relaxed atmosphere, it benefits the learner if he/she performs the skill with a similar emotional disposition.

## Making Decisions

There is a noticeable slowing in the decision-making process with aging. The primary source of this deficit is thought to be within the central nervous system in deciding what movements to make rather than in the execution of those movements. Another reason for making slower decisions is the greater tendency of elders to spend time (perhaps 150 to 200 msec) monitoring their previous response before switching their attention to a new signal. They are more cautious about making accurate, appropriate responses. Consequently, they make relatively more errors of omission and fewer errors of commission. Further, as Clark et al.

(1987) has shown, older learners are capable of improving their decision-making ability with practice.

**Instructional Strategies.** If the elderly tend to be concerned with performance accuracy, it makes sense to provide tasks, skills, and recreational endeavors in which *accuracy is more important for success than speed.* The type of skill that is most compatible with this need for performance accuracy and a slowing of decision-making is referred to as *self-paced or closed* (Marteniuk, 1976). As indicated earlier, closed, self-paced skills include a stable environment in which the performer controls response initiation and speed. Decision-making is slowed and deliberate; the opportunity exists to monitor responses prior to a subsequent attempt. This need partially explains the popularity of common physical activities of older people such as fishing, shuffleboard, billiards, dart-throwing, and bowling, among others.

## Responding To Pre-planned Movements Automatically

Two primary characteristics separate younger from older performers with respect to developing a motor program, i.e., executing a series of movements in the virtual absence of cognitive activity. First, as described earlier, the elderly tend to check their actions more than the young. Second, this additional post-response monitoring time causes an over-anticipation of the next arriving stimulus. Consequently, older performers: (1) need more time to reorganize their "expectancy set" (Brinley, 1965), (2) are less able to program a series of movements (Welford, 1979), and (3) have a limited capacity to program their movements for only a short sequence and in a relatively short time period. This ability becomes increasingly difficult for older persons with a more complex, prolonged series of actions. Despite these limitations, motor programming in older performers is certainly feasible under the proper conditions.

**Instructional Strategies.** Considerations to facilitate the development and execution of motor programs in older performers include: (1) providing instruction in the correct movement sequence so that the learner is able to organize, practice, and later speed up the rate of responding to appropriate levels, and (2) making the individual aware of response-produced feedback, especially derived from the sense modalities. This heightened awareness will contribute to subsequent changes in automated response. This can be accomplished by: (a) focusing the performer's attention on particular bodily movements just before, during, and/or after executing an action, (b) asking the person questions about the sensations that accompanied the response, and (c) providing knowledge of performance - precise, qualitative feedback on the correctness of the movements.

*TEACHING MOTOR SKILLS*

## Internal and External Feedback (KP and KR)

It has been shown conclusively that motor skill acquisition and retention are virtually nonexistent without some form of feedback, either external (KR) or internal (KP) (Salmoni et al., 1984). Older adults differ from their younger counterparts in their need to seek and obtain more information about a task both before and after it is performed (Cratty, 1973). This coincides with their concern for accuracy, even at the expense of speed. The elderly engage in far more self-monitoring during and after motor responses than younger persons. They rely more heavily on, and feel a greater concern for KR as a source of information about future performance than the younger learner. However, KP is given less of the older persons' attention. This is likely due to their use of cognitive and behavioral strategies - specifically their preoccupation with performance outcomes rather than the internal sensations that accompany movement execution. One would think, therefore, that older adults would consider KR as a priority in the learning process. Apparently this isn't necessarily so. There is some evidence that older people make less use of KR as well as KP than younger individuals, particularly in speeded, externally-paced tasks (Brinley, 1965; Welford, 1966).

Welford (1977) proposed two possible explanations for the tendency of elders not to make better use of KR and KP. First, whereas younger subjects program and monitor a regular series of stimuli as wholes, older performers tend to react to and monitor each stimulus individually. This preoccupation with segments of a task minimizes the person's ability to obtain and use information about the whole task after it has been performed. Older subjects "are less able - or less willing to omit such monitoring" (p. 475). Second, the rate at which information is transmitted and stored slows with aging. Therefore, elders use KP and KR less efficiently because they need more time to process and apply it toward future performance. It should be remembered that feedback is used in STM where it is rehearsed and stored in LTM and/or used in decision/making. The capacity and efficiency of STM becomes lower with age.

**Instructional Strategies.** Elderly learners do not differ markedly from younger persons with respect to the importance of receiving KP and KR, especially at the initital stages of learning. According to Magill (1985), Singer (1980), and Salmoni et al. (1984), verbal feedback on performance should include the following components. It should be: (a) *positively stated* (we retain information better when it's based on what we *should*, rather than should not do), (b) *specific* ("Nice going" has it's place in teaching, but it's non-informative), (c) *behaviorally-based* (the feedback should reflect observable actions), (d) *quantitative* ("You were off target by two feet to the right"), (e) *verbally-presented* (according to Salmoni, et al. 1984, if it's not verbal, it's not KR), (f) offered soon after a response followed by another attempt (referred to as a *short post-KR interval*), and (g) be offered *consistently* (i.e., not constantly after every trial, but on a regular basis).

## SUMMARY

Older persons need to learn motor skills for purposes of meeting recreational needs, overcoming the effects of a stroke or other medical disabilities, or learning and performing tasks that ensure adequate health care in a home environment, free of the restraints and costs accrued in a nursing care facility. Although the ability to learn, remember, and perform motor skills is directly affected by the aging process, it is important to realize that aging does not affect all individuals similarly. For example, relatively recent research indicates that physical activity can prevent premature aging. The implications are that categorizing and stereotyping older adults based on age per se as to their abilities and capacities often can be inaccurate at best and, at worst, debilitating to the individual. Older people who remain physically active can, and often do, have far more capability in performing cognitive and motor tasks than their inactive counterparts and sometimes are even equal to young performers. Nevertheless, it would be erroneous to assume that age does not alter the individual's ability to process and act upon information in an expeditious and accurate manner.

The ability to take in, selectively filter out, rehearse, store, retrieve, and physically respond rapidly and correctly to environmental stimuli slows to some degree in the elderly. Tasks which are relatively more cognitively demanding in terms of the amount and speed of processing input create larger age discrepancies than less-demanding tasks. For example, researchers have concluded that tasks involving complex decision-making demands produce slower reaction times than those requiring less difficult stimulus-response transmissions. Although performance is superior for older adults who remain physically active, differences between the exercised and sedentary groups on tasks requiring higher forms of information processing have not been examined extensively.

To compensate for slowing in cognitive and motor processes, older persons prefer activities in which task demands: (1) are self-initiated rather than externally-imposed (i.e., closed, rather than open tasks), (2) allow sufficient time to monitor responses before making a subsequent response, (3) require one to attend to one stimulus and response at a time instead of dividing attention between two or more stimulus-response actions occurring in rapid succession, (4) require relatively few decisions, and (5) do not necessitate extensive filtering of irrelevant or redundant verbal and/or visual information. In addition, older learners prefer environments that are free of excess noise and visual stimuli that are unrelated to the task.

The population of persons ages 65 and older continues to grow as advances in medical science and research prolong life. As the proportion of elderly increases with each decade, it becomes increasingly important to utilize their abundant experience, skill, and knowledge as a contribution, rather than a burden, to society. It is the job of gerontologists, medical personnel, recreation specialists, and, indeed, any person in a teaching situation with whom an older person interacts, to receive the proper training and help each person reach their potential. Finally, additional research is needed in the psychomotor area to solidify, and surpass, what is already known about the unique needs of older performers and to further develop instructional strategies to meet these needs.

## REFERENCES

Adamowicz, J.K. (1976). Visual short-term memory and aging. *Journal of Gerontology, 31,* 39-46.

Anshel, M.H. (1978). Effect of aging on acquisition and short-term retention of a motor skill. *Perceptual and Motor Skills, 47,* 993-994.

Anshel, M.H. (April, 1980). Learning, performing, and remembering motor skills as a function of age. A paper presented at the Ohio Conference on Aging. Cleveland State University, Cleveland, OH.

Birren, J.E., & Botwinick, J. (1955). Age differences in finger, jaw, and foot reaction time to auditory stimuli. *Journal of Gerontology, 10,* 429-432.

Brinley, J.F. (1965). Cognitive sets, speed and accuracy of performance in the elderly. In A.T. Welford & J.E. Birren (Eds.), *Behavior, aging, and the nervous system* (p. 114-149). Springfield, IL: Charles C. Thomas.

Brown, R.H. (1961). Visual sensitivity to differences in velocity. *Psychological Bulletin, 58,* 89.

Buccola, V.A., & Stone, W.J. (1975). Effects of jogging and cycling programs on physiological and personality variables in aged men. *Research Quarterly, 46,* 134-139.

Butler, R.N., & Lewis, M.I. (1977). *Aging and mental health: Positive psychosocial approaches* (2nd ed). St. Louis: Times Mirror/Mosby.

Clark, J.E., Lanphear, A.K., and Riddick, C.C. (1987). The effects of videogame playing on the response selection processing of elderly adults. *Journal of Gerontology, 42,* 82-85.

Craik, F.I.M. (1977). Age differences in human memory. In J.E. Birren & K.W. Schaie (Eds.), *The handbook of the psychology of aging* (pp. 384-420). New York: Van Nostrand Reinhold.

Cratty, B.J. (1973). *Movement behavior and motor learning* (3rd ed). Phila: Lea & Febiger.

Cremer, R., and Zeef, E.J. (1987). What kind of noise increases with age? *Journal of Gerontology, 42,* 515-518.

Fitts, P.M., & Posner, M. (1967). *Human performance.* Belmont, CA: Brooks/Cole Gagné, R.M. (1977). *The conditions of learning* (2nd ed). New York: Holt, Rinehart & Winston.

Gagne, R.M. (1977). *The Conditions of learning* (2nd ed). New York: Holt, Rinehart and Winston.

Haaland, K.Y., Vranes, L.F., Goodwin, J.S., & Garry, P.J. (1987). Wisconsin card sort test performance in a healthy elderly population. *Journal of Gerontology, 42,* 345-346.

Harris, D.V., & Harris, B.L. (1984). *The athlete's guide to sports psychology: Mental skills for physical people.* Champaign, IL: Human Kinetics.

Haywood, K.M. (1980). Coincidence-anticipation accuracy across the life span *Experimental Aging Research, 6,* 451-462.

Heitmann, H.M. (1982). Older adult physical education: Research implication for instruction. *Quest, 34,* 34-42.

Hulicka, I.M., & Weiss, R. (1965). Age differences in retention as a function of learning. *Journal of Consulting Psychology, 29,* 125-129.

Magill, R.A. (1985). *Motor learning: Concepts and applications* (2nd ed.) Dubuque, IA: Wm. C. Brown.

Marteniuk, R.G. (1976). *Information processing in motor skills.* New York: Holt, Rinehart and Winston.

Mayer, R. (1963). Nerve conduction studies in man. *Neurology, 13,* 1021-1030.

McPherson, B.D. (Ed.), (1986). *Sport and aging: The 1984 Olympic Scientific Congress Proceedings,* (Vol. 5). Champaign, IL: Human Kinetics.

Nideffer, R.M. (1981). *The ethics and practice of applied sport psychology.* Ithaca, NY: Mouvement.

Orlick, T. (1986) *Psyching for sports: Mental training for athletes.* Champaign, IL: Human Kinetics.

Ostrow, A.C. (1984). *Physical activity and the older adult.* Princeton, NJ: Princeton Book Co.

Paivio, A. (1971). *Imagery and verbal processes.* New York: Holt, Rinehart and Winston.

Rabbit, P.M.A. (1965). An age-decrement in ability to ignore irrelevant information. *Journal of Gerontology*, *20*, 233-238.

Salmoni, A.W., Schmidt, R.A., & Walter, C.B. (1984). Knowledge of results and motor learning: A review and critical appraisal. *Psychological Bulletin*, *95*, 355-386.

Salthouse, T.A., & Lichty, W. (1985). Tests of the neural noise hypothesis of age-related cognitive change. *Journal of Gerontology*, *40*, 443-450.

Schmidt, R.A. (1982). *Motor control and learning*. Champaign, IL. Human Kinetics.

Schonfield, D., Trueman, V., & Kline, D. (1972). Recognition tests of dichotic listening and the age variable. *Journal of Gerontology*, *27*, 487-493.

Shephard, R.J. (1978). *Physical activity and aging*. Chicago: Year Book Medical Publishers.

Shephard, R.J., & Sidney, K.H. (1979). Exercise and aging. In R.S. Hutton (Ed.), *Exercise and sport science reviews*, *6*, (pp. 1-58). Philadelphia: Franklin Institute Press.

Singer, R.N. (1980). *Motor learning and human performance* (3rd ed). New York: Macmillan.

Singleton, W.T. (1954). The change of movement timing with age. *British Journal of Psychology*, *45*, 166-172.

Spirduso, W.W. (1975). Reaction and movement time as a function of age and physical activity level. *Journal of Gerontology*, *30*, 435-440.

Spirduso, W.W. (1987). Physical activity and the prevention of premature aging. In V. Seefeldt (Ed.), *Physical activity and well being* (pp. 141-160). Reston, VA: AAHPERD.

Spirduso, W.W., & Clifford, P. (1978). Replication of age and physical activity effects on reaction and movement time. *Journal of Gerontology*, *33*, 26-30.

Suominen-Troyer, S., Davis, K.J., Ismail, A.H., & Salvendy, G. (1986). Impact of physical fitness on strategy development in decision-making tasks. *Perceptual and Motor Skills*, *62*, 71-77.

Welford, A.T. (1958). *Ageing and human skill*. London: Oxford University Press.

Welford, A.T. (1962). Changes in the speed of performance with age and their industrial significance. *Ergonomics*, *5*, 139-145.

Welford, A.T. (1966). Industrial work suitable for older people: Some British studies. *The Gerontologist*, *6*, 4-9.

Welford, A.T. (1968). *Fundamentals of skill*. London: Methuen.

Welford, A.T. (1977). Motor performance. In J.E. Birren & K.W. Schaie (Eds.), *Handbook of the psychology of aging* (pp. 450-495). New York: Van Nostrand Reinhold.

Welford, A.T. (1979). Motor skill and aging. In C.H. Nadeau, W.R. Halliwell, K.M. Newell, & G.C. Roberts (Eds.), *Psychology of motor behavior and sport-1979* (pp. 16-29). Champaign, IL: Human Kinetics.

Welford, A.T. (1984). Between bodily changes and performance. Some possible reasons for slowing with age. *Experimental Aging Research*, *10*, 73-88.

Young, R.J. (1979). The effect of regular exercise on cognitive functioning and personality. *British Journal of Sports Medicine*, *13*, 110-117.

# Part VII
# Methodological Issues

# 14

## Evaluating the Influence of Physiological Health on Sensory and Motor Performance Changes in the Elderly

WOJTEK J. CHODZKO-ZAJKO

ROBERT L. RINGEL

## ABSTRACT

This study investigated relationships between the physiological status of seventy elderly male subjects (age 63 $\pm$ 12 years) and selected sensory and motor abilities. A simple non-invasive instrument was developed for the evaluation of physiological status in elderly subjects. The Index of Physiological Status (IPS) differs from traditional measures of physiological fitness to the extent that participation in exercise stress protocols is not required for the computation of the IPS. Rather, the IPS is based on a combination of pulmonary, hemodynamic, biochemical, and anthropometric measures. The results of the study support the hypothesis that declines in sensory and motor performance are associated with both advancing age and deteriorating physiological fitness. The data underscore the importance of evaluating physiological differences between subjects when studying functional changes which occur in senescence.

## INTRODUCTION

By convention, age is most frequently expressed by the length of time lived. However, simple measures of chronology do not take into account factors which may mediate the consequences of the passage of time. Evidence that the passage of time, per se, is not a sufficiently adequate measure by which to explain changes in behavior is seen in the literature which shows that individuals with identical chronological ages often exhibit markedly different levels of sensory, motor, and cognitive performance (Montgomery & Ismail, 1977; Ramig & Ringel, 1983). While there are undoubtedly many factors which interact with time to produce such variability, it is clear that physiological components play a major role in determining the degree of behavioral change which accompanies advancing age (Finch & Schneider, 1985).

Numerous investigators have attempted to develop measures of senescence which are capable of taking into account physiological differences between subjects (Benjamin, 1947; Comfort, 1969; Ludwig & Smoke,

1980). The most common approach has been to estimate the "biological" or "functional" age of an individual using multiple regression analysis. In this procedure, a series of physiological variables are selected which are thought to be related to changes in behavior in old age. The linear combination of these physiological variables which maximizes the prediction of chronological age is used to estimate the biological age of participants in a study. In general, subjects whose biological age exceeds their chronological age are considered "old" for their age, whereas, those whose biological age is less than their actual age are considered physiologically "young".

A number of objections have been raised with regard to this approach, the most critical of which is the requirement that chronological age be selected as the criterion against which the biological age is to be defined (Costa & McRae, 1980; Ingram, 1983). This objection to the multiple regression approach is particularly difficult to overcome since there is no immediately apparent alternative external criterion to substitute for chronological age.

Several authors have adopted factor analytic approaches in an attempt to define biological age in the absence of an external criterion (Bell, 1972; Dirken, 1972; Heron & Chown, 1967; Hofecker et al., 1980; Jalavisto, 1965). The major focus of these studies has been the identification of a general factor of biological aging in which a number of physiological variables load together with chronological age in a single independent factor. Although some authors have claimed that a unitary factor of biological aging can be identified (Heron & Chown, 1967; Jalavisto, 1965), the general consensus is that aging is a multidimensional process and that efforts to reduce physiological variables to a single factor of biological aging are unlikely to meet with success (Borkan, 1978; Costa & McRae, 1980; Ingram, 1983).

Regardless of whether multiple regression or factor analytic procedures are adopted, indices of biological age are seldom very efficient predictors of age-related functional changes in behavior. Indeed most studies suggest that the single most powerful predictor of functional changes which occur in senescence remains chronological age (Ingram, 1983). Consequently, it is probably of only limited value for research to concentrate on the development of biological indices which are intended as substitutes for chronological age, and more useful to develop methods for evaluating physiological function in elderly subjects which are intended to be *complementary* to chronological age.

In our research we have attempted to develop a simple, minimally invasive procedure for the objective evaluation of overall physiological status in elderly subjects. These procedures mark a significant departure from more common approaches to the measurement of physiological health. Physiologists have traditionally evaluated the integrity of biological systems by gauging their ability to respond rapidly and appropriately to an external perturbation. In keeping with this philosophy, cardio-vascular responses to exercise tests have frequently been selected for the evaluation of physical fitness in elderly subjects (Buskirk, 1985).

There are a number of objections to the adoption of cardiovascular measures such as maximal oxygen consumption ($\dot{V}O_2$ max) for the evaluation of overall physiological status in elderly populations. Sidney and Shephard (1977) have shown that both direct and indirect measurement of $\dot{V}O_2$ max from submaximal data have been shown to underestimate direct measurements by as much as 25 percent. Sidney and Shephard conclude that valid measures of maximal oxygen consumption can only be obtained in approximately two-thirds of an elderly population.

In addition to these problems, there is still another serious objection to the reliance on exercise-stress test data for the evaluation of physiological status in elderly populations. Large numbers of elderly subjects are unable to meet the relatively stringent medical criteria required for participation in even submaximal exercise stress tests (American College of Sports Medicine, 1986). Consequently, most studies of physiological fitness in the elderly have been restricted to a relatively healthy segment of the population capable of meeting the above criteria (Buskirk, 1985; Shephard, 1978). The dependence on exercise-based testing for the evaluation of physiological status has effectively precluded more infirm subjects from participation in research, and has thus limited the extent to which findings can be generalized to the total aged population.

It is with recognition of this problem that Ludwig and Smoke (1980) suggested that variables selected for the evaluation of biological deterioration in aging should be readily observable in all individuals in the population under study. Furthermore they suggest that these variables should also be sufficiently diverse so as to be unrelated to a single physiological process.

The goal of the present study is to develop an Index of Physiological Status (IPS) which can be adopted as a convenient, objective procedure for the evaluation of physiological status in elderly subjects. The IPS is not intended to be an index of biological age and should not be regarded as an alternative to chronological age. Rather, our aim is to develop a simple, non-invasive instrument for the evaluation of physiological status which can be used with virtually all elderly subjects, which is a sufficiently sensitive measure for the detection of relationships between physiological health and a variety of auditory, visual, somatosensory, speech, and reaction time measures known to be important for health and effective functioning in old age, and which have previously been shown to be sensitive to age-related changes in physiological status (Ismail et al., 1973; Ramig & Ringel, 1983; Spirduso, 1975).

# METHOD

## Subjects

Seventy male subjects (age range 40 to 84 years, mean age 63 ± 12 years) volunteered to participate in the study. The subjects were recruited from the local community and a variety of residential institutions and senior citizens organizations. Since the tests chosen for the evaluation of physiological status were only minimally stressful, it was not necessary for subjects to meet overly stringent medical criteria in order to participate in the study. Less than 5 percent of the elderly subjects initially contacted were unable to complete the tests required for participation in the study. In all cases medical clearance was obtained from the subject's physician and informed consent was obtained.

## Procedures for the Collection of Physiological and Biochemical Data

In recognition of the previously discussed criteria suggested by Ludwig and Smoke (1980), in the present study, we restricted our measurement of physiological variables to those which could be readily observed in almost all the individuals in the population under study. The following physiological and biochemical variables were selected because (1) they are known to be good indicators of general physiological health, (2) they have been shown to be sensitive to modification by physiological training (Lamb, 1984; Shephard, 1978), and (3) they can be obtained with virtually no risk in almost all elderly subjects: Lean Body Weight (LWT), Systolic Blood Pressure (SBP), Diastolic Blood Pressure (DBP), Forced Vital Capacity (FVC), Forced Expiratory Volume (FEV1), Serum Triglyceride (TRIG), and Serum Total Cholesterol/High Density Lipoprotein (RISK).

Height, weight, and skinfolds were recorded, lean body weight was computed from these data in accordance with previously published procedures (Wilmore & Behnke, 1969). Following the collection of anthropometric data, subjects were requested to recline on a bed for 10 minutes after which resting heart rate, systolic and diastolic blood pressure were recorded. Finally, pulmonary performance was determined by computerized spirometric analysis (MCG Microloop) using sterile disposable mouthpieces and standard experimental procedures. In excess of 20 pulmonary variables were generated by this procedure, from which Forced Vital Capacity (FVC) and Forced Expiratory Volume (FEV1) were selected for inclusion in this study due to their well established relationship with age (Darby, 1981; Shephard, 1978).

The collection of blood for the biochemical analyses was performed on a separate day from the physiological testing. One hundred ml. of blood were collected between 7:00 and 8:00 while the subjects were in a 12-hour fasting state. Serum analyses of cholesterol and triglycerides were determined using a commercial serum metabolite autoanalyzer (Technicon SMA II). Serum high density lipoprotein analyses were performed using standard reagents (A-Gent, Abbott Labs).

Factor analytic procedures were used to reduce information from the seven physiological variables to a series of orthogonal factors. Subject scores on these factors were subsequently weighted and summed to generate a single composite score, the IPS.

## Selection of Sensory and Motor Performance Variables

One of the primary aims of the study was to determine the extent to which the IPS is able to discriminate between elderly subjects exhibiting different levels of performance on a variety of auditory, visual, somatosensory, speech, and reaction time tests. These tests were selected for their general importance to health and effective functioning in old age. In this study a relatively small number of tests were selected from within each of the above performance domains. A description of the measures and protocols is presented below.

## Audiometric Analyses

Pure tone conduction sensitivity was determined using a standard clinical audiometer. Air conduction thresholds were obtained at 1000, 2000, and 4000 Hz for left (L1, L2, L4) and right (R1, R2, R4) ears using an ascending threshold determination technique (Carhart & Jerger, 1959).

## Visual Analyses

Lens accommodation (LA) was selected for the evaluation of visual acuity. Lens accommodation was determined in accordance with the "push-up" method (Michaels, 1980) in which the subject was instructed to focus on a white printed target card which was moved toward the observer down a ruled slide until blurring was reported. Lens accommodation was defined as the total distance in centimeters throughout which the target could be kept in focus.

## Somatosensory Analyses

Two-point touch discrimination procedures were used to determine tactile sensitivity in the pad of the middle finger of the dominant hand. A sensory esthesiometer was used for the determination of two-point discrimination in accordance with previously established procedures (Ringel & Ewanowski, 1965). Stimuli were presented in both ascending and descending order in discrete steps of 0.5 mm. The probe was left in contact with the skin surface for approximately a two-second period. Both ascending and descending procedures were repeated three times and the mean value was determined to be the two-point discrimination threshold.

## Acoustic Analyses

Voice samples were collected in a sound-treated booth with the subjects seated at the constant distance from the microphone. Subjects were instructed to phonate the vowel "a" for as long as possible at a comfortable pitch and intensity level.

Acoustic analyses of the voice samples were performed using a computerized acoustic analysis program—GLIMPES (Glottal Imaging by Processing External Signals, Titze, 1984). The following acoustic measures were computed for a 300 cycle window occurring at the mid-point of the extended vowel phonation:

**Mean Fundamental Frequency (Fo):** the preferred vibratory frequency of the vocal folds.

**Vocal Jitter:** the cycle-to-cycle variation in vocal fold vibration frequency. Jitter is a particularly sensitive measure of temporal and mechanical irregularities in the vibratory cycle of the vocal folds and has been shown to be significantly correleated with both chronological age and physiological status (Ramig & Ringel, 1983).

**Vocal Shimmer:** the cycle-to-cycle amplitude perturbation of the glottal signal. Vocal shimmer has been shown to increase significantly with advancing chronological age and to decrease with improved physical health (Ramig & Ringel, 1983).

**Harmonic-to-Noise Ratio (H/N):** the spectral harmonics-to-noise ratio is a composite measure of vocal regularity which is affected by amplitude, period, and waveshape differences between cycles. This measure has also been shown to be particularly sensitive to temporal and mechanical disruptions of the vibratory cycle of the vocal folds (Scherer et al., 1986).

## Reaction Time Analyses

An 80 trial choice reaction time task was conducted in which subjects were instructed to discriminate between different colored stimuli presented as squares displayed on a screen (Offenbach, 1974). Forty of the trials constituted a relatively easy discrimination task—red/yellow stimuli (RTeasy), while the other forty trials constituted a more difficult discrimination task—blue/green stimuli (RTdiff). Each participant was seated in front of a box that had three 7.6 × 10.2 cm. windows in a row (7.6 cm apart, center to center). The task was self-paced, with the subject initiating the trial by pressing a start button 3 cm below the center window. Upon depression of the button, two colored squares (arranged vertically) appeared in the central window. The task was to press the left or right response window depending on which color square was in the top position of the center window. Each subject was asked to use the same hand throughout the experiment and the same finger to press the start button and response window. Stimulus presentation orders were randomized among subjects. The instructions given to the subjects emphasized both speed and accuracy. In this chapter, response latencies (msec) are reported for correct responses on both red/yellow and blue/green stimulus pairs.

## RESULTS

### Descriptive Data

Means and standard deviations for the seven physiological measures and 14 sensory and motor variables are presented in Table 14-1. Examination of these data reveals that the mean scores reported for the subjects in this study are generally in agreement with those reported in previous studies using similar elderly populations (Finch & Schneider, 1985; Shock et al., 1984).

TABLE 14.1. *Descriptive Data.*

| Variable | | M | SD |
|---|---|---|---|
| Physiological Variables | | | |
| Age | (yrs) | 62.94 | 12.79 |
| SBP | (mmHg) Systolic Blood Pressure | 134.61 | 14.03 |
| DBP | (mmHG) Diastolic Blood Pressure | 80.52 | 8.58 |
| LWT | (Kg) Lean Body Weight | 67.59 | 7.94 |
| FVC | (1) Forced Vital Capacity | 3.91 | .86 |
| FEV1 | (1/sec) Forced Expiratory Volume | 3.08 | .75 |
| TRIG | (mg) Triglycerides | 122.17 | 58.98 |
| RISK | (Chol/HDL) Cardiac Risk Index | 5.02 | 1.31 |
| Sensory and Motor Variables | | | |
| L1 | (dB) Auditory Thresholds Left | | |
| | 1000 Hz | 22.6 | 8.26 |
| L2 | 2000Hz | 26.83 | 11.81 |
| L4 | 4000Hz | 42.57 | 18.93 |
| R1 | Right 1000Hz | 24.04 | 11.63 |
| R2 | 2000Hz | 27.35 | 13.99 |
| R4 | 4000Hz | 41.32 | 18.41 |
| LA | (cm) Lens Accommodation | 77.80 | 51.90 |
| TP | (mm) Two Point Touch | 2.95 | .90 |
| Fo | (Hz) Fundamental Frequency | 118.24 | 39.53 |
| Jitter | (%) Frequency Perturbation | 2.60 | 1.50 |
| Shimmer | (dB) Amplitude Perturbation | 3.31 | 1.94 |
| H/N | Harmonics-to-Noise Ratio | 18.22 | 4.28 |
| RTeasy | (msec) Reaction Time | | |
| | Red/Yellow | .70 | .14 |
| RTdiff | (msec) Blue/Green | .79 | .17 |

# Derivation of the Index of Physiological Status (IPS)

As noted earlier, in order to reduce the seven physiological and biochemical variables to a single composite score indicative of overall physiological status, the correlation matrix for the physiological variables was factor analyzed. The principle axis form of solution was employed and the factors for each solution were rotated according to the varimax procedure (Kaiser, 1963). A minimum eigen value of one was adopted as the criterion for factor extraction.

Examination of Table 14-2 reveals that three factors met the minimum eigen value criterion and these three factors accounted for seventy-nine percent of the variability associated with the initial physiological variables. Factor 1 has high loadings on FVC and FEV1 and accordingly was named *Pulmonary Function.* Factor 2 is characterized by primary loadings on TRIG and RISK and secondary loadings on LWT. This factor was named *Blood Lipids and Body Weight.* The third factor which loaded almost exclusively on SBP and DBP was named *Blood Pressure.*

Factor scores were computed for each subject on each of the three factors. To account for the relative contribution of each of the three factors to the total factor solution, the pulmonary, blood lipid, and blood pressure factor scores were weighted in accordance with their respective eigen values (Ismail, Falls, & MacLeod, 1965). The weighted combination of the three factor scores was summed to generate the IPS according to the following equation:

$$IPS = E_1F1 + E_2F2 + E_3F3$$

where,

$E_i$ + the Eigen value associated with the ith factor

IPS scores were computed for each participant in the study and normalized to T-scores.

**TABLE 14.2.** *Factor Analysis of the Initial Physiological Variables.*

| Variable | F1 | F2 | F3 | h² |
|---|---|---|---|---|
| LWT | .16 | −.43 | −.14 | .22 |
| SBP | −.21 | −.05 | −.72 | .55 |
| DBP | .02 | .01 | −.80 | .64 |
| FVC | .96 | .04 | .11 | .92 |
| FEV1 | .97 | .08 | .10 | .96 |
| TRIG | −.14 | −.84 | .10 | .73 |
| RISK | −.16 | −.73 | .02 | .56 |
| Eigen Value | 2.18 | 1.36 | 1.07 | 4.61 |
| Percent Variance | 33.3 | 25.0 | 20.9 | 79.2 |

## Relationships Between Sensory and Motor Performance and Chronological Age

Table 14-3 presents the Pearson correlations between the performance items and chronological age. The correlational data confirm our expectations that performances on sensory and motor tasks generally deteriorate with age. The choice reaction time measures were most strongly correlated with age. Examination of the audiometric data reveals that the relationship between decreased auditory sensitivity and age was greatest for high frequency tones. Both two-point touch discrimination and lens accommodation also deteriorated with age. Finally, although vocal fundamental frequency was not significantly correlated with age, the most sensitive measures of voice perturbation (jitter, shimmer, H/N) were found to be more strongly related to chronological age.

## Relationships Between Sensory and Motor Performance and Physiological Status

Pearson correlations were computed to determine the association between subject scores on the performance tests and IPS scores. Table 14-4 presents the correlations between these sensory and motor items and the IPS. Examination of these data reveal significant correlations between IPS scores and many of the performance items. Faster reaction times for both easy and difficult discrimination tasks were associated

**TABLE 14.3.** *Correlations Between Sensory-Motor Performance Variables and Chronological Age.*

| Variable | r | n | p |
|----------|------|-----|------|
| L1 | .19 | 68 | .05 |
| L2 | .26 | 68 | .01 |
| L4 | .45 | 68 | .001 |
| R1 | .13 | 68 | .13 |
| R2 | .25 | 68 | .02 |
| R4 | .34 | 68 | .01 |
| TP | .35 | 68 | .001 |
| LA | −.42 | 70 | .001 |
| Fo | .14 | 79 | .16 |
| Jitter | .22 | 49 | .06 |
| Shimmer | .25 | 49 | .04 |
| H/N | −.26 | 49 | .03 |
| RTeasy | .53 | 64 | .001 |
| RTdiff | .61 | 64 | .001 |

Note: The number of subjects in the individual correlations varies since a few subjects did not participate in all of the sensory and motor tests. In particular, due to the cost of the acoustic analyses, voice data are restricted to 49 subjects.

**TABLE 14.4.** *Correlations Between the Sensory and Motor Variables and the Index of Physiological Status.*

| Variable | r | n | p |
|----------|------|----|------|
| L1 | −.17 | 68 | .07 |
| L2 | −.20 | 68 | .04 |
| L4 | −.37 | 68 | .001 |
| R1 | .00 | 68 | .49 |
| R2 | −.26 | 68 | .01 |
| R4 | −.36 | 68 | .001 |
| TP | −.07 | 70 | .26 |
| LA | .30 | 70 | .01 |
| Fo | −.13 | 49 | .17 |
| Jitter | −.21 | 49 | .06 |
| Shimmer | −.25 | 49 | .03 |
| H/N | .30 | 49 | .01 |
| RTeasy | −.36 | 64 | .001 |
| RTdiff | −.40 | 64 | .001 |

with improved physiological status. Similarly, increased lens accommodation was also associated with high scores on the IPS. Despite its significant decline with age, two-point touch discrimination was not significantly correlated with physiological status. The association between auditory sensitivity and the IPS was strongest for high frequency tones (L4, R4) and not significant at the lowest frequency (L1, R1). As with the chronological age data, mean fundamental frequency was not a sufficiently sensitive measure for the detection of performance differences between subjects. However, both shimmer and H/N ratios were significantly correlated with IPS scores and jitter measures approached statistical significance. In general, high scores on the IPS were associated with improved performances on the sensory and performance tests.

It is tempting to suggest that the above data indicate that high levels of physiological health are associated with a reduction in the detrimental effects of age on sensory and motor performance. Unfortunately, the correlational data alone cannot be accepted as evidence for the importance of physiological status since performance differences between subjects may have been confounded by chronological age.

The most common procedure for the control for chronological age differences between subjects is the computation of partial correlation coefficients. Table 14-5 presents partial correlation coefficients between IPS scores and the sensory and performance items controlling for chronological age. Examination of the partial correlation matrix reveals that relationships between IPS scores and the performance items are considerably reduced when statistical procedures are adopted to control for chronological age. The only variables which achieve or approach statisti-

**TABLE 14.5.** *Partial Correlations Between Sensory and Motor Variables and the Index of Physiological Status Controlling for Age.*

| Variable | r | n | p |
|---|---|---|---|
| L1 | -.08 | 68 | .25 |
| L2 | -.08 | 68 | .25 |
| L4 | -.17 | 68 | .07 |
| R1 | .08 | 68 | .25 |
| R2 | -.16 | 68 | .09 |
| R4 | -.22 | 68 | .03 |
| TP | -.11 | 68 | .18 |
| LA | .10 | 68 | .19 |
| Fo | -.09 | 49 | .28 |
| Jitter | -.14 | 49 | .16 |
| Shimmer | -.17 | 49 | .12 |
| H/N | .22 | 49 | .06 |
| RTeasy | -.10 | 64 | .21 |
| RTdiff | -.09 | 64 | .22 |

cal significance are hearing acuity at high frequencies (L4, R4) and spectral harmonics-to-noise ratios.

Since the partial correlation procedure is a relatively low powered statistical procedure, it is probably premature to dismiss the importance of physiological factors on the basis of these data alone. Accordingly, a multiple discriminant function procedure was adopted to determine whether a linear combination of sensory and motor performance items could discriminate between two groups of high and low IPS subjects matched for chronological age. In this procedure, selected subjects from the study were divided into two groups on the basis of physiological status. Subjects in group one ($n$ = 10, mean age = 65.7 yrs) scored at least one-half a standard deviation above the mean on the IPS, whereas, subjects in group two ($n$ = 10, mean age = 65.4 yrs) scored at least one-half a standard deviation below the mean. This subject matching procedure resulted in two groups which were virtually identical in age, yet markedly different with regard to physiological status.

The results of the discriminant function analyses are presented in Table 14-6. These data reveal that a linear combination of visual, auditory, somatosensory, reaction time, and speech measures significantly discriminated between subjects in the good and poor condition groups. The subjects in better physiological health exhibited less behavioral slowing, improved lens accommodation, greater tactile sensitivity, and greater phonatory control. Furthermore, when the discriminant function canonical was used for classification purposes, one hundred percent accurate classification of subjects into the high and low IPS groups was achieved.

**TABLE 14.6.** *Discriminant Function Analysis Between High and Low Physiological Status Groups Matched for Age.*

| Variable | Standardized Canonical Discriminant Function Coefficients |
|---|---|
| TP | .7397 |
| LA | 1.0105 |
| Jitter | −.5252 |
| H/N | .4684 |
| RTeasy | −2.0987 |
| RTdiff | 1.6244 |
| R4 | .0796 |

Chi Square = 18.30
Canonical Correlation = .87
Wilke's Lambda = .2312
Probability = .01
Percent Correct Classification = 100%

## DISCUSSION

As expected, performance on virtually all of the sensory and motor items was shown to be associated with an appreciable decline with advancing age. The strongest correlations were between age and the reaction time measures, underscoring the importance of behavioral slowing which has frequently been referred to as one of the strongest and most ubiquitous characteristics of old age (Salthouse, 1985). Similarly, lens accommodation and tactile sensitivity exhibited patterns of deterioration with age which were consistent with those reported by other investigators (Gellis & Pool, 1977; Michaels, 1980; Morgan & Fevens, 1972). Examination of the auditory data revealed that age-related hearing impairment was greatest for the high frequency tones, a finding which has also been frequently reported elsewhere (Corso, 1963; Harford, 1980). Finally, jitter, shimmer, and H/N ratios were found to be significantly correlated with age. These findings are similar to those reported by Ramig & Ringel (1983), who have suggested that fundamental frequency may be an insufficiently sensitive measure for the detection of age-related changes in the voice and that it is frequently necessary to sample finer aspects of vocal behavior in order to detect age changes in vocal performance (Ramig, 1983; Ramig & Ringel, 1983). In summary, for virtually all of the tests reported in this study, the observed relationships between chronological age and sensory and motor performance were consistent with those previously reported in the literature.

The data were more difficult to interpret with regard to the role of physiological status on sensory and motor performance. Initial examination of the Pearson correlation matrix seemed to indicate significant associations between physiological health and functional performance. High scores on the IPS were associated with faster reaction times, improved hearing at high frequencies, greater phonatory control, and improved lens accommodation. A somewhat surprising finding was that although tactile sensitivites decreased significantly with age, there was no relationship between two-point touch scores and IPS levels.

As previously stated, to demonstrate the influence of physiological factors on sensory and motor performance, it is insufficient to simply report correlations between the IPS and the performance items, since these relationships are potentially confounded by chronological age differences between subjects. In this study, two approaches were adopted in an attempt to dissociate age effects from physiological condition effects.

In the first procedure, correlations were computed between IPS scores and the performance items partialling out the effects of chronological age. Examination of these data revealed only very modest relationships between physiological status and sensory and motor performance. These results suggest that much of the relationship between physiological fitness and sensory and motor performance can be explained in terms of age differences between subjects. This conclusion is supported by the relatively high correlation between the IPS and age ($r = -.53$, $p < .001$).

However, examination of the aging literature suggest that in individuals for whom the traditional association between physical fitness and chronological age does not hold, physical fitness levels independent of chronological age may be important predictors of functional performance. For example, Spirduso (1975) has shown that the reaction times of physically active elderly subjects resemble those of inactive younger individuals and fail to exhibit the classic age-related declines which are observed in sedentary elderly individuals. In a more recent experiment, Dustman et al. (1984) demonstrated that the performance of elderly subjects on a variety of neuropsychological tests can be significantly improved by a 12-week program of aerobic physical training. (See chapter three.)

These studies suggest that it may be possible to dissociate the effects of physical fitness and chronological age on sensory-motor performance by either manipulating fitness levels through exercise training, or by comparing individuals of similar age but differing physical fitness levels.

Accordingly, a second procedure was adopted in an attempt to clarify the nature of relationships between the IPS and the sensory and motor performance tests. In this procedure, subjects were divided into discrete high and low IPS groups which were matched for chronological age. Discriminant function analysis revealed significant sensory and motor performance differences between the two groups. When the discriminant function canonical was applied for classification purposes, subjects could be classified into the appropriate health group on the basis of their sensory and motor performance scores with one hundred percent classification accuracy.

The discriminant function analyses emphasize the importance of physiological health measures by focusing on performance differences between individuals with relatively extreme physiological profiles. Although it is clear that auditory, visual, somatosensory, speech, and reaction time performances, in general decline with advancing age, there can be little doubt that subjects in good physiological condition exhibit less age-related sensory and motor impairment than those in poorer physiological health.

The reasons why physiologically healthy subjects should experience less sensory and motor impairment are undoubtedly complex. However, it does not seem unreasonable to suggest that individuals who experience generalized cardiovascular, pulmonary, metabolic or biochemical insufficiencies, are in turn likely to also exhibit more specific sensory and motor inadequacies, perhaps due to factors such as impaired circulation, insufficient supply of nutrients, and disrupted neural innervation.

Evidence which supports the existence of such an association between general physiological health and the effects of aging is afforded by examination of the human larynx. Significant cellular, structural, and neurological changes in the larynx can be shown to be present not only in old age, but also in subjects with deteriorating physiological health (Darby, 1981). Degenerative changes present in both elderly subjects and diseased patients include, muscle atrophy (Hirano, Kurita, & Nakashima, 1983), ligamental deterioration (Kahane, 1983), cartilagenous calcification, and neuronal atrophy (Segre, 1971). The acoustic consequences of the above changes are essentially similar in both aged and diseased patients. Both groups frequently exhibit inappropriate fluctuations of vocal intensity and significant disturbances in phonatory control (Aronson, 1985; Darby, 1981).

We believe that the data presented in this study underscore the importance of the evaluation of physiological health variables when studying functional changes in sensory and motor performance, not only in diseased patients, but also in elderly subjects without overt manifestations of pathology.

It is questionable whether physiological measures can be developed into indices of biological age which will be able to replace chronological age. However, it is clear that our understanding of senescent processes influencing sensory and motor performance benefits from a knowledge of both age and physiological status, and the omission of either of these parameters significantly reduces our ability to understand the nature of the phenomenon.

Having argued in favor of the inclusion of measures of physiological status in experiments with aging populations, our final task is to evaluate the propriety of the IPS as a valid approach for the estimation of physiological status in elderly subjects. Much of our thinking in this area has been influenced by the work of Borkan and his colleagues who have argued that a profile of biological parameters is required to adequately describe the physiological characteristics of senescence (Borkan & Norris, 1980). Borkan's profile acknowledges the multivariate nature of physiological aging but is primarily descriptive and does not easily lend itself to quantification for experimental purposes.

In our approach, we have attempted to recognize the multidimensional nature of physiological health while at the same time attempting to reduce these measures to a single convenient estimate of physiological status. The IPS was found to be a sufficiently sensitive measure for the detection of relationships between physiological health and sensory and motor performance abilities. Subjects with high scores on the IPS exhibited less behavioral slowing, improved lens accommodation, greater tactile sensitivity, and greater phonatory control than less healthy subjects of the same age.

It is recognized that because the IPS has been established on a relatively small number of subjects it represents a preliminary solution and should not be regarded as a comprehensive measure of physiological integrity. Nonetheless, it is our belief that the procedures reported in this study provide the researcher with a convenient, pragmatic, and valid approach to the estimation of physiological status in elderly subjects.

Although in the current study the IPS was used exclusively for cross-sectional analyses, the index also has considerable potential for use with longitudinal designs. In longitudinal studies it is frequently necessary to obtain repeated measures on subjects whose physical condition deteriorates significantly over the time course of a study. Subjects who are able to satisfy medical criteria for participation in exercise-stress protocols at the beginning of a study may not always meet these criteria at subsequent data collection points. In such instances, the exclusive reliance on exercise-based measures for the evaluation of physiological health necessitates the elimination of these subjects from the study. Since the physiological protocols required for the computation of the IPS can be easily and safely applied to almost all subjects regardless of physical condition, the procedure avoids many of the sample bias problems associated with stress-based measures and thus is well suited for the evaluation of longitudinal changes in physiological health.

In summary, the evidence we have presented supports the hypothesis that sensory and motor abilities decline progressively with both advancing age and deteriorating physiological health. Although it is not always possible to clearly dissociate the influence of physiological factors from chronological age effects, there can be little doubt of the importance of evaluating physiological differences between subjects when studying functional changes which occur in senescence. A simple, non-invasive procedure is proposed for the evaluation of physiological status in elderly subjects. The IPS has shown promise as a measure of physiological condition appropriate for use with elderly subjects, and the adoption of similar procedures in future research designs could contribute significantly to our understanding of the aging process.

## REFERENCES

American College of Sport Medicine. (1986). *Guidelines for graded exercise testing and exercise prescription.* New York: Lea & Febiger.

Aronson, A.E. (1985). *Clinical voice disorders.* New York: Thieme, Inc.

Bell, B. (1972). Significance of functional age for interdisciplinary and longitudinal research in aging. *International Journal of Aging and Human Development, 3,* 145-147.

Benjamin, H. (1949). Biologic versus chronologic age. *Journal of Gerontology, 2,* 217-227.

Borkan, G.A. The assessment of biological age during adulthood (Doctoral dissertation, University of Michigan, 1978). *Dissertation Abstracts International, 39,* 06-A, 3682. (University Microfilms No. 78228-61).

Borkan, G.A., & Norris, A.H. (1980). Assessment of biological age using a profile of physical parameters. *Journal of Gerontology, 35,* 177-184.

Buskirk, E.R. (1985). Health maintenance and longevity: Exercise. In L.E. Finch & E.L. Schneider (Eds.), *Handbook of the biology of aging,* (pp. 894-924), New York: Van Nostrand Reinhold.

Carhart, R., & Jerger, J. (1959). Preferred method for clinical determination of pure-tone thresholds. *Journal of Speech and Hearing Disorders, 24,* 330-345.

Comfort, A. (1969). Test battery to measure aging rate in man. *Lancet, 27,* 1411-1415.

Corso, J.F. (1963). Age and sex differences in pure tone thresholds. *Archives of Otolaryngology, 77,* 385-405.

Costa, P.T. & McCrae, R.R. (1980). Functional age: A conceptual and empirical critique. In S.G. Haynes & H. Feinleib (Eds.) *Epidemiology of Aging,* U.S. Dept. of Health and Human Services, Washington, D.C., pp. 23-49.

Darby, J.K. (1981). *Speech evaluation in medicine.* New York: Grune & Stratton.

Dirken, J.M. (1972). *Functional age of industrial workers.* Groningen, Netherlands: Woolters—Noordhoff.

Dustman, R.E., Ruhling, R.O., Russell, E.M., Shearer, D.E., Bonekat, H.W., Shigeoka, J.W., Wood, J.S., & Bradford, D.C. (1984). Aerobic exercise training and improved neuropsychological function of older individuals. *Neurobiology of Aging, 5,* 35-42.

Finch, E.E., & Schneider, E.L. (1985). *Handbook of the biology of aging.* New York: Van Nostrand Reinhold.

Furukawa, T., Inave, M., Kijiya, F., Inada, H., Takasugi, S., Fukui, S., Takeda, H., & Abe, H. (1975). Assessment of biological age by multiple regression analysis. *Journal of Gerontology, 30*(4), 422-434.

Gellis, M., & Pool, R. (1977). Two-point discrimination distances in the normal hand and forearm. *Plastic and Reconstructive Surgery, 59*(1), 57-63.

Harford, E.A. (1980). Hearing aid amplification for adults. *Monographs in Contemporary Audiology, 4, 1,* 123-147.

Heron, A., & Chown, S., (1967). *Age and function.* Boston: Little, Brown & Company.

Hinchcliffe, R. (1973). Epidemiology of sensorineural hearing loss. *Audiology, 12,* 446-452.

Hirano, M., Kurita, S., & Nakashima, T. (1983). Growth, development and aging of human vocal folds. In D.M. Bless, & J.H. Abbs (Eds.), *Vocal fold physiology. Contemporary research and clinical issues* (pp. 22-43). San Diego, CA: College Hill Press.

Hofecker, G., Skalicky, M., Kment, A., & Niedermuller, H. (1980). Models of the biological age of the rat. A factor model of age parameters. *Mechanisms of Aging and Development, 14,* 345-359.

Ingram, D.K. (1983). Toward the behavioral assessment of biological aging in the laboratory mouse: Concepts, terminology and objectives. *Experimental Aging Research, 9,* 225-238.

Ismail, A.H., Falls, H.B., & MacLeod, D.F. (1965). Development of a criterion for physical fitness tests from factor analysis results. *Journal of Applied Physiology, 20,* 991-999.

Jalavisto, E. (1965). The role of simple test measuring speed of performance in the assessment of biological vigor: A factorial study in elderly women. In A.T. Welford & J.E. Birren (Eds.), *Behaviour, aging & the nervous system* (pp. 353-365). Springfield, IL: Charles C. Thomas.

Kahane, J.C. (1983). A survey of age-related changes in the connective tissues of the human adult larynx. In D.M. Bless & J.H. Abbs (Eds.), *Vocal fold physiology. Contemporary research and clinical issues* (pp. 44-49). San Diego, CA: College Hill Press.

Kaiser, H.F. (1963). The varimax criterion for analytic rotation in factor analysis. *Psychometrika, 23,* 187-200.

Lamb, D.R. (1984). *Physiology of exercise: Responses and adaptations* (pp. 138-169). New York: Macmillan.

Ludwig, F.C., & Smoke, M.E. (1980). The measurement of biological age. *Experimental Aging Research, 6*, 497-521.

Michaels, D.M. (1980). *Visual optics and refraction: A clinical approach.* New York: C.V. Mosby.

Montgomery, D.L., & Ismail, A.H. (1977). The effect of a four-month physical fitness program on high and low-fit groups matched for age. *Journal of Sports Medicine and Physical Fitness, 17, 3,* 327-333.

Morgan, R.F., & Fevens, S.K. (1972). Reliability of the adult growth examination: A standardized test of aging. *Perceptual and Motor Skills, 34,* 415-419.

Offenbach, S.I. (1974). A developmental study of hypothesis testing and the selection strategies. *Developmental Pyschology, 10,* 484-490.

Ramig, L.A. (1983). Effects of physiological aging on vowel spectral noise. *Journal of Gerontology, 38,* 223-225.

Ramig, L.A., & Ringel, R.L. (1983). Effect of physiological aging on selected acoustic characteristics of voice. *Journal of Speech and Hearing Research, 26,* 22-30.

Ringel, R.L., & Ewanowski, S.J. (1965). Oral perception: Two-point discrimination. *Journal of Speech and Hearing Research, 8*(4), 389-398.

Salthouse, T.A. (1985). Speed of behavior and its implications for cognition. In J.E. Birren & K.W. Schaie (Eds.). *Handbook of the Psychology of Aging* (pp. 400-422). New York: Van Hostrand Reinhold Company.

Scherer, R.C., Titze, I.R., Raphael, B.N., Wood, R.P., Ramig, L.A., & Blager, F.B. (1986). Vocal fatigue in a professional voice user. In L. Lawrence, *Transcripts of the Fourteenth Symposium on the Care of the Professional Voice.* New York: Voice Foundation.

Serge, R. (1971). Senescence of the voice. *Eye, Ear, Nose and Throat Monthly, 50,* 223-233.

Shephard, R.J. (1978). *Physical activity and aging.* Chicago: Croom Helm.

Shock, N.W., Greulich, R.C., Andres, R., Arenberg, D., Costa, P.T., Lakatta, E.G., & Tobin, J.D. (1984). *Normal human aging: The Baltimore longitudinal study of aging.* Washington, DC: NIH, U.S. Government Printing Office.

Sidney, K.H., & Shephard, R.J. (1977). Maximum and submaximum exercise tests in men and women in the seventh, eighth and ninth decades of life. *Journal of Applied Physiology, 43,* 280-287.

Spirduso, W.W. (1975). Reaction and movement time as a function of age and physical activity level. *Journal of Gerontology, 30,* 435-440.

Titze, I.R. (1984). Parameterization of the glottal area, glottal flow and vocal fold contact area. *Journal of the Acoustical Society of America, 75,* 570-580.

Wilmore, J.H., & Behnke, A.R. (1969). An anthropometric estimation of body density and lean body weight in young men. *Journal of Applied Physiology, 27,* 25-31.

*PHYSIOLOGICAL HEALTH*     **323**

# 15

## A Longitudinal Analysis of Anticipatory Judgment in Older Adult Motor Performance

KATHLEEN M. HAYWOOD

### ABSTRACT

Anticipatory motor responses are important in skill performance, but little is known about their retention in older adulthood. It was hypothesized that older adults could retain their accuracy on an anticipatory motor task once they became familiar with the task. This investigation tested 12 older adults, 62 to 73 years old, four times over a period of seven years. They performed a coincidence-anticipation task with various speeds of movement in the frontal plane. Participants also repeated testing one week after their third session to establish the range of session-to-session variation, and responded to sagittal plane movement after their fourth session. Performance on the coincidence-anticipation task was measured by asking participants to press a button coincident with the arrival of a stimulus light at a target point, permitting assessment of both the accuracy and direction of the response. Univariate, repeated measures ANOVAs were conducted on absolute, constant, and variable ratio error.

The older adults anticipated inaccurately by responding very late in the initial session, but were able to better center their responses around coincidence thereafter. Absolute error declined with advancing years. The participants responded similarly to sagittal plane movement the first time they encountered this task variation. The retention and even improved skill recorded here could be attributed to task familiarity as well as learning, and stresses the importance of multiple testing sessions with older adults.

### INTRODUCTION

Sport activities sought out by older adults are more likely to require accuracy and precision of movement than maximum speed or strength. Undoubtedly, this reflects maintenance of skill on self-paced motor tasks coupled with a deterioration of performance on speeded or maximal strength tasks in older adulthood. A rather large number of sports and everyday tasks (like driving an automobile), in fact emphasize accuracy as well as speed. For example, racquet sports demand anticipation of a moving ball such that an arm movement can be matched precisely to the object's path and the object struck. The criterion is more for accuracy than speed unless the speed of movement approaches the individual's performance limitations. When opponents are matched approximately on physical strength and power, the speed of the object to be intercepted is manageable to the performer and accuracy of judgment becomes critical to successful performance. Hence, anticipatory skills are an important aspect of motor performance in the aging, and study of these skills contributes to an understanding of aging.

The importance of anticipatory judgment in skills has long been recognized and studied under the terms coincidence-anticipation, coincident timing, and interception. Poulton (1957) distinguished among several types of anticipation. Effector anticipations are acquisitions of stationary stimuli, such as moving rapidly to aim at a target. Receptor anticipations are made to a moving stimulus whose future pathway is displayed ahead. This is the type of action undertaken when driving a car within a lane. Finally, perceptual anticipations are made to a moving stimulus when its path is predictable by known properties but not displayed ahead. Such is the case when a tennis player intercepts an approaching ball with backspin. In laboratory simulations of such skills, however, the task has typically been simplified to a prediction of time or place, but not both. The direction of object movement has been in the sagittal or frontal plane, rarely in an oblique plane. The most common anticipation task used in laboratory studies is provided by the Bassin Anticipation Timer (Lafayette Model 50-575). This apparatus uses sequentially lit L.E.D.s mounted on a black trackway to simulate moving objects of various speeds. The spatial dimensions of stimulus movement are obviously fixed. The performer is typically given a hand-held button and instructed to press it at the exact time the light arrives at a designated point. The performer's error in timing the motor response to the light's arrival can be determined in both amount and direction.

A considerable amount of research has been conducted on various aspects of coincidence-anticipation performance by children and young adults. Some investigators have emphasized the effects of varying the visual display, such as speed of movement, direction of movement, distance and/or exposure time, size of object, etc. (Dunham, 1977; Dunham & Glad, 1985; Ridenour, 1977). Others have focused on the effects of learning variables, particularly knowledge of results (Haywood, 1975; Wiegand & Ramella, 1983). A few have varied the type of motor response to the object (Grose, 1976; Haywood, 1977). Such study has contributed to a better understanding of the factors influencing skill performance.

Coincidence-anticipation performance in older adulthood has received limited attention in the literature, but the study of this topic contributes to a general understanding of skill performance with aging. Initially, it is of interest to know how older adults' coincidence-anticipation performance compares to that of younger performers. Haywood (1980) studied coincidence-anticipation accuracy in four age groups: 7 to 9-year-olds, 11 to 13-year-olds, younger adults, and physically active older adults (60 to 76 years of age). Stimulus speed was varied between two and five miles/hour from trial to trial, and movement was in the frontal plane. An analysis of absolute error scores showed no significant differences in the accuracy of younger and older adults, although the older adults had a higher mean error. In terms of constant error, which reflects the tendency to respond early or late, the older adults responded early as a group while the younger adults tended to be late. There was no significant difference in variability of performance. Overall, the performance profile of the older adults was most similar to that of the 11 to 13-year-olds. A second analysis with a group of slightly older (64 to 86 years) and more sedentary older adults yielded significantly less accurate and more variable performance on the part of older adults. This group also demonstrated a late directional bias, particularly at the fastest stimulus speed. These findings indicate that something associated with maintaining an active lifestyle might also be associated with better performance on a timing task.

A second study by Haywood (1982) used slightly faster stimulus speeds (three, five, and seven miles/hour) on the Bassin apparatus but yielded similar findings. A group of active older adults (62 to 78 years of age) was less accurate and more variable than a group of young adults, but showed similar directional bias. It should be recognized that the older adults in both studies were significantly less accurate than younger adults, but by a relatively small amount. Mean absolute error scores ranged (in the two studies) from 49 to 62 ms in the younger groups and from 75 to 90 ms in the older groups, a difference of 26 to 28 ms. There was a much larger difference in mean error between young children and the younger adults, 82 ms. The same was generally true for variable error, so there was no indication that older adult performance regressed to a level exhibited by children.

In studying the effect of practice and temporal location of knowledge of results, Wiegand and Ramella (1983) also tested both younger and older adults on the Bassin Anticipation Timer. A constant stimulus speed of five miles/hour was used. The older adults in this study also were less accurate (approximately 38 ms) and more variable (approximately 23 ms) than younger adults. Additionally, the older adults here tended to be late while the younger adults showed only a slight bias to be early. Wiegand and Ramella further documented an improvement in performance with practice on this task by both age groups. The improvement ratio was similar for younger and older adults.

In summary, previous studies reveal significantly poorer performance by older adults than younger adults on coincidence-anticipation tasks, although by a small margin. Such cross-sectional studies as these, however, do not indicate whether accuracy of performance declines throughout adulthood or is maintained at a level slightly less accurate than the peak achieved in young adulthood. In addition, the performance of the same older adults is not observed in subsequent sessions when the participants could be more familiar with the experimental procedure and therefore more relaxed.

The purpose of this longitudinal investigation was to study the coincidence-anticipation performance of the same group of older adults over a number of years. Participants in an earlier study of performance in 1980 and 1981 (Haywood, 1982) were invited to be measured again in 1985 and 1987. It was hypothesized that the accuracy of performance would be maintained at the level demonstrated in 1981, but that performance in 1985 would be characterized by late responses, as in 1980, reflecting the time interval between 1981 and 1985. That is, the participants would approach the task in 1985 as if it were new and the speed of the stimulus very fast, rather than familiar and manageable. Further, it was hypothesized that asking the older adults to perform the task with stimulus movement in a new orientation would result in performance levels similar to those in the first, 1980 testing session.

## METHOD

### Subjects

The subjects participating in this study were 12 older adults, six men and six women, who had been attending a fitness program for older adults at the University of Missouri in St. Louis. Participation required each adult to have seen a medical doctor within the year and to have filed a physician's approval for participation. The group was first tested in 1980 at an average age of 66.9 years (range 62.4 to 73.3). They were tested one year later (1981), three-and-one-half years following that session (1985), and finally in 1987 at an average age of 73.5 years (range 69.0 to 80.0). Each participant was paid $5.00 per experimental session. All 12 subjects returned for testing in 1981; 11 were available in 1985, with one undergoing cataract surgery; 10 returned in 1987.

Form 5-B of the Keystone Visual Skills Profile was administered to each participant at the first session. This screening test assured that participants had at least 96% usable distance vision, could fuse images, view objects with the two eyes simultaneously, and were free of phoria (turning of the eyeball). Every subject had prescribed glasses. At subsequent sessions each was queried about the frequency of visual checkups and were administered a visual screening test only if there was doubt that the existing prescription was adequate. Subjects wore their prescribed glasses during the experimental session if the prescription was intended for the distance used here.

## Apparatus

The coincidence-anticipation task performed by the subjects was presented on a Bassin Anticipation Timer. Speed was constant within trials but was varied across trials. The row of lights was positioned such that movement was from the subjects' left to right in the frontal plane over a distance of 150 cm at a viewing distance of 150 cm (see Figure 15-1). At the conclusion of the last testing session, additional trials were administered with the light approaching the participants in the mid-sagittal plane. Room lighting was fluorescent. In this study, the light moved at a speed of 46.5, 77.5, or 108.6 deg/s (three, five, or seven miles/hour, respectively). The subjects depressed a hand-held button with the preferred finger to indicate the moment they judged the light to arrive at the marked termination point on the right end of the row of lights. The timer provided the subjects' errors in ms early or late.

## Design and Procedure

The subjects were initially tested in 1980 and 1981 to determine the relationship between precise viewing of the stimulus light and task performance (Haywood, 1982). When the participants were tested in 1985 they were asked to return 5 to 14 days later to repeat the procedure. The purpose of this repetition was to establish the normal session-to-session variation in performance. Only data from the first session were used in the longitudinal analysis. The older adults were last tested in 1987. Testing procedures were identical in all sessions, except that additional trials with the Bassin apparatus oriented in the mid-sagittal plane were added to the end of the 1987 session to observe similarity of performance. This orientation is more like that encountered in sport and everyday activities.

Informed consent was obtained at the beginning of each session. After any necessary visual screening tests were administered, the subjects were given 9 practice trials. A set order of 12 trials with the 3 speeds randomly distributed was presented. A variable warning period of 1.5 or 2.0 s was used so that the subjects were not able to internally time the task and were required to monitor the stimulus speed on each trial. An

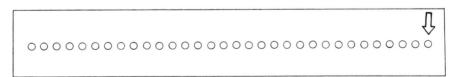

**FIGURE 15.1.** *The Bassin Anticipation Timer trackway. The first light on the left was an amber warning light. The last light on the right was marked by an arrow as the target.*

earlier analysis established that 9 warm-up trials are sufficient to reach a stable level of performance continuing over 20 additional trials in this age group (Haywood, 1982). The 1987 mid-sagittal trials used the same order of 3 stimulus speeds over 12 trials following a series of 9 warm-up trials.

Instructions to the subject stressed that the experimenter merely wanted to know how people watched the moving light and that no particular viewing strategy was "correct". It was suggested that attention be given to the task wherein subjects were directed to press the response button at the same time the light arrived at the target point. A reminder was included that the decision and response initiation would be necessary before the arrival of the light at the target. Each trial began with a verbal "ready" signal.

Task scores were prepared for analysis by first converting ms error to a percentage or ratio error. This allowed trials at different stimulus speeds to be treated equivalently. For each trial, the ms of error were divided by the time taken for the stimulus to traverse the track. Mean constant, absolute, and variable error were then calculated for each subject. Constant error indicates the subjects' directional bias, early (designated negative) or late (designated positive). Absolute error, the absolute value of the error score, reflects response accuracy regardless of direction. Variable error was calculated by obtaining the standard deviation around subjects' mean constant error, and indicates consistency of performance. Hence task scores were available for four time points in constant, absolute, and variable error.

The experimental design used to analyze the task scores was a repeated measures ANOVA with four repetitions on time of testing (1980, 1981, 1985, and 1987). Univariate analyses of absolute, constant, and variable error were conducted because of the small sample size. Scheffe post-hoc analyses were conducted following those ANOVAs yielding a significant $F$-ratio at the .05 level or better. Correlations and $t$-tests were used to examine the relationship between performance in the frontal and sagittal planes in 1987. Mean group error for time of testing was entered into the three missing data cells (Subject 5, 1985; subject 11, 1987; Subject 12, 1987) for the analyses of variance.

## RESULTS

### Retention of Skill

The ANOVA of absolute error with repeated measures on time of testing yielded a significant $F$ ratio at the .02 level (see Table 15-1 and Figure 15-2). A Scheffe post-hoc analysis determined that the 1980 and 1987 means were significantly different at the .05 level of significance. Hence, there was a trend to improved accuracy of performance over the

**TABLE 15.1.** *Repeated Measures ANOVAs Summary Table.*

| Error Term | ANOVA MS | df | F | p | 1980 M | SD | 1981 M | SD | 1985 M | SD | 1987 M | SD |
|---|---|---|---|---|---|---|---|---|---|---|---|---|
| Absolute Error | 7.47 | 3,33 | 3.73 | .02 | 17.8 | 4.8 | 15.3 | 5.3 | 13.8 | 4.4 | 11.8 | 5.7 |
| Constant Error | 71.81 | 3,33 | 19.11 | .00 | 17.8 | 4.8 | 1.3 | 10.7 | 3.9 | 10.6 | 3.5 | 8.0 |
| Variable Error | 8.33 | 3,33 | 3.80 | .02 | 10.3 | 3.7 | 16.5 | 6.5 | 13.7 | 4.0 | 12.0 | 6.7 |

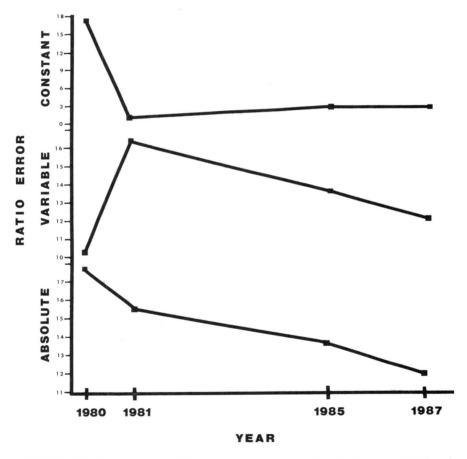

**FIGURE 15.2.** *Mean constant, variable, and absolute error for each time of testing from 1980 through 1987.*

ANTICIPATORY JUDGMENT

time span with performance being significantly more accurate by the fourth testing. Year-to-year improvement was better than 1%.

An identical ANOVA of constant error also yielded a significant $F$ ratio but at the .001 level of significance. A post-hoc analysis indicated that the 1980 mean was significantly different from all other means at the .05 level of significance. The 1981, 1985, and 1987 means were not significantly different from each other. The high positive mean of 1980 indicated that the group tended to respond late at the initial testing. In subsequent years the group was much better at centering their responses on the time of coincidence, with just a slight tendency to be late.

The ANOVA of variable error yielded a significant $F$ ratio at the .02 level. The post-hoc analysis of mean variable error at each time of testing demonstrated that only the 1980 and 1981 means were significantly different, at the .05 level. Performance among group members was significantly more variable at the 1981 testing than the 1980 testing but tended to be more consistent in subsequent years, although not significantly different.

## The 1985 Repetition

Participants returned 5 to 14 days after their initial 1985 testing to repeat the experimental session to establish the variation in session-to-session testing. A $t$-test was conducted to test for differences between the two session scores for each error measure. The $t(9)$ values were 1.10, 0.45, and 0.61 for absolute, constant, and variable error, respectively, all nonsignificant. The difference between session means was only 0.3%, 1.1%, and 0.8% for absolute, constant, and variable error, respectively. Therefore, session-to-session variation in performance was small and identified as approximately 1% error.

## Sagittal Plane Performance

Pearson product-moment correlations were calculated between 1987 performance in the frontal and sagittal planes for absolute, constant, and variable error. These correlation coefficients were .47, .75, and .12, respectively. Only the coefficient for constant error was significant, $p < .012$, indicating a relationship in the direction of response bias. A series of matched $t$-tests indicated that mean absolute, constant, and variable errors were not significantly different, although the sagittal-plane means were slightly lower, 10.0% ($\pm$ 2.4), 2.7% ($\pm$ 7.9), and 10.7% ($\pm$ 2.2), respectively.

## DISCUSSION

This longitudinal study examined the retention of coincidence-anticipation accuracy in older adults. Participants were tested four times over a period of seven years. The statistical analysis of their performance indicated that the group responded late in their initial testing, but were significantly better at centering their responses on the time of coincidence when they returned in 1981. This improved directional judgment was maintained in 1985 and 1987, refuting the hypothesis that participants would again respond late in 1985. The significantly late responses in 1980 and subsequent improvement might reflect an initial perception that the stimulus speeds were fast and the task difficult. In subsequent sessions, participants might have approached the task with increased confidence and familiarity, permitting responses better timed to stimulus speed.

The older adults lowered their mean absolute error in every subsequent year, with the last year's performance being significantly better than that of the initial year, supporting the hypothesis made earlier. For this task and this group of older adults, then, rather than performance deteriorating over the older adult years, skill was well retained and even improved.

Variable error increased significantly from the first to second sessions. This increase is associated with the large, parallel shift in response bias. While all of the older adults responded quite late in the first session, most were better able to center their responses on the time of coincidence in the second. A few continued to respond late in the second session. Mean variable error for the group was lower in the third and fourth session, but not significantly different than either the first or second sessions.

These findings suggest that the older adult participants of this study were not only able to retain their skill level over seven years, but to actually improve it. This improvement could reflect learning of the anticipation task with repetitive practice. If such learning occurred, the possibility exists that older adults indeed can train to improve on such eye-hand coordination tasks or develop coordination strategies to improve performance. Yet, it must be recognized that the amount of practice undertaken by the older adults in attending the experimental sessions was limited, particularly in relation to the elapsed time between sessions. Wiegand and Ramella (1983) documented improvement over 20 trials on a Bassin task among older adults. Improvement over the initial trials might have been a warm-up effect, and the investigators found no statistically significant improvement over the last eight trials. Haywood (1982) found older adults improved over an initial nine trials of a Bassin task then stabilized at their level of performance over the remaining 20 trials. While it was demonstrated here that older adults do not necessarily decline in anticipatory motor skill over a seven year interval, it cannot be definitely concluded that they learned the skill through repetitive practice.

The retention and improvement of skill recorded in this study might be associated with a variety of factors other than learning through repetitive practice. It is important to note that this group of participants was recruited from an exercise program for older adults. Eight were still program participants in the last year and the others were maintaining an active lifestyle. The retention of skill might be linked to the maintenance or improvement of fitness, either because the fitness activities themselves require speeded and timed movements or good health permits older adults to continue similar activities, such as driving. In addition, the potential of exercise to maintain physiological processes could be responsible for the maintenance of the central, neurological processes involved in anticipatory motor behavior. Improvement in the exercise program almost might have convinced the participants that they were capable of improving performance and learning new things (many had taken up new activities such as tap dancing and low-impact aerobics in their program). This group, then, might have approached participation in the present study differently than would another group of older adults. Additionally, the continuing association with the experimenter might encourage increased effort in contrast to a single testing session wherein no follow-up is anticipated.

Certainly in the short term, this study indicates that the true level of older adult motor performance might not be exhibited in an initial experimental session. Multiple testing sessions are desirable. In the long term, future research is needed to sort out the roles of social-psychological and physiological factors on improved anticipatory motor skill among older adults, and to document actual learning of anticipatory skills independent of performance variables.

This study also examined the relationship between performance in the frontal and sagittal planes in older adults. While many experimental settings have used the frontal plane for stimulus movement, approach in the sagittal plane is similar to more sport skills (batting, catching, striking). The earlier study which recorded eye movements (Haywood, 1982) necessitated movement in the frontal plane for those recordings. This study allowed observation of performance in both planes in 1987, although repetition of the earlier years' testing required frontal plane performance to precede sagittal plane performance for all subjects.

Mean scores of performance in response to movement in the two planes were not significantly different, refuting the hypothesis made earlier. This result is in agreement with Shea and Northam (1982) who found that orientation made little difference in young adults' ability to discriminate velocities on the Bassin Anticipation Timer. However, Dunham and Glad (1985) found significant differences in young adults' performance on another apparatus in favor of frontal plane movement. The older adults here apparently approached the new orientation as an

*AGING AND MOTOR BEHAVIOR*

alternate version of a well-known task. Their performance level in the mid-sagittal plane was similar to their 1987 performance at the familiar orientation, whereas their initial performance in the frontal plane was very late and inaccurate. In the absence of other literature indicating that the sagittal orientation typically yields significantly less error, performance level in the two planes is evidently equivalent in older adults. The same individuals were not necessarily the better performers in each plane, however, as evidenced by the low correlation for both absolute and variable error. The tendency to respond early or late was consistent between orientations.

In summary, this study demonstrated that active older adults can well maintain and even improve a motor skill after an initial session that was characterized by inaccurate or tentative performance as indicated by late responses. While this refutes the stereotyped notion of declining skill in the older adult years, it is not clear that the improvement was actually learning. Several social-psychological and physiological factors are equally tenable if not more plausible explanations of improved performance.

### REFERENCES

Dunham, P., Jr. (1977). Age, sex, speed and practice in coincidence-anticipation performance of children. *Perceptual and Motor Skills, 45,* 187-193.
Dunham, P. & Glad, H. (1985). Effect of plane of movement and speed of stimulus on anticipatory coincidence. *Perceptual and Motor Skills, 61,* 1191-1194.
Grose, J.E. (1976). Timing control and finger, arm and whole body movements. *Research Quarterly, 38,* 10-21.
Haywood, K.M. (1982). Eye movement pattern and accuracy during perceptual-motor performance in young and old adults. *Experimental Aging Research, 8,* 153-157.
Haywood, K.M. (1980). Coincidence-anticipation accuracy across the life span. *Experimental Aging Research, 6,* 451-462.
Haywood, K.M. (1977). Eye movements during coincidence-anticipation performance. *Journal of Motor Behavior, 9,* 313-318.
Haywood, K.M. (1975). Relative effects of three knowledge of results treatments on coincidence-anticipation performance. *Journal of Motor Behavior, 7,* 271-274.
Poulton, E.C. (1957). On prediction in skilled movements. *Psychological Bulletin, 54,* 467-478.
Ridenour, M.A. (1977). Influence of object size, speed, direction, height and distance on interception of a moving object. *Research Quarterly, 48,* 138-143.
Shea, C.H., & Northam, C. (1982). Discrimination of visual linear velocities. *Research Quarterly for Exercise and Sport, 53,* 222-225.
Wiegand, R.L., & Ramella, R. (1983). The effect of practice and temporal location of knowledge of results on the motor performance of older adults. *Journal of Gerontology, 38,* 701-706.

### ACKNOWLEDGMENTS

The assistance of Mignon Jutton, Julie Quibell, Janice Evers, Kathy Ferguson, Catherine Lewis, and Matt Shank with testing of the subjects is gratefully acknowledged. The help of Matt Shank in conducting the data analysis also is gratefully acknowledged.

This research was supported in part by the Missouri Gerontology Institute, University of Missouri, and the Gerontology Committee, the Office of Research, and the School of Education, University of Missouri-St. Louis.

RETURNED YOUR CALL

Message _____

_____

_____

_____

_____

_____

_____

_____

Operator _____

AMPAD
EFFICIENCY®

REORDER
#23-000

# Index

Acoustic analyses, 312
Affiliation, 225-226, 233, 240, 251
Age grading, 119, 135, 146
Ageism, 145-146
Age role stereotypes, 119, 135, 146, 220
Agoraphobia, 265
Alpha rhythms, 49
Anger, 141, 148, 195
Anticipation, 295, 325-335
Anxiety: cognitive, 179; competition and, 5-24; drug therapy and, 10, 28; exercise and, 141-143, 148, 159-172, 179, 195, 220; memory and, 11-15; somatic, 179; state anxiety, 179; trait anxiety, 1, 179. See also, Arousal
Arousal, 1, 4-24
Arthritis, 122, 132, 134, 140-141, 194, 203, 276
Atherosclerosis, 121
Attention, 1, 11-12, 16-24, 80, 289-290, 294
Attentional training, 28-29, 294
Attitudes: toward exercise, 145-146, 220-221
Audition, 70, 141, 202, 283, 287-288, 290, 311, 315
Automobile driving, 36, 325
Autonomous state (of motor learning), 291

Back pain, 276
Balance, 44, 124, 133, 135
Bandura, Albert, 261-265
Bassin Anticipation Timer, 325-335
Beck Depression Inventory, 145
Biofeedback, 141
Biological age, 184, 308
Blood lactate, 115
Blood pressure, 115, 121, 127, 141, 202, 205-206, 310, 314
Body fat, 115, 122, 129
Body image, 139-140, 151, 180, 185-186, 188, 196
Bowling, 196, 296, 299

Cancer, 140, 194
Cardiac rehabilitation program, 258, 267-268
Cattell 16 Personality Factor Questionnaire, 137-138
Central nervous system, 35, 37, 42; aerobic exercise and, 50-59, 67-80, 106; morphological changes, 43-44; neural noise and, 47; neurophysiological changes, 43-50
Cerebral blood flow, 46
Cholesterol, 311
Chronological age categories, 184-185
Closed motor task, 290, 299
Coincidence-anticipation. See Anticipation
Competition, 149, 225-226, 233, 240, 252
Competitive State Anxiety Inventory (CSAI), 162
Continuous motor task, 291-292
Cornell Medical Health Index, 207
Coronary heart disease, 140
Critical flicker fusion threshold (CFF), 70
Cross-cultural research, 235

Crystalized intelligence, 182. See also, Intelligence
Death, 126, 141
Decision-making, 290-291, 298-299. See also, Information processing
Dementia, 203
Dendrites, 44
Dependency, 127
Depression, 70, 73, 80, 124, 127, 141-142, 144-145, 148, 178-179, 192, 194-195, 207
Detraining, 159-172
Developmental stages, 126
Diabetes, 203-204
Dichotic listening performance, 105-113
Disengagement, 126, 146, 217, 220

Ecological validity, 24-25. See also, Research design
Electromyography, 143
Endorphins, 194
Eustress, 140
Exercise addiction, 148
Exercise adherence, 147, 152, 187-188, 208, 217, 222, 227, 230, 231, 241-242, 244, 252, 258-260, 268, 276
Exercise compliance, 135, 208-209, 212, 217, 249, 258
Exercise prescription, 132-135, 146-150; frequency, 133-134, 149-150, 188-189; intensity, 133-134, 150, 188-189, 222, 232; psychological principles, 146-149

Figure-ground discrimination, 293
Fitness Status Locus of Control Scale, 244
Flexibility, 122, 127, 133, 135, 160
Fluid intelligence, 182. See also, Intelligence

Geriatric Depression Scale, 207
Goal setting behavior, 147, 222, 230, 241, 244, 253, 269-273, 275, 277

Happiness, 139
Hawthorne effect, 191
Health locus of control, 268-269
Heart rate: arousal and, 5-24; detraining and, 159-172; rating of perceived exertion and, 160
Hopkins Symptom Check List, 192

Index of Physiological Status (IPS), 307-322
Information processing: acquisition and, 285-303; exercise and, 35
Institutionalized elderly, 182-183, 201-216
Instructional strategies, 293-302
Intelligence, 42, 56-58, 68, 70, 182-183, 207
Interactionist perspective, 222, 260
Intergenerational motor development program, 283
Inverted-U hypothesis, 1. See also, Anxiety

Kenny Self-Care Evaluation Scale, 208

Kenyon's Body Image Scale, 181
KinderSkills, 283
Kinesthetic feedback, 292, 300
Knowledge of results (KR), 292, 300-301

Labeling, 297
Larynx, 320
Lean body weight, 310
Lens accommodation, 311, 315-316
Life expectancy, 117, 130-131, 285
Life quality, 140
Life satisfaction, 126-127, 138-140, 151, 174, 178, 220, 229
Life span, 130-131, 160
Locus of control, 180, 185, 195, 220, 241, 264, 266, 268-269
Longevity, 125-126, 130-131; sex differences and, 131
Longitudinal research, 287, 321, 325-335
Long-term memory, 288, 290, 297, 298. See also, Memory

Maximal oxygen uptake, 120, 122-123, 127, 129, 159-172, 181, 309
Maximum heart rate, 100
McPherson's Real Me Test, 181
Memory, 26, 85-104, 124, 288-290; aerobic exercise and, 54, 57-58, 60, 70, 105-113, 183-184; encoding, 91-92; rehearsal strategies, 92-93; under stressful conditions, 11-15
Mental imagery, 297-298
Mental Status Questionnaire, 207
Modeling, 283
Motor learning, 333-334
Motor programming, 291
Motor set, 295
Muscular endurance, 122-133, 160, 291
Muscular strength, 122, 127, 133, 135, 160, 291
Myocardial infarction, 131

Neural noise, 288
Neuronal loss, 43-44. See also, Central nervous system
Neurotransmitters, 44-46; 78-79; 111; acetlycholine, 45; dopamine, 45, 79, 111, 123; noradenaline, 45; serotonin, 45-46, 50, 79, 111
Nideffer, Robert, 294
Nurses' Observation Scale (NOSIE), 208
Nutrition, 125

Obesity, 141
Osteoporosis, 121-122, 135, 151, 278
Oxygen deprivation, 48, 53-56, 68, 78-79, 111

Parkinson's disease, 45
Perceived exertion, 260, 265
Perception, 288-289
Performance Test of Activities, 202
Personal Incentives for Exercise Questionnaire, 227, 233, 243, 251-252
Personal Investment Theory: 217-256, 260; perceived options, 230-231, 242; personal incentives, 224-227, 240-241, 244-248, 251-253; sense of self, 227-230, 241-242, 248-249, 253-254
Personality: fitness and, 137-138

Pflaum Life Quality Inventory, 140
Physical self-efficacy scale, 243
Physical stature, 122, 129
Position computer tomography (PET), 47
Processing rate theory, 38-41, 56, 60
Profile of Mood States (POMS), 178-179, 185, 192
Progressive relaxation, 28
Psychological age, 184
Psychometric issues, 191-192, 214
Psychomotor slowing: 35-36, 39, 41-42, 123, 318; aerobic exercise and, 35, 50-56, 130; cerebral blood flow and, 46; neuronal transmission time, 49; neurophysiological explanations for, 47-50; oxygen deprivation, 48
Psychotherapy, 194

Racquet sports, 325
Rating of Perceived Exertion (RPE), 159-172
Raven's Progressive Matrices Test, 184
Reaction time: 49, 51-56, 123, 289-291, 312-313; choice, 51-52, 54-56, 71, 73, 105, 129, 289, 291, 312-313, 315; motor, 51, 123, 202; premotor, 51-52, 54-56, 71, 73, 105, 123, 129, 289, 291, 312-313, 315
Recall memory: 88-102, 290; task familiarity and, 91. See also, Memory
Reciprocal causation: 261. See also, Social cognitive theory
Recognition memory: 88-102; task familiarity and, 90-91. See also, Memory
Regression effect: 182. See also, Research design
Relaxation training. See also, Progressive relaxation
Research design: 189-191; cross-sectional design, 25; ecological validity, 24-25
Respiratory changes (with age), 121
Retirement, 126, 141, 195, 286
Rheumatism, 203
Running, 136, 182, 189

Salthouse, Tim, 35, 38-42, 60
Schema theory, 95, 97
Schizophrenia, 194
Schmidt, Richard, 95
Self-concept, 126, 137, 139-140, 148, 151, 180-181, 185-186
Self-efficacy, 139, 181-182, 186, 196, 228-229, 233, 253, 262-272
Self-monitoring, 222, 253
Sensory detection, 47
Sensory set, 295
Sex differences, 185-186
Sexual activity, 125-126
Short-term memory: 288-290, 293, 297. See also, Memory
Signal-to-noise ratio, 288-289, 291-292
Sleep disorders, 194
Smoking behavior, 266, 270
Social age, 185
Social cognitive theory: 257-279; efficacy expectations, 262-278; outcome expectations, 262-264; 270-273; 276-278
Social recognition, 225, 227, 233, 252
Social reinforcement, 195, 230, 240
Socioeconomics status, 188

*AGING AND MOTOR BEHAVIOR*

Sport Competition Anxiety Test (SCAT), 10, 14
Steinberg paradigm, 60
Stress: 3-4, 9-24, 140-141. See also, Anxiety, Arousal
Stress inoculation, 142, 146-150
Suicide, 127
Swimming, 182, 186, 189, 196, 259, 265, 296
Synapse, 44, 48, 50

Tactile sensitivity, 311, 319
Taylor Manifest Anxiety Scale, 142, 179
Tennis, 180

Theory of reasoned action, 270
Type A personality, 179, 185

Visual acuity, 70, 73, 141, 202, 283, 287, 290, 311, 328
Volunteer effect, 128, 186

Wechsler Adults Intelligence Scale, 182, 202
Wechsler Memory Scale, 184, 207
Weight loss, 266-267

Zung Self-Rating Depression Scale, 144